T0226543

Toxicology and Drug Testing

Editor

MARTIN H. BLUTH

CLINICS IN LABORATORY MEDICINE

www.labmed.theclinics.com

December 2016 • Volume 36 • Number 4

ELSEVIER

1600 John F. Kennedy Boulevard • Suite 1800 • Philadelphia, Pennsylvania, 19103-2899

http://www.theclinics.com

CLINICS IN LABORATORY MEDICINE Volume 36, Number 4
December 2016 ISSN 0272-2712, ISBN-13: 978-0-323-47796-3

Editor: Stacy Eastman
Developmental Editor: Colleen Viola

Reprints. For copies of 100 or more, of articles in this publication, please contact the Commercial Reprints Department, Elsevier Inc., 360 Park Avenue South, New York, New York 10010-1710. Tel. 212-633-3874, Fax: 212-633-3820, E-mail: reprints@elsevier.com.

Clinics in Laboratory Medicine (ISSN 0272-2712) is published quarterly by Elsevier Inc., 360 Park Avenue South, New York, NY 10010-1710. Months of issue are March, June, September, and December. Business and Editorial offices: 1600 John F. Kennedy Blvd., Suite 1800, Philadelphia, PA 19103-2899. Periodicals postage paid at NewYork, NY and additional mailing offices. Subscription prices are $250.00 per year (US individuals), $469.00 per year (US institutions), $100.00 per year (US students), $305.00 per year (Canadian individuals), $570.00 per year (Canadian institutions), $185.00 per year (Canadian students), $390.00 per year (international individuals), $570.00 per year (international institutions), $185.00 (international students). Foreign air speed delivery is included in all Clinics subscription prices. All prices are subject to change without notice. POSTMASTER: Send address changes to *Clinics in Laboratory Medicine*, Elsevier Health Sciences Division, Subscription Customer Service, 3251 Riverport Lane, Maryland Heights, MO 63043. **Customer Service: 1-800-654-2452 (US). From outside of the US and Canada, call 1-314-447-8871. Fax: 1-314-447-8029. E-mail: journalscustomerservice-usa@elsevier.com (for print support) or journalsonlinesupport-usa@elsevier.com (for online support).**

Clinics in Laboratory Medicine is covered in *EMBASE/Exerpta Medica, MEDLINE/PubMed (Index Medicus), Cinahl, Current Contents/Clinical Medicine, BIOSIS and ISI/BIOMED.*

Contributors

EDITOR

MARTIN H. BLUTH, MD, PhD
Professor of Pathology, Wayne State University School of Medicine, Detroit, Michigan; Chief Medical Officer, Consolidated Laboratory Management Systems, Southfield, Michigan

AUTHORS

HUSAM M. ABU-SOUD, PhD
Department of Obstetrics and Gynecology, The C.S. Mott Center for Human Growth and Development, Wayne State University School of Medicine, Detroit, Michigan

CHRISTOPHER ALOEZOS, MD
Department of Psychiatry and Behavioral Sciences, Montefiore Medical Center, The University Hospital for Albert Einstein College of Medicine, Bronx, New York

MARTIN H. BLUTH, MD, PhD
Professor of Pathology, Wayne State University School of Medicine, Detroit, Michigan; Chief Medical Officer, Consolidated Laboratory Management Systems, Southfield, Michigan

WELLMAN W. CHEUNG, MD, FACS
Clinical Professor of Urology, State University of New York Downstate Medical School, Brooklyn, New York

MATEUSZ CIEJKA, MD
Department of Emergency Medicine, Wayne State University School of Medicine, Detroit, Michigan

ELIZABETH DUBEY, MD
Department of Emergency Medicine, Wayne State University School of Medicine, Detroit, Michigan

HOWARD FORMAN, MD
Assistant Professor of Psychiatry, Department of Psychiatry and Behavioral Sciences, Montefiore Medical Center, The University Hospital for Albert Einstein College of Medicine, Bronx, New York

M.P. GEORGE, MS
Chief Toxicologist, VP US Laboratory Operations, Alere Toxicology, Austin, Texas

NATHAN J. GONIK, MD, MHSA
Assistant Professor, Department of Otolaryngology, Head and Neck Surgery, ENT Clinic, Children's Hospital of Michigan, Wayne State University School of Medicine, Detroit, Michigan

ROOHI JEELANI, MD
Department of Obstetrics and Gynecology, The C.S. Mott Center for Human Growth and Development, Wayne State University School of Medicine, Detroit, Michigan

RAUNO JOKS, MD
Associate Professor of Clinical Medicine, State University of New York Downstate Medical Center, Brooklyn, New York

FRANK ANTHONY MYERS Jr, MD
Department of Urology, State University of New York Downstate Medical Center, Brooklyn, New York

KHOA NGUYEN, MD
Department of Emergency Medicine, Wayne State University School of Medicine, Detroit, Michigan

MATTHEW R. PINCUS, MD, PhD
Professor of Pathology, State University of New York Downstate Medical Center, Brooklyn, New York

DANIEL A. SCHWARZ, MD
Director, The Center for Pain Recovery, Southfield, Michigan

MICHAEL P. SMITH, PhD
Assistant Professor of Pathology, Oakland University William Beaumont School of Medicine, Rochester, Michigan; Technical Director, Toxicology and Therapeutic Drug Monitoring Laboratory, Beaumont Laboratories, Beaumont Hospital-Royal Oak, Royal Oak, Michigan

JONATHAN M. WAI, MD
Department of Psychiatry and Behavioral Sciences, Montefiore Medical Center, The University Hospital for Albert Einstein College of Medicine, Bronx, New York

BIN WEI, PhD
Toxicology Laboratory, Michigan Surgical Hospital, Warren, Michigan

YAN VICTORIA ZHANG, PhD, DABCC
University of Rochester Medical Center, Rochester, New York

YANHUA ZHANG, PhD
Total Toxicology Labs, LLC, Southfield, Michigan

YU ZHU, PhD
Consolidated Laboratory Management Systems, LLC, Southfield, Michigan

Contents

Pain management is an evolving discipline. New formulations mature with promises of improved pain control, better dosing, and fewer side effects. These agents also have an equal risk for abuse. Street chemists are adept at manipulating drugs to more potent versions and creating new compositions of matter. The clinical assessment of the patient is paramount to developing an index of suspicion of overdose, toxicity, or illicit drug use; the clinical laboratory can be a resource to support investigations and guide therapy. The clinical toxicology laboratory needs to keep in step, adapting technology and methodology to facilitate detection of such substances.

In the last decade, liquid chromatography–tandem mass spectrometry (LC-MS/MS) has seen enormous growth in routine toxicology laboratories. LC-MS/MS offers significant advantages over other traditional testing, such as immunoassay and gas chromatography–mass spectrometry methodologies. Major strengths of LC-MS/MS include improvement in specificity, flexibility, and sample throughput when compared with other technologies. Here, the basic principles of LC-MS/MS technology are reviewed, followed by advantages and disadvantages of this technology compared with other traditional techniques. In addition, toxicology applications of LC-MS/MS for simultaneous detection of large panels of analytes are presented.

Interferences relating to laboratory toxicology testing refer to results which differ from their true value and are often encountered in the setting of a drug screen compared with confirmatory testing. Such interferences fall into two general categories; those that cause false positive results (when a drug screen is positive but confirmatory testing is negative) and those that cause false negative results (when a drug screen is negative when in reality the sample donor has ingested the tested substance). Such interferences can result from differences in laboratory testing methodology, reagent and analyte cross reactivity, limits of analyte detection, instrument resolution, reporting cutoff, sample processing, tissue type and sample adulteration among others. Awareness of the possible causes of such interferences are integral to proper laboratory result interpretation and patient management.

Toxicology testing in pain management has become the standard of care. The Center for Disease Control and Prevention published guidelines including urine drug testing prior to initiating opioid therapy and for monitoring prescription and illicit drugs. Physicians must know indications for toxicology testing, and the frequency based upon risk stratification. This includes personal and family history of alcohol or substance related disorders, mental illness and smoking. Knowledge of opioid metabolism and various matrices to test are described. Additional knowledge of presumptive vs definitive testing along with algorithms and medical necessity with evidence-based clinical standards are discussed.

Toxicology testing in addiction medicine varies across the spectrum, yet remains a powerful tool in monitoring addictive patients. There are many reference laboratories offering toxicology testing, and physicians should have some understanding of laboratory, methodology, testing portfolio, and customer support structure to aid them in selecting the best toxicology laboratory for their patients. Consultation with a clinical pathologist/toxicologist in conjunction with the consideration of monitoring large numbers of illicit and psychoactive drugs in the addictive patient may provide important clinical information for their treatment.

Precision medicine applies primarily to pharmacokinetics in toxicology. Mastering hepatic metabolism through an understanding of the genetics behind Phase I, or oxidation/reduction and some Phase II, or conjugation, enhances the scientific and clinical application of common drug toxicology. This review includes basic hepatic metabolism, the common substrates, inducers and inhibitors of cytochrome P450 along with genetic variants behind the enzymes. Detailed metabolism of commonly measured opioids in clinical practice is provided. Finally, evidence based research and clinical correlations conclude that knowledge of inducers and inhibitors, in conjunction with genetic variations, are integral components for applied precision medicine in toxicology.

Fertility relies on a series of time dependent events, which are largely regulated by hormones. Concentration and function of these hormones can be altered by exposure of consumed and environmental toxins. It is important to consider the dose and timing of toxin exposures in assessing the impact of them on reproductive health, however the utility of laboratory assessment in this regard is not well established. General laboratory assessment of reproduction and infertility includes hormone evaluation (hCG, prolactin, TSH, free thyroxin, FSH, LH and androgens among others) and treatment is via various assisted reproductive technologies. Reduction and abstinence from exposure to toxins is recommended to improve reproductive health.

In this review, the authors address the general principles of prescribing psychiatric medications and discuss how the clinical laboratory can be used to guide prescribing practices. Treatment considerations in different settings and for different medications are discussed. Because the clinical laboratory is advancing in its technology, so should the clinician's knowledge of how to use the clinical laboratory. The authors propose recommendations and a simple algorithm for how to use medication levels in blood and other fluids to guide care in medications without well-defined therapeutic windows.

Although both the prevalence of asthma and the prescription drug use, notably the opiate analgesic class, epidemics are increasing, there is a complex interplay between both disorders, with both protective and exacerbating factors involved in the effect of opiates on asthma pathogenesis and clinical severity. This review examines the airway effects, both immunologic and neurologic, of opiates, which may interact and result in protection or exacerbation of asthma.

CLINICS IN LABORATORY MEDICINE

Preface

Drug Testing and Toxicology: Redefining the Plague of Darkness

 CrossMark

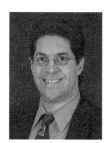

Martin H. Bluth, MD, PhD
Editor

The book of Exodus recounts the experience of the plague of darkness during Pharaoh's rule. The narrative discusses the imposing nature of the Darkness that occurred throughout the land of Egypt as a "darkness which may be felt… a thick darkness, where no one could see another person, and no one could rise from his place."[1]

What's old is new again. Although the narrative is thought to have occurred over three thousand years ago, modern day reports of increasing pain and treatment over the last two decades may offer another insight into this experience. As the plague imposed a sense of complete and utter isolationism where one afflicted could not interact with another nor shed the enveloping sense of imprisonment, so too can the pain experience impose similar overtones.

Pain is becoming a pervasive state of being. It has garnered its own cadre of diagnostic codes, given rise to multiple treatment modalities, pain specialties and subspecialties, devices, and—since 2005—has recruited September to be its own awareness month.[2] Pain can be likened to darkness. Numerous books, publications, and narratives have described the experience of pain as fostering intense isolationism, hopelessness, worthlessness, despondency, nonacceptance, lack of productivity, familial discord, social outcast state, and other intimations of a lone and dark existence.[3–5] In addition, the social and physical relationships of pain are thought to share underlying biological processes.[3]

Over the past two decades, the number of people suffering from some manner of pain, and the narcotic prescriptions that are tethered to pain symptoms, has increased four- to tenfold depending on how data are collected and/or stratified and can account for over 80% of physician visits.[6,7] Many of these initial acute pain experiences progress to chronic pain conditions, which afflicts patients for years. Recent data estimate that as many as one in three individuals suffer from some manner of pain; over

Clin Lab Med 36 (2016) xi–xx
http://dx.doi.org/10.1016/j.cll.2016.09.003   labmed.theclinics.com
0272-2712/16/© 2016 Published by Elsevier Inc.

125 million people (US) reported some pain over a 3-month period and that approximately 50 million Americans, and over half of various populations in general, suffer from chronic pain.[8,9] As health care providers, we feel obligated to mitigate the suffering of our patients. Oftentimes, treating pain goes hand in hand with the treatment of disease and, of late, frequently it is the only presentation pertaining to the patient's chief complaint.

As conscientious caregivers, we have been able to select from an ever-increasing arsenal of narcotic analgesics, each with its own unique claims for its ability to assuage pain. Indeed, numerous classes of benzodiazepines, opiates, amphetamines, and others have availed themselves as wellsprings of pain obviation. However, these medications come with their own side effects, which require secondary prescriptions. For example, opioid administration has been reported to precipitate adverse effects, including but not limited to sedation, physical dependence, tolerance, hyperalgesia, and notably, constipation.[10] In fact, opioid-induced constipation (OIC) has become such a common and expected gastrointestinal sequelae of patients on opioids, that the rescue pharmacopeia for OIC were repeatedly advertised during the recent Super Bowl 50 commercial spots,[11] further demonstrating the prevalent, almost household, use of narcotic analgesics in our society.

The literature has concordantly mirrored this explosion of pain relief options in that a PubMed search for the limited query of "pain medication review" publications in 1992 would yield 45 review-type articles published in that year, whereas a similar query 20 years later in 2012 would provide a >five-fold increase of over 250 publications per annum, the total number that can be exponentially increased if one removed the limitation of a "review" article from the search query.

In light of increasing pain, the commensurate increase in pain medication prescriptions, and subsequent side effects of select pain medications, many emerging drug offerings promote reduction of side effects, improved dosing and dependency, as well as increased potency and effectiveness. Many such claims have not held up and were likely the result of overzealous advertising campaigns to capture the ever-increasing pain-centric market share in the way Postum coffee alternative marketed itself as an coffee-like beverage that, unlike the villainous coffee bean, would not stunt the growth of children, cause divorce, promote business failures, or be the etiological agent responsible for the completely fictitious disease known as "coffee heart."[12,13]

The current *Pain Paradox*™ poses additional challenges. The ability to note, qualify, and quantify a patient's pain is largely a subjective exercise. Numerous psychosocial variables, including but not limited to age, gender, personality, and ethnicity, among others, affect the manner in which a patient relates to pain,[14] and certain such variables have been reported to help predict responses to pain treatment.[15] To this end, various psychosocioeconomic questionnaires and screening tools (ie, Screener and Opioid Assessment for Patients with Pain, the Opioid Risk Tool, the Oswestry Disability Index, the NIH Patient-Reported Outcomes Measurement Information System) have been employed to attempt to create objective quantification of pain scores and risk stratification for pain patients in how they relate to pain and pain medication prescriptions as well as the risks of succumbing to drug addiction or abuse.

Furthermore, in light of the molecular age of *personalized* or more recently dubbed discipline of *precision medicine*, we may be able to more effectively tailor which analgesic should be preferably prescribed to a patient—based on their genetic polymorphisms—that impact drug absorption, distribution, metabolism, and excretion (ADME). To this end, Genome Wide Association Studies (GWAS) were culled from many individuals being prescribed analgesia (ie, opioids) to identify optimal genetic inputs, which would ideally characterize how a patient's genetic constitution would translate into an individual's unique enzymatic footprint and thus affect ADME, drug efficacy and function, and help guide prescribing habits.

A caveat to this approach, however, is the understanding that polygenic rather than single major gene effects will foster and translate the likelihood of a patient's response to opiates or other analgesia. In addition, patients enrolled in GWAS studies may be on polypharmacy (drugs, herbs, nutraceuticals, other) for pain and/or other maladies, which may introduce additional variables as well as exert epigenetic effects that contribute or influence genomic and proteomic results.[16] Nonetheless, genetic influences that may be common across different opioid analgesics include polymorphisms in the CYP2D6 gene and findings that the A118G single-nucleotide polymorphism (SNP) of the mu opioid receptor gene and the V158M SNP of the catechol-o-methyl-transferase gene may alter both analgesic responsiveness and opioid abuse risk,[17] although the value of identifying such polymorphisms in moderating drug-prescribing habits is not without debate.[18]

The *Pain Paradox*™ has given rise to the behemoth aptly dubbed the *Pain Problem*™. This "problem" encompasses all the sequelae that have become an epidemic of national and global concern, including but not limited to death, addiction, diversion, pill pushing, doctor shopping, abuse, and all the damage that this juggernaut leaves in its wake. The morbidity and mortality associated with such behavior have reached epic proportions. Recent reports demonstrate that drug-induced deaths have been on the rise for the last decade, steadily increasing from ~30,000 deaths per year in 2003 to over 45,000 deaths in 2013, which surpasses homicide-, motor vehicle-, and firearm-related deaths, nationally.[19,20] Drug overdose claims the lives of approximately 120 people each day. Disturbingly, the number of deaths attributable to controlled prescription drugs has outpaced those for illicit drugs such as cocaine and heroin combined. Furthermore, with regard to prescription drugs, it is alarming to note that over the last few years, select prescription drugs for pain have precipitated untoward mortality. To this end, the schedule II synthetic opioid fentanyl and its analogues have been responsible for more than 700 deaths across the United States.[19]

The increase in pain combined with the increase in pain prescriptions, many of which can be dispensed without discretion and in considerable quantities at each visit, has availed a unique market for supply and demand. For example, a 30-mg Oxycodone tablet can cost ~$2 at the clinic but can be resold for up to $30 ($1/mg) on the street; at 120 to 150 pills per prescription, the street value for a few refills is enough for a decent used car, or other useful commodities.[20]

In addition to patients-turned-addicts being punished by law enforcement for criminal activity, doctors are being subjected to such as well. A recent ruling from the Supreme Court has provided *patients the ability to sue their physicians*, under "wrongful conduct," for getting them addicted to pain medications,[21] thus fostering distance between physicians and their patients. Additional physician narcotic prescription monitoring initiatives have also been instituted. Some states have created mandatory educational/monitoring initiatives, also known as "pill mill" legislation,[22] requiring all pain management clinics to be certified by their Medical Board on a biennial basis and to be owned and operated by a licensed physician, whereas other states encourage physicians to require opioid education and proactive addiction counseling for patients who are prescribed schedule II or III controlled substances for chronic pain for extended periods,[23] whereas other states keep a watchful eye on how MDs prescribe in that simultaneously prescribing opioids and benzodiazepines can precipitate an audit.[24] Furthermore, *Prescription-Drug Monitoring Programs* (PDMP) are statewide electronic databases that serve to help clinicians identify patients obtaining controlled substances from multiple prescribers (ie, "doctor shopping") for appropriate pain management. To this end, over 40 states currently have a PDMP program in operation.[25]

So what's a doc to do? Prescribe? Not prescribe? It seems bleak on either front. Then again, maybe not.

It is reasonable to assume that no individual chooses to become an addict. Most start out as your "average Joe" who are prescribed narcotics after surgery, giving birth, sports or back injury in the appropriate manner. In some, the meds stop working efficiently, whether as a result of individualized modulation of pain receptor cell density, tolerance, and the like, thereby fostering the need to seek out (a) increased dosing of the same medication, (b) adding polypharmacy of other classes of pain medication, and/or (c) non-prescribed sources of pain relief. The latter can include illicit drugs as well as alcohol for their sedative synergy. In short order, when one becomes an addict, one is no longer subject to logic, reason, or rationality as their brain chemistry has changed.

But how does the physician know where the patient before him lies on the spectrum of "patient to addict" without the aid of a crystal ball? The clinical laboratory can be very helpful in this regard in that it has matured in step with this conundrum and can provide objective drug compliance and monitoring assistance to aid the physician in managing the patient. The application of toxicology and drug monitoring to one's practice can be very helpful in aiding the physician in answering two basic questions as he/she assesses the patient:

1. Is the patient taking what has been prescribed?
2. Is the patient taking something else?

The rudimentary value of these queries is not to be underscored. Knowing if one's patient is taking what is being prescribed provides an objective determination of pain management as told by the patient's physiology and his/her body fluid prose of parent and metabolite drug signatures. The value of the patient taking something else—and the something else can be prescription medications not disclosed or prescribed by another health care provider, as well as illicit drugs—is also compelling. To this end, recent studies have shown that an unscheduled toxicology assessment of patients scheduled for maxillofacial surgery highlighted that 47% of those patients yielded illicit drug results that were inconsistent with the information obtained by the treating physician/surgeon[26]; almost one-half of patients tested had drugs in their system that were not known to their health care provider. It is likely that any conscientious physician would want to know if the patient they were about to operate on had a sedative/narcotic/illicit on board before subjecting them to anesthesia or other drugs that may interact with the patient's systemic drugs, fostering deleterious outcomes.

Urine drug testing (UDT) has been unfortunately utilized by some to paint proverbial "cross-hairs" on the backs of their patients. Recent studies have reported that physicians use "inconsistent" UDT to "fire" their patients from their clinics.[27] However, this is not unexpected. Part of this binary "flip the switch" attitude is that clinicians themselves are under ever-increasing scrutiny by accrediting, governmental, societal, and federal bodies, among others as outlined earlier, thus adding a relatively new defensive gestalt, which has been ingrained into the health care provider who dispenses such medication. It makes relative sense that a patient who is not squeaky clean in a busy pain clinic to be "let go" by the physician who only has an average of 8 minutes to see his/her patient,[28] rather than take the time to discuss, and/or repeat the UDT on the patient. Such an act theoretically obviates further risk to the clinician's practice and license and can be documented in the patient's chart as the reason for termination of care.

However, UDT may actually improve adherence[29,30] and provide a two-way street for trust, compliance, and management. An objective UDT may be employed to rule out problematic drug use for patients under specific monitoring programs, allow the clinician to search for other causes for pain, lend support to patient self-reporting which can be otherwise unreliable,[31,32] as well as provide objective evidence for increasing pain dosing and/or switching drug classes. The value of properly utilizing UDT is compelling. One can search the Web and easily find all manner of professional and lay press on how UDT results were used to fire employees and sever doctor-patient relationships.[27,33] In contrast, UDTs can be also be appropriately implemented as part of a patient workup to provide objective approaches to drug prescribing and monitoring.[34]

A major issue is understanding what the UDT actually can and cannot do. Many clinicians wrestle with the interpretation of results[35,36] and may inappropriately conclude that, although UDT can detect use of illicit drugs or nonuse of prescribed opioids, it can also diagnose prescription opioid abuse, addiction, or diversion, when in fact it cannot provide such in the routine health care setting.[29] To this end, below are a few guidelines to appropriately approach and interpret a UDT:

First, a health care provider must know what he or she is prescribing to his/her patient. There are those who are habituated to prescribe select narcotics based on clinic formularies, training history, and/or drug representative narrative excerpted from drug manufacturer's boilerplate information packaging.[37] Support systems can be employed for the benefit of the physician by fostering continuing education initiatives, which can modify prescribing habits, by employing support of evidenced-based medicine, expert advisement, and/or institutional support.[37]

Second, one must be well versed in the characteristics of the drug, such as its half-life, parent/metabolite relationships, and drug-drug interactions. Although this practice applies to all drugs, the narcotic analgesic space is unique in that these drugs should be considered lethal weapons if not prescribed properly: a sensitivity to be mindful of and not shared with many other medications. It is unlikely for one to open the newspaper and read a news story on how someone on omeprazole was driving impaired, jumped a divider, and killed drivers in the oncoming traffic lane. Such an event is unfortunately common for those on schedule I or II controlled substances.[38]

Third, one must understand (a) what laboratory assay they are ordering (eg, immunoassay employed in drug _screening_ technology versus gas/liquid chromatography/mass spectrometry utilized for drug _confirmatory_ testing), (b) which tissue fluid they are submitting for testing (ie, blood, oral swab, urine, and so forth), and (c) be familiar with the expected drug detection timing windows, which often differ among fluids tested. For example, a very common source of confusion can be depicted by a patient that tests negative on an a drug _screen_ from an oral swab but positive on a _confirmatory_ test from a urine sample, often precipitating disparaging overtones from the physician's clinic regarding the competency of one lab over another. This testing competency argument would be similar to comparing apples to cats. One should be familiar with the understanding that detection windows are routinely shorter for saliva than for urine (ie, 6 hours vs 72 hours), and that the detection sensitivity is greater when assessed via mass spectrometry (gas chromatography or liquid chromatography) than for immunoassay screens (ie, 20 ng/mL versus 300 ng/mL). Furthermore, toxicology assessment on different fluids (blood vs urine), even if collected within minutes of each other, can have different results based on differences in processing methodology, carrier proteins, half-life, and ADME for drugs in unique fluid compositions, and as such, cannot necessarily be linearly compared with each other.[39,40])

Fourth, it is important to understand and respect the fact that clinical toxicology laboratories, and laboratories in general, are accredited entities that are regulated, audited, and inspected by governmental regulatory bodies (FDA, CAP, COLA, and so forth). There are rules that a lab must abide by to remain in good standing, accredited, competent, and reimbursable by third-party payors for the services they render to the clinician for patient management. A common misunderstanding is the issue of test or retest inconsistencies, which can seem frustrating to the health care provider. Laboratory quantitative values are determined by establishing a standard curve utilizing controls, which will set the minimum and maximum reportable concentration values (ie, 50-500 ng/mL), which a lab is then legally permitted to result to the clinician. Anything above the maximum validated value will often be depicted as "greater than" (ie, >500 ng/mL) no matter what the value. The reason for such is that without validation of reportable concentration values by a verifiable control source, the extrapolated data above the validated maximum may be subject to bias (positive or negative drift, and so forth) and be grossly inaccurate. Conversely, a value below the validated cutoff will often be reported as "less than" (ie, <50 ng/mL) as well as "negative" depending on the standard operating procedure employed by the lab. This approach is necessary for the same reasons as above with the additional caveat that a value below the cutoff may be due to background, processing, and/or method-specific noise. Thus, pressing a laboratory to provide raw data above or below the cutoff that is not in-line with standard controls is doing a disservice to the laboratory as well as the patient.

Moreover, if inconsistencies are found in *different* samples even if taken close in time, those samples can be profoundly different from one another in detection of the analyte of interest; such differences can be due to catabolism of said drug, liver, kidney function, other meds, and hydration status among other items.[41] The conclusion for any inconsistency is merely the most likely reason as a result of eliminating all putative/known causes, yet there are some variables that are out of the lab's control as well as areas that are not easily identified. Thus, sending a fresh sample, where the patient sample procurement is scheduled or unscheduled, can more often than not shed light on such reporting quandaries.

Fifth, UDT results should not be considered gospel to precipitate a decision to terminate, believe, or admonish a patient. Common scenarios that pose difficulty for a clinical service include (a) patients having tested negative for prescribed medication, (b) positive for a nonprescribed medication, (c) presence of illicit drugs, (d) and/or a change in positive/negative status upon retesting. The UDT laboratory results are intended to provide the health care provider with laboratory supplemental data for discretionary use, in conjunction with other clinical patient profiles, presentations, signs, symptoms, history, and physical findings obtained by the patient's primary care provider and do not necessarily reflect timing or dosage of administration. Parent drug or metabolite concentrations are subject to many metabolic factors, including but not limited to hydration, kidney and liver function, time and dose of drug ingestion as stated above,[41] in addition to other factors, including pharmacogenomics and poly-pharmacy, and so forth. Ideally, in scenarios where there is confusion, suspicion, or inconsistency, the physician should obtain a fresh sample from the patient, preferably at random for additional testing. This will provide a trail of objective UDT data to identify trends of patient drug administration behavior in conjunction with other clinical findings and provide content for a cogent dialogue with the patient. If the physician does decide to terminate care of his/her patient, serial UDT results will also serve to provide the documentation to justify such a decision when other interventions (addiction clinic, detox referral, and so forth) fail.

It is also important to note that standard UDT is not the same as forensic testing, which requires chain of custody and specific forensic protocols regarding sample collection, which ascertain the fidelity of the sample from patient voiding to result. Standard UDT is often collected in the physician's office and subsequently shipped to the testing lab via courier which does not employ forensic protocols or require forensic lab accreditation.[42]

Sixth, prior to sending a UDT, the clinician should document when the patient last took the medication being tested for. If the patient has not taken the medication (ie, opioid) for the past 72 hours, it may not be detected, depending of the detection window. Furthermore, the level of concern and subsequent management would be different if a patient disclosed that he had **not** taken his opioid prior to his/her negative test result rather than in the context of a strained overtone of an unexpected or inconsistent test result. The rationale of requiring a UDT should always be discussed openly with patients. It is less about catching patients doing something wrong and more about assessing increased prescription misuse risk, patient compliance, and trust in the patient-physician relationship.

In light of the aforementioned complexities encountered with UDT interpretation, clinicians may need access to a laboratory toxicologist to help with both UDT ordering and assessment.[34–36] To this end, recent data[35] suggest that primary care clinicians' lack of education and training to interpret and implement urine toxicology tests may impact their management of patient opioid misuse and/or substance use. The issue for clinicians is how to implement urine toxicology tests as a routine clinical procedure. While tests have become more frequent with the many new medical association guidelines, many clinics do not have sufficient staff or resources to systematically address how often clinicians should test, which substances to test for, and how to implement standardized urine toxicology tests. Clinicians who described using urine toxicology tests routinely to monitor misuse had difficulty interpreting results due to insufficient education and training. As such, clinicians may benefit from additional education and training about the clinical implementation and use of urine toxicology tests. Many such avenues (courses, symposia, associations) are becoming available in e-tutorial format, thereby creating up-to-date information of UDT ordering and management with the click of a mouse.

In summary, the adage, "With great power comes great responsibility," which helped forge Spiderman as a superhero, can be applied to physicians who have the noble task of alleviating pain. Medication can be a powerful ally for the doctor who uses such appropriately to treat the patient. Pain meds are powerful, effective, physiologically altering entities, and as such, require pause prior to putting pen to prescription pad. Such pause includes working with the patient to foster a *subjective* empowering relationship, which includes their personal understanding and recounting of pain as well as an *objective* empowering relationship, which includes disclosing to the patient the value and buy-in for the physical exam, imaging, and other ancillary services, notably the clinical laboratory. The ability to perform a urine toxicology screen and/or confirmation creates an objective baseline snapshot of the patient's on-board pharmacopeia, which should foster trust between the patient and physician as a unit. This Patient-Physician Unit (PPU)™ ideally works together to maintain mutual trust, integrity, and transparency to achieve pain relief and improved health. Although not simple, the Pain Problem™ can be improved upon through appropriately engaging the services, support, and resources of the clinical toxicology laboratory along with other health care support structures. This collective health care "village" can work synergistically to empower the PPU™, obviate pain, end the plague, and bring light to the darkness.

Martin H. Bluth, MD, PhD
Department of Pathology
Wayne State University School of Medicine
540 East Canfield
Detroit, MI 48201, USA

Consolidated Laboratory Management Systems
24555 Southfield Road
Southfield, MI 48075, USA

E-mail addresses:
mbluth@med.wayne.edu; martin.bluth@consolidatedlabsmgt.com

REFERENCES

1. Exodus 10:21–29.
2. Available at: https://www.govtrack.us/congress/bills/109/hr1020/text/ih. Accessed April 1, 2016.
3. Macdonald G, Leary MR. Why does social exclusion hurt? The relationship between social and physical pain. Psychol Bull 2005;131:202–23.
4. Foreman J. A nation in pain. New York: Oxford University Press; 2014.
5. Relieving Pain in America. A Blueprint for Transforming Prevention, Care, Education, and Research. Institute of Medicine (US) Committee on Advancing Pain Research, Care, and Education. Washington (DC): National Academies Press (US); 2011.
6. Voscopoulus C, Lema M. When does acute pain become chronic? Br J Anaesth 2010;105(Suppl 1):i69–85. http://dx.doi.org/10.1093/bja/aeq323.
7. US Department of Health and Human Services; 2011.
8. Harstall C. How prevalent is chronic pain? IASP Pain Clin Updates 2003;XI:1–4.
9. Nahin RL. Estimates of pain prevalence and severity in adults: United States, 2012. J Pain 2015;16:769–80.
10. Nelson AD, Camilleri M. Opioid-induced constipation: advances and clinical guidance. Ther Adv Chronic Dis 2016;7:121–34.
11. Kroll D. OIC is different: the drug behind the Super Bowl 50 constipation ad. 2016. Available at: Forbes.com. Accessed April 1, 2016.
12. Shockey L. Foods with fake health benefits. Village Voice. May 16, 2011. Available at: http://www.villagevoice.com/restaurants/foods-with-fake-health-benefits-its-been-the-case-for-years-just-look-at-breakfast-cereals-6515525. Accessed May 1, 2016.
13. Stromberg J. It's a myth: there's no evidence that coffee stunts kids' growth. 2013. Available at: SMITHSONIAN.COM. Accessed April 1, 2016.
14. Eccleston C. Role of psychology in pain management. Br J Anaesth 2001;87:144–52.
15. Carroll I, Gaeta R, Mackey S. Multivariate analysis of chronic pain patients undergoing lidocaine infusions: increasing pain severity and advancing age predict likelihood of clinically meaningful analgesia. Clin J Pain 2007;23:702–6.

16. Li J, Bluth MH. Pharmacogenomics of drug metabolizing enzymes and transporters: implications for cancer therapy. Pharmacogenomics Pers Med 2011;4: 11–33.
17. Bruehl S, Apkarian AV, Ballantyne JC, et al. Personalized medicine and opioid analgesic prescribing for chronic pain: opportunities and challenges. J Pain 2013;14:103–13.
18. Walter C, Lötsch J. Meta-analysis of the relevance of the OPRM1 118A>G genetic variant for pain treatment. Pain 2009;146:270–5.
19. Available at: http://www.dea.gov/docs/2015%20NDTA%20Report.pdf. Accessed April 1, 2016.
20. Available at: http://www.deadiversion.usdoj.gov/mtgs/pharm_awareness/conf_2013/august_2013/prevoznik.pdf. Accessed April 1, 2016.
21. Available at: http://www.courtswv.gov/supreme-court/docs/spring2015/14-0144.pdf. Accessed April 1, 2016.
22. Available at: http://www.legis.state.tx.us/tlodocs/81R/billtext/pdf/SB00911I.pdf#navpanes=0. Accessed April 1, 2016.
23. Available at: http://www.legis.ga.gov/Legislation/20152016/145217.pdf. Accessed April 1, 2016.
24. Available at: www.NAMSDL.org. Accessed April 1, 2016.
25. Perrone J, Nelson LS. Medication reconciliation for controlled substances—an "ideal" prescription-drug monitoring program. N Engl J Med 2012;366(25): 2341–3.
26. McAllister P, Jenner S, Laverick S. Toxicology screening in oral and maxillofacial trauma patients. Br J Oral Maxillofac Surg 2013;51:773–8.
27. Owen GT, Burton AW, Schade CM, et al. Urine drug testing: current recommendations and best practices. Pain Physician 2012;15:ES119–33.
28. Chen PW. For new doctors, 8 minutes per patient. NY Times. May 30, 2013. Available at: http://well.blogs.nytimes.com/2013/05/30/for-new-doctors-8-minutes-per-patient/. Accessed May 1, 2016.
29. Starrels JL, Becker WC, Alford DP, et al. Systematic review: treatment agreements and urine drug testing to reduce opioid misuse in patients with chronic pain. Ann Intern Med 2010;152:712–20.
30. Pesce A, West C, Rosenthal M, et al. Illicit drug use in the pain patient population decreases with continued drug testing. Pain Physician 2011;14:189–93.
31. Sakai LM, Esposito TJ, Ton-That HH, et al. Comparison of objective screening and self-report for alcohol and drug use in traumatically injured patients. Alcohol Treat Q 2012;30:433–42.
32. Williams RJ, Nowatzki N. Validity of adolescent self-report of substance use. Subst Use Misuse 2005;40:299–311.
33. Available at: https://www.nationaldrugscreening.com/show-blog.php?id=234. Accessed April 1, 2016.
34. Manchikanti L, Atluri S, Trescot AM, et al. Monitoring opioid adherence in chronic pain patients: tools, techniques, and utility. Pain Physician 2008;11:S155–80.
35. Ceasar R, Chang J, Zamora K, et al. Primary care providers' experiences with urine toxicology tests to manage prescription opioid misuse and substance use among chronic non-cancer pain patients in safety net health care settings. Substance Abuse 2016;37:154–60.
36. Reisfield GM, Webb FJ, Bertholf RL, et al. Family physicians' proficiency in urine drug test interpretation. J Opioid Manag 2007;3:333–7.
37. Sbarbaro JA. Can we influence prescribing patterns? Clin Infect Dis 2001;33: S240–4.

38. Available at: https://www.whitehouse.gov/sites/default/files/ondcp/issues-content/fars_report_october_2011.pdf. Accessed April 1, 2016.
39. Sklerov JH, Magluilo J Jr, Shannon KK, et al. Liquid chromatography-electrospray ionization mass spectrometry for the detection of lysergide and a major metabolite, 2-oxo-3-hydroxy-LSD, in urine and blood. J Anal Toxicol 2000;24:543–9.
40. Knittel JL, Holler JM, Chmiel JD, et al. Analysis of parent synthetic cannabinoids in blood and urinary metabolites by liquid chromatography tandem mass spectrometry. J Anal Toxicol 2016;40:173–86.
41. Cone EJ, Caplan YH, Moser F, et al. Normalization of urinary drug concentrations with specific gravity and creatinine. J Anal Toxicol 2009;33:1–7.
42. Available at: www.samhsa.gov. Accessed April 1, 2016.

Narcotic Analgesics and Common Drugs of Abuse
Clinical Correlations and Laboratory Assessment

Martin H. Bluth, MD, PhD[a,b], Matthew R. Pincus, MD, PhD[c],*

KEYWORDS

- Drugs • Toxicology • Addiction • Pain • Clinical • Laboratory • Abuse • Analgesia

KEY POINTS

- Pain management is an evolving discipline; new formulations of narcotic analgesics mature to the marketplace with the promises of availing improved pain control, better dosing, and fewer side effects.
- These agents also avail an equal risk for abuse, which may mature as a result of physiologic tolerance, polypharmacy, metabolic factors, phramacogenomics, and economic concerns.
- Street chemists are adept at manipulating current and evolving drugs to more potent versions and creating new compositions of matter for consumption in the medical and illicit marketplaces.
- Clinical assessment is paramount to developing an index of suspicion of overdose, toxicity, or illicit drug use; the laboratory can support such investigations and guide therapy.
- As new agents pervade the health care system, the clinical toxicology laboratory keeps in step with adapting its technology and methodology to facilitate detection.

EXTENT OF USE OF DRUGS OF ABUSE

Over the last decade, there has been a general increase in the use of all drugs of abuse in the US population aged 12 years and over. The reported difference in illicit drug use from 2013 to 2014 has demonstrated an increase from 41.6 million users to 44.2 million, representing a greater than 6% increase, or 2.6 million new drug abusers, over 1 year alone. These agents include common illicit drugs including heroin, cocaine, and hallucinogens as well as nonmedical use of prescription drugs, sedatives, tranquilizers, pain relievers, and other agents.[1] The highest number of drug

[a] Department of Pathology, Wayne State University School of Medicine, 540 East Canfield, Detroit, MI 48201, USA; [b] Consolidated Laboratory Management Systems, 24555 Southfield Road, Southfield, MI 48075, USA; [c] Department of Pathology, SUNY Downstate Medical Center, 450 Clarkson Avenue, Brooklyn, NY 11203, USA
* Corresponding author.
E-mail address: mrpincus2010@gmail.com

Clin Lab Med 36 (2016) 603–634
http://dx.doi.org/10.1016/j.cll.2016.07.013
0272-2712/16/© 2016 Elsevier Inc. All rights reserved.
labmed.theclinics.com

abusers occurs in the 15- to 39-year-age range, at almost 75%. Interestingly, individuals in the 40- to 59-year bracket comprise most of the remainder, comprising more than 20% of the overall number of drug abusers, a sizable fraction. Drug abuse does spare any age, race, gender, socioeconomic, employment, or educational status. In fact, illicit drug use in 13-year-old children increased by approximately 30% from 2013 to 2014 (275,000 to >350,000 nationwide), and persons aged 26 and older have a 20% to 25% lifetime probability of using cocaine no matter whether they be full time, part time, or unemployed.[1] Because all persons are at risk for drug abuse, including prescribed, nonprescribed, and illicit substances, understanding the general and specific biological and physiologic effects of such pharmacopeia, in addition to absorption, distribution, metabolism, and excretion can help health care providers to select appropriate medications, either alone or in concert with other agents, as well as use appropriate ancillary clinical toxicology laboratory testing approaches to manage their patient populations.

APPLICATION OF THE CLINICAL TOXICOLOGY LABORATORY

The role of the clinical toxicology laboratory provides substantial support to patient pain management. It can facilitate objective information on whether the patient is (1) taking what the physician prescribed and (2) if he or she is taking something else. However, the laboratory results are not to be considered the be all and end all of whether a patient is adhering to clinical instruction or compliant with medication prescribing habits. As with most drugs, it is important to understand that the results of routine urine drug testing are not intended for use to diagnose, manage, treat, cure, or prevent any disease as a sole independent ancillary support application in lieu of the patient–physician relationship nor for application to forensic, employment, or court proceedings unless orchestrated through appropriate channels (www.samhsa.gov). Appropriate clinical management resides solely with the patient's primary care provider. However, laboratory results are intended and appropriately situated to provide laboratory supplemental data for discretionary use, in conjunction with other clinical patient profiles, presentations, signs, symptoms, history, and physical findings obtained by the patient's primary care provider. Furthermore, to this end, parent drug or metabolite concentrations are subject to many metabolic factors, including but not limited to hydration, kidney and liver function, time and dose of drug ingestion, and pharmacogenomics. For example, it is plausible that a patient who was prescribed codeine for pain management resulted in a urine test negative for codeine but positive for hydromorphone. It could be that this patient, who is a "rapid metabolizer" ingested codeine as prescribed, and catabolized codeine to morphine by O-demethylation, which also exerts its effects on its congeners—dihydrocodeine, ethylmorphine, hydrocodone, or oxycodone—but carried the polymorphically variant CYP2D6 allele or multiple alleles thereof, thereby fostering rapid conversion to hydromorphone, which is what was resulted in the patient's urine test.[2] In such an instance, varying the time of last ingestion to collection, in addition to being mindful of the other factors listed above, could shed light on identifying personalized testing that should be considered in performing urine drug testing. Understanding the results of such tests, which can differ from one patient from another, are necessary even when both are prescribed the same drug regimen. To this end, studies by Smith and colleagues[3] demonstrated that volunteers who ingested opiates and were assessed for urine parent drug and their metabolites (hydrocodone, hydromorphone, oxycodone, and oxymorphone) differed considerably from one another based on dose, time of collection, and analysis method used.

Regarding the methodology used in the clinical toxicology laboratory, there are different approaches that can be used to obtain pain medication analyte measurements in body fluids (blood, urine, saliva) including chromatographic (thin layer chromatography [TLC]; high-performance liquid chromatography), enzyme immune assay–based (enzyme-mediated immunologic technique; florescence polarization immunoassay), and gas or liquid chromatography based mass spectrometry (GS/MS or LC/MS, respectively). In general, basic enzyme and chromatographic tests are used for drug screening and are sometimes found in the point of care or clinical office setting. However, screening technologies are not very specific. Therefore, when screens are positive they are subsequently confirmed for the presence of specific drugs via GC/MS or LC/MS because these technologies use high complexity methodologies that assess the mass to charge ratio of each analyte, which can serve a "molecular fingerprint" for various entities including specific drugs of abuse (see Yan Victoria Zhang and colleagues article, "Liquid Chromatography–Tandem Mass Spectrometry: An Emerging Technology in the Toxicology Laboratory," in this issue).

GENERAL ASPECTS OF THE MECHANISMS OF ACTION

The major drugs of abuse include those prescribed in analgesia.[4] They can be generally divided into the natural and semisynthetic opioids (codeine, morphine, hydrocodone, hydromorphone, oxycodone, oxymorphone, heroine, buprenorphine, norbuprinorphine, meperidine), synthetic opioids (fentanyl, norfentanyl, methadone and EDDP [2-ethylidene-1,5,dimethyl-3-3-diphenylpyrrolidine; a methadone metabolite], tapentadol, tramadol, and other new composition of matter).[5,6] These drugs, with the exception of the barbiturates and the cannabinoids, are all basic amino group–containing compounds, most of which also contain benzene rings. The steric relationship of the amino group with respect to the aromatic benzene rings is rather similar, especially in cocaine, the opiates, and methadone. As might be expected, these compounds can cross-react, although with lower affinities, with each other's target receptors, and as such may also cross-react in toxicology screens that use immunoassay detection methodologies, yet are resolvable through mass spectrometry confirmatory testing approaches.[7]

The primary physiologic mechanisms of action of these drugs are not completely understood, but some rudimentary knowledge has been gained as to some of the main targets of these drugs. Many of these drugs act directly on dopaminergic and norepinephrinergic neurotransmitter systems, especially the limbic system, which is associated with general pleasure seeking and can precipitate behavior to that end.[8]

Fig. 1 depicts the likely mechanism of action of several of the most important drugs in the system. The class of amphetamines, closely related structurally to dopamine and the catecholamines, and cocaine seem to cause release of dopamine from the vesicles at the axonal side of the synapse, which may partially be responsible for the production of a pleasant sensation (so-called "high") in many individuals.[9] The tricyclic antidepressants stimulate pathways that use norepinephrine as the neurotransmitter. These pathways, like the dopaminergic pathways, are involved in arousal and pleasure seeking. In this case, the tricyclic antidepressants, rather than promoting release of the neurotransmitters, block the reuptake of norepinephrine into the vesicles on the axonal side of the synapse. They also may exert nonspecific reuptake blockade of dopamine in the dopaminergic pathways.[10] It is of great interest that, paradoxically, the tricyclic antidepressants such as imipramine (Tofranil) have been used successfully to treat the effects of cocaine, although success with benzodiazepine tranquilizers (oxazepam) in conjunction with cortisol synthesis inhibitors

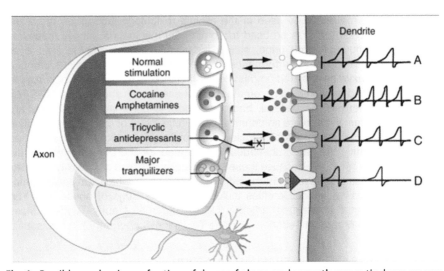

Fig. 1. Possible mechanisms of action of drugs of abuse and some therapeutic drugs on sym-pathomimetic amine (dopamine and norepinephrine) pathways. (A) Normal neural trans-mission. A nerve impulse is conducted down the axon to the terminal boutons at the nerve ending. Vesicles, represented by the round gray structure, release their contents of neurotransmitter, here dopamine, represented by small white circles. Dopamine molecules traverse the synaptic cleft and bind to dendritic receptors, initiating action potentials (*at right under "dendrite"*) in the dendrites. Notice the *arrows* showing that dopamine is both released and taken up by the vesicles. (B) In the presence of cocaine and amphet-amines, enhanced release of neurotransmitter (*red circles*) from vesicles occurs, increasing the rate of firing in the dendrites. (C) Tricyclic antidepressants block (*arrow with "X" in yellow box*) reuptake of the neurotransmitter (*purple circles*), in this case norepinephrine and, less specifically, dopamine, causing more neurotransmitter to "recycle" to the dendritic receptors, resulting in increased firing. (D) Some of the neuroleptics act by blocking (*gray wedge*) postsynaptic dendritic receptors for dopamine (*blue circles*), causing decreased firing. (*From* Pincus MR, Bluth MH, Abraham NZ. Toxicology and therapeutic drug moni-toring. In: Pincus MR, McPherson RA, editors. Henry's clinical diagnosis and management by laboratory methods. 23rd edition. Elsevier; 2017. p. 333.e2; with permission.)

(metyrapone) have been described.[11] Further use of benzodiazepines have been posited to enhance γ-aminobutyric acid (GABA) responses either via increasing re-ceptor expression density or channel gating efficiency.[12] To this end, major tranquil-izers such as haloperidol (Haldol) and chlorpromazine, used to treat psychotic states such as schizophrenia, seem to block attachment of dopamine to the dendritic receptors in the synapse, thereby blocking the stimulatory effects of dopamine. Asso-ciated with many dopaminergic neurons are inhibitory neurons that use GABA as their neurotransmitter. It seems that many benzodiazepine receptors exist on these neu-rons, causing potentiation of GABA at the synapses in this system, reducing the dopa-minergic effects of the stimulatory pathways on the limbic system. Thus, some of the tranquilizing effects of diazepam (Valium) and other benzodiazepines can be explained.

Widely distributed throughout the central nervous system (CNS) and periphery are a variety of opioid receptors classified mainly as μ-, δ-, κ-, and ε-receptors.[13] The μ-receptors seem to be rather specific for morphine and heroin, both of which produce a general analgesic state. Many of the drugs of abuse also act on 2 other major pathways in the brain: those using serotonin (serotonergic) and those using N-methyl-D-aspartate (NMDA) as their neurotransmitter. Neurotranmission by serotonin occurs by its binding to the 5-hydroxytryptamine (5-HT) receptor on the dendritic side of the synapse. There is a rather wide range of 5-HT receptors, not all of which produce the same physiologic effects. The major ones seem to be the 5-HT_1 and 5-HT_2 receptors. The serotonin pathways encompass a rather wide swath of the brain and even the spinal cord. This neurotransmitter is the principal one for the limbic system and, in addition, the basal ganglia, especially the amygdala that is involved in aggressive behavior. As mentioned, the limbic system is involved in pleasure seeking and pleasure reinforcement. Serotonergic pathways also extend to the hippocampus and are involved in memory. As a neurotransmitter in the spinal cord, serotonin induces muscle contraction. NMDA pathways are more involved in nociceptive (pain) pathways and are involved in memory and neuronal plasticity.[14] They have been found to be involved in chronic pain reinforcement. Blockade of NMDA pathways by drugs of abuse can therefore remove this perceived undesirable effect.

DRUG METABOLISM

Many drugs are converted to metabolites, some of which are pharmacologically active and some inactive. Much of this conversion occurs in the extramitochondrial, microsomal system present in hepatocytes. This metabolic system is mainly an oxidative one that uses a series of oxidative enzymes that, in turn, use a special cytochrome system: cytochrome P450.[15] This extremely critical cytochrome system, and genetic polymorphism of the cytochrome P450 enzymes, affects an individuals particular response to a drug, including toxicity and an adverse drug reaction. It is now possible to test individuals for their ability to metabolize specific drugs by amplification of their genes encoding cytochrome P450. Certain amino acid substitutions in this protein cause it to be very active in drug metabolism (ie, rapid inactivation of the drug). This implies that the patient may need substantially higher doses to achieve a therapeutic level, or that it may be necessary to use another less rapidly metabolized drug (see Daniel A. Schwarz, M.P. George, Martin H. Bluth's article, "Precision Medicine in Toxicology," in this issue).

Because the excretion of many drugs depends on the integrity of the liver and the cytochrome P450 system, in patients with liver failure owing to passive congestion, hepatitis, cirrhosis, and the like, the effective half-life of the drug is increased, making it necessary to lower the divided dose of the drug. Conversely, some drugs induce the intracellular synthesis of the microsomal enzymes, leading to diminished half-life values, so that it may be necessary to increase the divided dose. In certain cases drugs can induce microsomal enzymes to facilitate its own metabolism (ie, phenobarbital, phenytoin) so that its concentration levels do not obey first-order kinetics, as well as others that are differentially catabolized through phase I and/or phase II metabolic pathways.[16] In instances in which the levels of a drug metabolized in the liver are higher than the highest therapeutic value, reductions in the levels may be induced by administering low levels of such a drug to induce the microsomal system. Furthermore, although many narcotic analgesics are principally metabolized by the liver, there are those (ie, gabapentin, pregabalin) that are metabolized by nonhepatic organ pathways.[17]

These summaries of some of the general principles of drug administration should be helpful in the interpretation of values clinically and should permit a better understanding of the subsequent discussion of specific analgesic drugs, most frequently prescribed for pain management, yet are also subject to abuse potential.

COCAINE

Cocaine is derived from the coca plant and has enjoyed much popularity as an additive to certain foods. At the beginning of the 20th century, it was used in Coca-Cola, but owing to its addictive effects, this practice was discontinued. Cocaine is a derivative of the alkaloid ecgonine (ie, the methyl ester of benzoylecgonine) and can metabolize to benzoylecgonine, as shown in **Fig. 2**. The normal route of administration of cocaine is nasal (ie, inhalation, snorting), such that the drug passes through the nasal membranes. A particularly potent form of cocaine, called "crack," is the free-base form that passes rapidly across the nasal membranes such that, for a given dose, most or all of it enters the bloodstream rapidly. The half-life of cocaine is 1 to 2 hours, and the parent compound and its metabolites are usually cleared from the body within 2 days.

It is estimated that as many as 25 million people in the United States have used cocaine at least once[18]; fortunately, most of these individuals do not continue. Fatalities from cocaine abuse are of 2 types: direct toxicity of the drug and crime related to the illicit acquisition of the drug. Up to 25% of myocardial infarctions in patients between the ages of 18 and 45 have been attributed to cocaine abuse.[18]

Cocaine has been used medically to induce local anesthesia during nasopharyngeal surgery. However, in large doses, it induces a euphoric state (the "high" experienced by the user) and may also induce hallucinatory states. It can also promote violent behavior.[19] Many of these results can be explained by cocaine's dopaminergic effects. One study[20] suggests that cocaine induces increased calcium ion influx in dopaminergic neurons. The increased intracellular calcium activates phospholipases that possibly act as second messengers in causing ultimate release of dopamine in synapses. Prolonged action of phospholipases, however, ultimately causes cell death. In the previously mentioned study, in fact, cocaine was found to be neurotoxic. It also has a general cytotoxic effect from formation of an N-oxide free radical produced in the metabolism of this compound in the liver. It seems then that, over time, cocaine induces neuronal loss. In addition, binding of cocaine to cell receptors in the limbic system induces synthesis of cyclic adenosine monophosphate that seems to be critical in activating cell processes involved in dopamine release.[21] Cocaine may also block the reuptake of dopamine at the axonal side of the synapse, similar to tricyclic antidepressants (see **Fig. 1**). As if becoming toxic from cocaine abuse was not sufficient, many cocaine abusers consume this drug together with alcohol. Ethanol becomes esterified to cocaine in the liver to form cocaethylene, which blocks reuptake of dopamine in dopaminergic pathways more effectively than does cocaine and causes pronounced

DOPAMINERGIC PATHWAY STIMULANTS

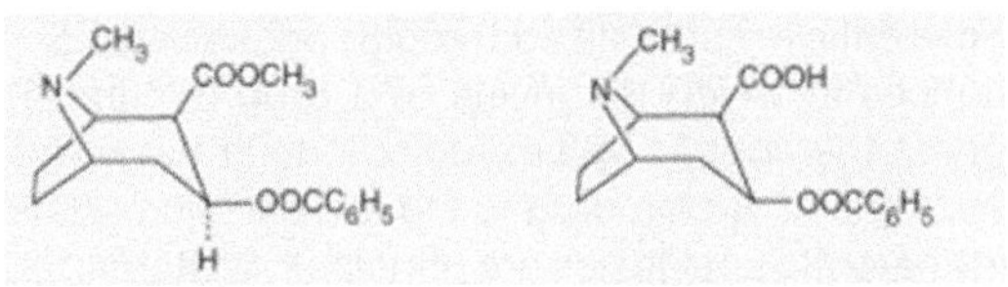

Cocaine

Benzoylecgonine
(less active metabolite)

Fig. 2. Chemical structures of dopaminergic pathway stimulants. (*From* Pincus MR, Bluth MH, Abraham NZ. Toxicology and therapeutic drug monitoring. In: Pincus MR, McPherson RA, editors. Henry's clinical diagnosis and management by laboratory methods. 23rd edition. Elsevier; 2017. p. 332.e2; with permission.)

vasoconstriction of the coronary arteries, inducing increased myocardial oxygen demand. This cocaine derivative is deadlier than either cocaine or ethanol alone.

Other studies[18] further indicate that prolonged use of cocaine results in cardiotoxicity—that is, cocaine can cause progressive atherosclerosis and causes constriction of the coronary arteries that can, in turn, induce myocardial ischemia and sometimes frank infarction. Cocaine has been found to induce sympathomimetic effects on the myocardium by increasing heart rate. At the same time, it induces increased vasoconstriction. The net effect is increased chronotropy and afterload, resulting in increased oxygen demand by the myocardium. At the same time, cocaine induces platelet aggregation and stimulates production of plasminogen activator inhibitor. These events all predispose to development of myocardial infarction.

One highly disturbing aspect of cocaine abuse is that cocaine passes readily across the placenta and also into the lactating mammary gland and is readily passed from mothers to nursing infants. Often in the hospital setting, mothers receive the drug from dealers and breastfeed their newborn babies, who are therefore maintained on this drug. Cocaine causes mental retardation, delayed development, and strong drug dependence in newborns. It can also produce malformations in utero. According to the 2012 Survey on Drug Use and Health, 5.9% of pregnant women use illicit drugs, resulting in more than 380,000 offspring exposed to illicit substances.[22]

Cocaine has not been considered classically to be an addictive drug, because it does not cause the true physical dependence typical of abusers of barbiturates and opiates. However, the high produced by the drug is extraordinarily reinforcing, so that the drug-seeking behavior of the cocaine and opiate abuser is similar. Evidence in experimental animals suggests that cocaine can induce the release of β-endorphins that bind to μ-receptors in the limbic system. This induces a pleasant and positive feeling of reinforcement. Clinically, patients who are overdosed with cocaine may become violent and irrational, requiring sedation. One such treatment for patients in hyperexcitable states with cardiac symptoms such as palpitations is one of the benzodiazepines. Thus, it is not uncommon to find cocaine and a benzodiazepine (ie, oxazepam) in the urine of cocaine addicts.[11] Occasionally, overdosed patients will become obtunded or comatose. The treatment for these patients is usually supportive. Additionally, antidepressants, including the tri/tetracyclics, selective serotonin reuptake inhibitors, and the cortisol synthesis inhibitor metyrapone have been found in certain studies to inhibit some of the undesirable effects of cocaine and have been used in the treatment of cocaine abuse.

The half-life of cocaine, as stated, is approximately 1 to 2 hours. It is metabolized to more polar compounds that have significantly less potency than the parent compound. These metabolites have longer half-lives and, with techniques such as GC/MS, can be detected up to 48 hours after administration of the drug. The immunoassay methods can detect the drug for about 24 to 36 hours after administration. Certain metabolites (benzoylecgonine cocaine derivative) can be detected in urine for 3 to 5 days after administration. If a patient has inhaled cocaine free-base ("crack"), it is possible to detect the parent compound, cocaine, by TLC up to several hours after administration, owing to the high doses of drug present.

THE OPIATES

The primary medicinal use of opiates such as codeine and morphine is to diminish or eliminate pain in a patient. As noted, there are several classes of opiate receptors that are involved in the modulation of pain. These receptors are classified as μ, κ, δ, and ϵ. The endogenous ligands for each of these receptors are the antinociceptive peptides: endomorphin (Tyr-Pro-Trp-Phe-NH$_2$) for μ receptors, dynorphins A (Tyr-Gly-Gly-Phe-Leu-Arg-Arg-Ile-Arg-Pro-Lys-Leu-Lys) and B (Tyr-Gly-Gly-Phe-Leu-Arg-Arg-Gln-Phe-Lys-Val-Val-Thr) for κ receptors, Met- and Leu-enkephalin (Tyr-Gly-Gly-Phe-Met and Tyr-Gly-Gly-Phe-Leu) for ϵ receptors and deltorphin (Tyr-D-Met-Phe-His-Leu-Met-Asp-NH$_2$) and Met and Leu-enkephalin for δ receptors. Note that the first 5 amino acids of dynorphin are identical to those of Leu-enkephalin, suggesting a possible reason for the binding of enkephalin to κ receptors. The exogenous opiates, that is, morphine, codeine, fentanyl, and others, whose structures are shown in **Fig. 3**, are known to be agonists, primarily, for μ receptors. As can be seen in this figure, morphine, codeine, heroin, oxycodone, and buprenorphine have similar structures. In fact, morphine is a metabolite of heroin, the diacetyl precursor of morphine.

A major target for each of the endogenous opiate peptides and for the exogenous agents is the main pain pathway, that is, the spinothalamic tract. This neural pathway carries nerve impulses from peripheral pain receptors to the peripheral nerves that innervate them to the posterior horn of the spinal cord where the nerves synapse to ascending fibers in the spinothalamic pathway. These nerves travel to the next spinal level where they cross the midline and then travel to the medulla as the lateral lemniscus that synapses in the thalamus (mainly in the ventroposterior nucleus) and then projects to the cortex where pain perception takes place. Activation of the opioid

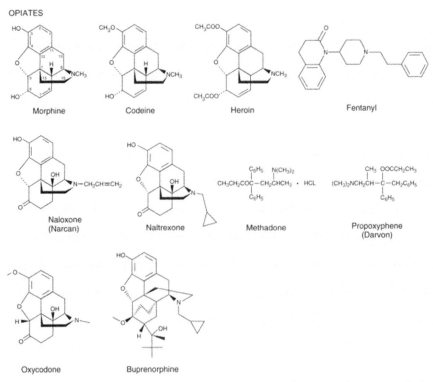

Fig. 3. Chemical structures of opiates. (*From* Pincus MR, Bluth MH, Abraham NZ. Toxicology and therapeutic drug monitoring. In: Pincus MR, McPherson RA, editors. Henry's clinical diagnosis and management by laboratory methods. 23rd edition. Elsevier; 2017. p. 331.e2; with permission.)

receptors that occur at these synapses results in hyperpolarization of the dendritic side of the synapses, blocking nerve conduction, thereby diminishing the sensation of pain.

In addition, it seems that the opioid receptors also play another major role in pain modulation via the activation of descending tracts that emanate from the midbrain in the periaqueductal gray area and travel to nuclei in the median raphe of the medulla. After synapsing with these nuclei, these tracts synapse at interneurons in the posterior horn of the spinal cord where they activate the release of GABA, resulting in inhibition of nerve conduction in the spinothalamic tract. Normally, these pathways are quiescent, but release of any of the endogenous antinociceptive peptides or introduction of exogenous drugs such as morphine or codeine, results in removal of inhibition of these pathways, again resulting in inhibition of nerve conduction in the spinothalamic pathway with diminished perception of pain.

Morphine and Heroin

Morphine, a μ receptor agonist, in addition to acting on pain pathways as described, further acts by binding to μ-receptors in the limbic system (CNS), mainly in the nucleus accumbens and the ventral tegmental area, resulting in an analgesic state. Binding of morphine and the other opiates to the μ-receptor inhibits the release of GABA from the nerve terminal, reducing the inhibitory effect of GABA on dopaminergic neurons. The resulting increased activation of dopaminergic neurons results in sustained activation of the postsynaptic membrane, causing a sense of euphoria. On the molecular level, binding of morphine to these receptors activates a cell signaling cascade via G-protein activation that results in elevated expression of many transcriptionally active proteins such as ERK, jun, and fos, and superactivation of adenyl cyclase resulting in high intracellular levels of cyclic adenosine monophosphate.[23] Besides being used as a major analgesic, morphine (ie, Dilaudid) is important in treating acute congestive heart failure by lowering venous return to the heart (ie, it is a powerful preload reducer by causing increased splanchnic pooling of blood).

Heroin induces a pleasant, euphoric state and is highly addictive both physically and psychologically. As can be seen in **Fig. 3**, heroin is a diacetyl form of morphine. This characteristic facilitates heroin's crossing the blood–brain barrier, allowing it to reach higher concentrations in the CNS. Withdrawal from this drug is exceedingly difficult, with a myriad of symptoms such as hypothermia, palpitations, cold sweats, and nightmares. This is a true physical dependence, the molecular basis for which is not fully understood. It seems that the dependence is strongly linked to the number of cell surface μ-receptors.[23]

This class of compounds exhibits certain important paradoxic effects on the parasympathetic nervous system. These drugs exert a procholinergic effect on the eyes and on blood vessels in the periphery (ie, they cause constriction of pupils ["pinpoint pupils"] and peripheral vasodilation). In contrast, in the gut they lower gastrointestinal (GI) motility (ie, they exhibit anticholinergic effects in the GI tract). This fact enables rapid diagnosis of heroin or, in general, opiate abuse in a patient brought to the emergency room in an obtunded or comatose state. These patients typically have severe miosis (pupillary constriction). Although the sign is not useful in acute diagnosis, constipation commonly occurs.

Administration of heroin occurs via the intravenous route. Addicts are readily recognized by the presence of needle tracks on their arms and hands and by extensive thrombosis of their peripheral veins. The half-life of heroin via the intravenous route is about 3 minutes, and the effects of the drug last approximately 3 hours. Heroin is almost immediately hydrolyzed by cholinesterase and arylesterase to

6-monoacetylmorphine (6-MAM), which occurs in plasma, erythrocytes, and liver. 6-MAM, is reported to have a half-life of 10 to 40 minutes and can be detected in urine up to 24 hours after intake. Heroine, via 6-MAM, is further metabolized to morphine, which has a half-life of 2 to 4 hours and can has a detection window in urine for approximately 2 to 4 days after ingestion. Morphine can be further conjugated to yield morphine-3-glucoronide (M3G), which can be detected in urine for up to 5 days, and other glucoronidated forms (ie, morphine-6-glucuronide). In general, 60% to 80% of heroin is excreted as morphine or M3G.[24] Thus, urine toxicology testing for heroin and its metabolites (6-MAM, morphine) are often performed in concert to determine the plausibility of heroin administration in the context of urine drug testing, which results as positive for morphine and its metabolites (**Fig. 4**). This approach has also been beneficial for those ingesting poppy seeds, which also convert to morphine, to clarify confusion of suspected heroin ingestion in this regard.[25,26]

Overdoses of heroin are extremely dangerous and can cause severe obtundation, coma, respiratory arrest, hypotension (secondary to histamine release), and cardiac arrhythmias. One of the most common acute therapeutic modalities for heroin overdose is intravenous treatment with naloxone (Narcan; see **Fig. 3**), a strong competitive antagonist to the action of heroin. Naloxone can be detected in urine approximately 2 days after ingestion.

Methadone

Heroin addiction, as a chronic problem, is treated pharmacologically with a partial agonist of heroin—methadone. This interesting compound, whose structure is shown in **Fig. 3**, binds competitively with morphine to μ-receptors in the brain. However, although it can become addictive, the addictive effects are less than those of

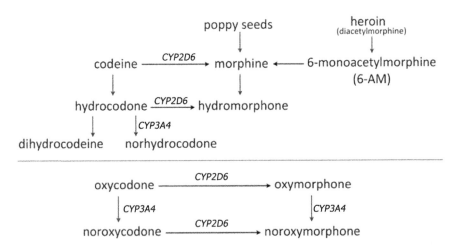

Fig. 4. Opiates and opioid metabolism. Shown in *italic* are the major cytochrome P450 enzymes involved in phase I metabolism; patterns of drug metabolites may reflect the metabolic phenotype of the patient. Actual proportions of individual metabolites will vary. Phase II reactions (eg, glucuronide conjugation) are not shown but are prominent for most compounds. (*From* ARUP Consult https://arupconsult.com/https://arupconsult.com, an ARUP Laboratories test selection tool for healthcare professionals.)

equivalent concentrations of heroin, possibly because its binding affinity is lower, so that it induces less of an effect than heroin. Thus, administration of methadone to heroin addicts allows them to experience the effects of heroin but in a modulated manner. By gradually lowering the methadone dose, physical dependence becomes reduced, and it seems that a trough serum methadone level greater than 100 ng/mL is adequate for effective methadone maintenance.[27]

However, it should be noted that addiction to methadone can also occur. In toxicology laboratories, the most common request received for methadone screens comes from methadone clinics to test whether a patient is administering methadone or has relapsed into taking heroin. Methadone can be distinguished from the opiates by many detection methods—TLC, enzyme-mediated immunologic technique, and florescence polarization immunoassay detects each drug with high specificity. Confirmation via GC/MS and LC/MS is also used and can detect methadone in urine approximately 3 to 5 days after ingestion. Methadone is further metabolized to EDDP. Recent studies have reported the usefulness of methadone-to-EDDP ratios to monitor for patient compliance.[28]

Another opiate antagonist is naltrexone, whose structure is shown **Fig. 3**. The primary effect of this drug is to lower the euphoria experienced by opiate abusers. However, it has no effect on opiate craving by drug abusers. In contrast, it has been found to be effective in reducing the physical dependence of patients treated with the drug; however, to achieve abstinence, psychosocial support of the patient is required. Surprisingly, naltrexone has been found to be effective in the treatment of alcohol dependence; in particular, it has been found to reduce relapse rates after abstinence and to reduce heavy drinking to lower levels of consumption. The half-life of naltrexone is about 4 hours. Treatment of opiate abuse generally requires daily administration (ie, 50 mg/day) and excretion is via urine with a detection window, similar to naloxone, of 2 days post ingestion.

Codeine and Analogs

The structure of codeine is similar to that of morphine and heroin (see **Fig. 3**). Codeine acts in a manner similar to that of morphine and is used as a milder analgesic and as an antitussive. Codeine metabolism is complex and can yield metabolites that are prescribed drugs themselves, which can be synergistically administered for maximal pain relief. As shown in **Fig. 4**, codeine can metabolize to morphine or hydrocodone. Hydrocodone in turn can be metabolized to hydromorphone as well as dihydrocodiene and norhydrocodone. Of interest is that morphine can also further metabolize to hydromorphone. Thus, it is not uncommon for a clinician to prescribe codeine to a patient whose urine drug test results as negative for codeine but positive for hydromorphone. This result can easily introduce suspicion of diversion of codeine and/or surreptitious ingestion of morphine. Therefore, appropriate understanding of opiate pathway metabolism can mitigate such concerns.

Dextromethorphan

Dextromethorphan (D-3-methoxy-N-methylmorphine), an analog of codeine, is the active component of cough syrups because of its antitussive effects. Recently, there has been a "run" on cough medicines by addicts, who can obtain them legally and then consume quantities sufficient to reach their desired euphoric state. Unlike codeine, dextromethorphan is believed generally not to be addictive, although cases of drug dependency have been documented. For therapeutic use, the recommended dose of dextromethorphan is 15 to 30 mg given 3 to 4 times per day. Moderate intoxication is achieved at about 100 to 200 mg, and heavy intoxication is reached at around 1500 mg.[29] It is surprising to note that dextromethorphan does not have analgesic properties because of its lack of affinity for μ-, κ-, and δ-receptors. It has been found to induce the release and to block the reuptake of serotonin. Similar to the action of phencyclidine (PCP), discussed elsewhere in this article, dextromethorphan has also been found to block NMDA receptors that are critical for neuronal plasticity and memory and are involved in central pain pathways in the brain.[14] Dextromethorphan is readily absorbed from the GI tract and, in about 85% of individuals, is rapidly metabolized to dextrophan, an active metabolite, and D-hydroxymorphinane via the 2D6 cytochrome P450 isozyme. It is dextrophan that has a high affinity for NMDA receptors, so that most individuals experience PCP-like effects (ie, euphoria; tactile, auditory, and visual hallucinations; paranoia, altered time perception; and general disorientation). For the 15% of individuals who are slow metabolizers of dextromethorphan, these effects are much less pronounced and are replaced by sedation and dysphoria.[29] Overdoses of dextromethorphan can result in mainly neurologic effects, such as lethargy, or, conversely, hyperexcitability, ataxia, slurred speech, tremors and fasciculations, hypertonia and hyperreflexia, and nystagmus, as well as either pupillodilation or pupilloconstriction. Diaphoresis may also occur. In addition, cardiovascular sequelae include tachycardia and hypertension. Unfortunately, a number of antitussives contain, in addition to dextromethorphan, anticholinergic agents such as chlorpheniramine. Thus, abuse of antitussive medication can give rise to such symptoms as tachycardia, mydriasis, flushed skin, urinary retention, and constipation. Megadoses of dextromethorphan can occasionally produce a false-positive screening test for PCP or opiates, which can be confirmed with GC/MS or LC/MS.[30] Dextromethorphan can be detected in urine after ingestion with a detection window of 1 to 2 days.

Oxycodone

This drug is effective in reducing pain, especially pain associated with malignancy. Its structure is shown in **Fig. 3**, where it can be seen to be similar in structure to codeine with the difference that there is a keto rather than a hydroxyl group at the 7-position (lower cyclohexone ring) and a hydroxyl group rather than a hydrogen atom at the carbon between the 2 bridgehead carbons. On an empty stomach, pain diminution commences within about 15 minutes after oral drug administration. Peak serum levels are achieved in about 1 hour. The slow release form of oxycodone is oxycontin that achieves peak serum levels in about 3 hours. Although there is some controversy about the site of action of oxycodone, that is, primary action on κ, rather than μ, receptors, oxycodone does bind to μ receptors and one of its metabolites, oxymorphone, is known to have a high affinity for μ receptors.[31] The half-life for oxycodone is about 3.2 hours and for oxycontin is 4.5 hours. Metabolites of oxycodone are α- and β-oxycodol, oxymorphone, α- and β-oxymorphol, noroxymorphone, noroxycodone, α- and β- noroxycodol, and noroxymorphone (N-desmethyloxycodone). Most of the parent compound, as with other opioids, and its metabolites are excreted in the urine with a detection window of 2 to 4 days after ingestion.

As with morphine and codeine, oxycodone, especially at high doses, can induce euphoria and a sense of well-being, and, like the other opiates, it induces a true physical dependence. At high doses, side effects are particularly pronounced, and these include fatigue, dizziness, constipation, vomiting, anxiety, shallow breathing and apnea, hypotension, meiosis, circulatory collapse, and death. Withdrawal from oxycodone includes such symptoms as myositis, anxiety, nausea, insomnia, fever, hypogonadism, and hormonal imbalance. Given the side effects and the physical consequences of withdrawal, it is difficult to fathom the appeal of abuse of this drug.

Nonetheless, abuse of oxycodone has grown to the point where it has now been added to the roster of drugs of abuse that are routinely assayed for mainly in urine.

Buprenorphine

Although, like oxycodone, this prescription drug has become a drug of abuse, buprenorphine exerts a mixed agonist–antagonist effect on opiate receptors. It has some opiate activity on μ receptors, but it is purely an antagonist on κ and δ receptors. Its major use is the same as for methadone in treating addiction to opiates, but is also used in the treatment of pain. Because it has partial agonist activity, it does not cause life-threatening respiratory depression as is true of the agonists like morphine. It undergoes extensive metabolism in the liver and, therefore, excretion is via the hepatobiliary system in contrast with oxycodone, whose excretion is almost completely via the urinary tract. Thus, renal failure does not result in accumulation of buprenorphine in serum, although it does cause increased levels of oxycodone. Treatment of patients with buprenorphine for addiction is carried out in programs where the patient has access to private and group counseling during and after the treatment period. Suboxone is a combined drug of buprenorphine and naloxone (see **Fig. 3**). Naloxone is an antagonist at μ receptors and is administered with buprenorphine to block its toxic effects in patients who try to inject suboxone intravenously as a drug of abuse. The antagonism is limited because the affinity of buprenorphine for the μ receptor is about 5 times that of naloxone.

Buprenorphine is also available as a transdermal patch (Butrans), is used to treat chronic, rather than acute, pain, and has been found to be effective for this purpose. However, the transdermal patch route has posed some challenges with regard to urine and oral drug testing because (1) it does not require the same first-pass metabolism through the liver as with sublingual (Subutex, Suboxon) ingestion and (2) releases micro doses compared with the pill form. Buprenorphine is metabolized via the CYP3A4 enzyme to norbuprenorphine via the liver and both analytes are often included in a standard urine drug test to demonstrate ingestion of the parent drug. The presence of both buprenorphine and its metabolite norbuprinorphine in the urine can help to obviate suspicion of diversion in a patient suspecting of adding straight buprenorphine directly to the urine, which would not yield norbuprinorphine in such a case.

Buprenorphine has been found to be more effective than methadone in treating patients with depressive traits,[32] a phenomenon that is thought to be associated with its pure antagonistic effects on κ receptors. Because it, like oxycodone, has become popular as a drug of abuse, screening for its presence in urine has become common. Toxic effects of this drug include nausea, vomiting, drowsiness, dizziness, headaches, memory loss, perspiration, dry mouth, miosis, orthostatic hypotension, impotence, decreased libido, and urinary retention. Constipation can occur, but is less frequent than with morphine. Hepatic necrosis and hepatitis with jaundice, as with the major tranquilizers/neuroleptic drugs, have further been observed in patients with high levels of buprenorphine. The half-life of buprenorphine is 23 to 42 hours, whereas that of naloxone is 2 to 12 hours. The detection window for urine drug testing for buprenorphine is 4 to 5 days and for naloxone it is approximately 2 days.

Fentanyl

This opiate analgesic (see **Fig. 3**), is about 80 times more potent than morphine in blocking pain. It can be taken orally as so-called fentanyl lollipops, smoked, inhaled, or administered by transdermal fentanyl patches.[29] Overdose effects of this drug are the usual ones seen for opiate abuse and include respiratory depression and miosis. Treatment may involve irrigation of the bowel, and antiopiates such as naloxone may be administered. Hypotension is less common than with other opiates like morphine, because of the lack of histamine release. The detection window for fentanyl in urine is about 3 to 4 days after ingestion.

AMPHETAMINES

These compounds, as can be seen in **Fig. 5**, bear a close resemblance to the adrenergic amines such as epinephrine and norepinephrine, and may be expected to exert sympathomimetic effects. They also resemble dopamine and may be expected to have effects on dopaminergic pathways. The amphetamines cause euphoria and increased mental alertness that may be attributed to their effects on these pathways. This group of drugs, however, also exerts pronounced stimulatory

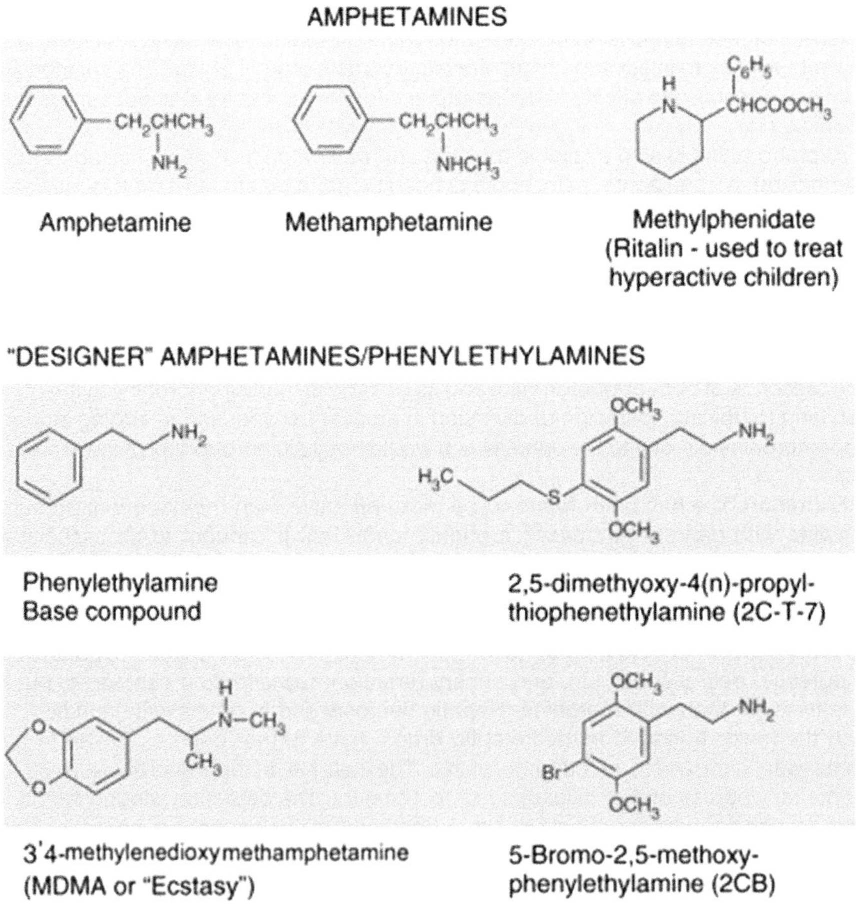

Fig. 5. Chemical structures of amphetamines and "designer" amphetamines/phenylethylamines. (*From* Pincus MR, Bluth MH, Abraham NZ. Toxicology and therapeutic drug monitoring. In: Pincus MR, McPherson RA, editors. Henry's clinical diagnosis and management by laboratory methods. 23rd edition. Elsevier; 2017. p. 332.e2; with permission.)

effects on γ- and β-receptors in the cardiovascular system and in the kidney to cause pronounced adrenergic effects such as increased heart rate, increased blood pressure, palpitations, bronchodilation, anxiety, pallor, and tremulousness. Studies indicate that amphetamines are also competitive inhibitors of the enzyme monoamine oxidase, which inactivates adrenergic neurotransmitters by oxidatively removing their amino groups. Blockage of this enzyme prolongs the effects of epinephrine and norepinephrine, with the attendant neurologic and cardiovascular sequelae.

One particular amphetamine, 3,4-methylenedioxymethamphetamine (MDMA or ecstasy), a derivative of methamphetamine (see **Fig. 5**), has become popular as a recreational drug of abuse because it has euphoric and psychedelic effects but minimal hallucinogenic effects.[29] Various other methamphetamine derivatives (N-methyl-1-phenylpropan-2-amine) also referred to as Crystal Meth, Speed, Ice, and Chalk, among others, are continuously emerging as new drugs of abuse. Methamphetamine can be also be found in over-the-counter cold remedies and inhalers, which can cause confusion on drug testing.[33] However, in general, over-the-counter formulations contain the L-isomer [$R(-)$], which has mild dopaminergic effects and can be found in nasal decongestants (ie, Vicks VapoInhaler). In contrast, drugs containing the D-isomer [$S(+)$] (ie, Desoxyn used for attention deficit disorder) are strong CNS stimulants releasing dopamine from storage vesicles and interfering with dopamine transporter function, thereby affording high abuse liability owing to increased dopamine release in the extracellular synapse. Both Toxi-Lab (Irvine, CA) and enzyme-mediated immunologic technique (Syva, San Jose, CA) procedures are effective as a screening method in detecting these drugs of abuse. Occasionally, on the Toxi-Lab A strip, amphetamines may be confused with antihistamines like diphenhydramine. Confirmation of amphetamine and methamphetamine can be determined by GC/MS or LC/MS of patient's urine. When assessed by this method, methamphetamine and its D and L isomers have a detection window of approximately 2 to 3 days after ingestion. The presence of greater than 30% D isomer in the absence of prescription drugs that contain or metabolize to D-methamphetamine (Desoxyn, selegiline, benzphetamine) can raise suspicion of illicit drug use. Methamphetamine is converted to amphetamine, which has a detection window for urine drug testing of 3 to 5 days after ingestion.

The pharmacologic action of amphetamines includes CNS and respiratory stimulation and sympathomimetic activity (eg, bronchodilation, pressor response, mydriasis). Loss of weight may also occur as the result of an anorectic effect, which has been the reason for amphetamine and similar derivatives (ie, phentermine) for use and abuse in certain cases.[34] Psychic stimulation and excitability, leading to a temporary increase in mental and physical activity, can occur; anxiety and nervousness can also be produced.

Tolerance may be produced within a few weeks, and physical or psychological dependence may occur with prolonged use. Symptoms of chronic abuse include emotional lability, somnolence, loss of appetite, occupational deterioration, mental impairment, and social withdrawal. Trauma and ulcer of the tongue and lip may occur as a result of continuing chewing or teeth-grinding movements. A syndrome with the characteristics of paranoid schizophrenia can occur with prolonged use at a high dose. Aplastic anemia and fatal pancytopenia are rare complications.

No specific antidote for amphetamine overdose is known, and treatment of overdose is symptomatic with general physiologic supportive measures immediately implemented. When cardiovascular symptoms are noted, propranolol (Inderal) can be used as an antidote.

The quest for euphoria-producing drugs has resulted in the advent of synthetic phenylethylamines, so-called designer drugs, like MDMA, several further examples of which are shown in **Fig. 5**. With all of these drugs, the price for the sought-after effects of euphoria and hallucinations consists of headaches, nausea, vomiting, anxiety, agitation, violent behavior, tachycardia, hypertension, respiratory depression, and seizures, as discussed in the case of standard amphetamines.

Other phenylethylamine derivatives shown in **Fig. 5**, especially 2C-T-7 and 2CB, bind to 5-HT$_2$ receptors and induce hallucinogenic effects.[29] These drugs have been taken orally or have been insufflated, smoked, administered intravenously, and even taken rectally. Death from overdose of these designer drugs has been reported and varies based on newer compositions that become available over time. Unfortunately, thus far no specific assays are available for most of these drugs in urine. Their presence must be ascertained by history and/or symptoms reported in the absence of positive urine tests for standard amphetamines. On occasion, GC/MS LC/MS can be used to detect their presence.

TRYPTAMINES

Tryptamines are derivatives of serotonin, whose structure is shown in **Fig. 6**. These tryptamines, some of which occur in plants, are relatively simple to obtain and are also being assessed for select conditions (ie, xaliproden for chemotherapy-induced peripheral neuropathy). An example is *N,N*-dimethyltryptamine (DMT), which has strong hallucinogenic properties. Smoking DMT results in the rapid onset of hallucinogenic effects that are short-lived, giving rise to the term, "businessman's lunch." Other tryptamines contain modifications of the indole ring. These also allow them to interact with 5-HT receptors,[29] and this interaction is thought to result in their hallucinogenic effects. However, the mechanism of action of this class of drugs is not well understood. Psilocin shown in this figure is a component of the so-called Psilocybe, called magic mushrooms because of their hallucinogenic effects. The hallucinogenic effects of these drugs are enhanced by the presence of monoamine oxidase inhibitors such as β-carbolines. The mixture of these 2 compounds is present in a South American

TRYPTAMINES

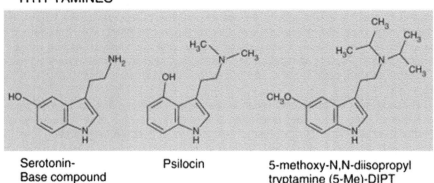

Serotonin-   Psilocin   5-methoxy-N,N-diisopropyl
Base compound   tryptamine (5-Me)-DIPT

Fig. 6. Chemical structures of tryptamines. (*From* Pincus MR, Bluth MH, Abraham NZ. Toxicology and therapeutic drug monitoring. In: Pincus MR, McPherson RA, editors. Henry's clinical diagnosis and management by laboratory methods. 23rd edition. Elsevier; 2017. p. 333.e2; with permission.)

tea called *ayahuasca*, which combines 2 plants—one containing DMT and the other carbolines, which themselves can induce nausea and vomiting. Like the amphetamines and other phenylethylamine derivatives, the tryptamines cause, in addition to the "desired" effects of euphoria and empathy, auditory and visual hallucinations, nausea, vomiting, diarrhea, and emotional distress. Symptoms further include agitation, tachycardia, hypertension, diaphoresis, salivation, dystonia, mydriasis, tremors, confusion, seizures, and, in a few cases, rhabdomyolysis and paralysis. Currently, no routine assays are available for these compounds. As with the amphetamines, many of the psychogenic and physiologic effects of the tryptamines can be countered with supportive therapy and the administration of benzodiazepines.

PIPERAZINES

The structure of the parent compound, piperazine, is shown in **Fig. 7**. Several of the derivatives of piperazine are also shown. Many of these piperazines were used as antihelminthics during the 1950s, but were subsequently discontinued. However, their euphoria-producing effects were discovered, leading to a "legal" way of obtaining drugs of abuse. Two classes of piperazine derivatives have been identified: *N*-benzylpiperazines, the parent compound of which is *N*-benzylpiperazine (BZP), and phenylpiperazines. The former group includes 1-(3,4-methylenedioxybenzyl)piperazine, and the latter group includes 1-(3-chlorophenyl)piperazine, 1-(4-methoxyphenyl)piperazine, and 1-(3-trifluoromethylphenyl)piperazine (TFMPP). BZP (known as "A2") and TFMPP (known as "Molly") are among the most popular piperazines. Studies have shown that these piperazines produced effects that were similar to those of the amphetamines, suggesting that the target receptors of these drugs are the same. Both classes of piperazines have been found to increase dopamine and serotonin levels. TFMPP has been found to act as a partial agonist at 5-HT$_{2A}$ receptors and

PIPERAZINES

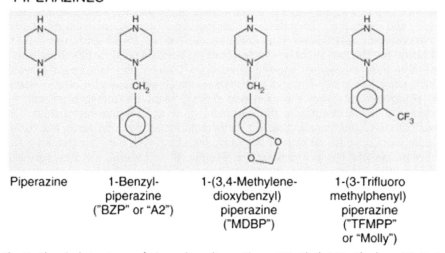

| Piperazine | 1-Benzyl-piperazine ("BZP" or "A2") | 1-(3,4-Methylene-dioxybenzyl) piperazine ("MDBP") | 1-(3-Trifluoro methylphenyl) piperazine ("TFMPP" or "Molly") |

Fig. 7. Chemical structures of piperazines. (*From* Pincus MR, Bluth MH, Abraham NZ. Toxicology and therapeutic drug monitoring. In: Pincus MR, McPherson RA, editors. Henry's clinical diagnosis and management by laboratory methods. 23rd edition. Elsevier; 2017. p. 333.e2; with permission.)

is a full agonist at other 5-HT receptors. Although TFMPP is 3 times less potent than MDMA, it produces a full MDMA effect when combined with BZP, with which it is synergistic.[29] The TFMPP-BZP combination at low doses induces euphoria with decreased motor action, making the euphoric "experience" more pleasurable. The acute undesirable effects of piperazines are similar to those of the amphetamines and MDMA (ie, hallucinations, psychomotor agitation, increased heart rate and blood pressure, and increased body temperature). Deaths from BZP have been reported when combined with another drug like MDMA. Both TFMPP and BZP have skin irritant properties, causing sore nasal passages and throats; treatment is generally supportive. As with select tryptamines and designer amphetamines, currently no standard assay method detects these drugs in urine, although recent methods to detect these drugs using LC/MS have been described.[35]

BENZODIAZEPINES

Among this group of drugs, shown in **Fig. 8**, the most prominent is diazepam (Valium); they are used therapeutically, as so-called minor tranquilizers. Their mechanisms of action seem to be potentiation of GABA, a neurotransmitter that inhibits conduction in dopaminergic neurons, and facilitation of its binding to GABA receptors.[36] Benzodiazepines bind to the α subunit of the $GABA_A$ receptor at a site that is distinct from that for GABA itself and cause an increase in the frequency of chloride ion channel opening at the $GABA_A$ receptor. Usually used as a therapeutic drug to produce calming effects at doses between 2.5 and 10 mg and to produce muscle-relaxing effects at higher doses, diazepam has been used by drug addicts in high dosage to counter the excitatory effects of other drugs of abuse or as a means of inducing tranquil states. Among some drug abusers, benzodiazepines are used to potentiate the effects of heroin.[37] A number of drug abusers have become addicted to diazepam when using high doses several times each day. Acutely, benzodiazepine overdose may produce somnolence, confusion, seizures, and coma. Rarely, hypotension, respiratory depression, and cardiac arrest may occur. Chronically, physical and psychological dependence occur. Sudden discontinuance of the drug may lead to anxiety, sweating, irritability, hallucinations, diarrhea, and seizures. Treatment is supportive. Gradual diminution of the benzodiazepine removes physical dependence. The half-life for diazepam is 20 to 70 hours, but the half-life of one of its active metabolites is 50 to 100 hours. Other common benzodiazepines include alprazolam (Xanax) and lorazepam (Ativan), which differ in the half-life and are often administered based on clinical needs (ie, alprazolam for panic disorder) and dosing. Many benzodiazepines can be detected in urine directly as the parent drug or as selective metabolites. For example, diazepam can be detected via its metabolites of nordiazepam and temazepam, both of which catabolize to oxazepam; alprazolam can be detected by its active metabolite α-hydroxyalprazolam (see **Fig. 8**). In general, the detection window for urine sampling after ingestion is approximately 5 to 7 days after ingestion or 6 weeks with chronic ingestion (>1 year of use). Recent studies have reported greater ease and speed of sample extraction methods thereby affording a broader range of compounds that can be analyzed with shorter run times using LC/MS technology.[38]

PHENCYCLIDINE

This interesting tricyclic compound, shown in **Fig. 9**, has numerous effects on a variety of different neural pathways. Used almost exclusively as a drug of abuse, this

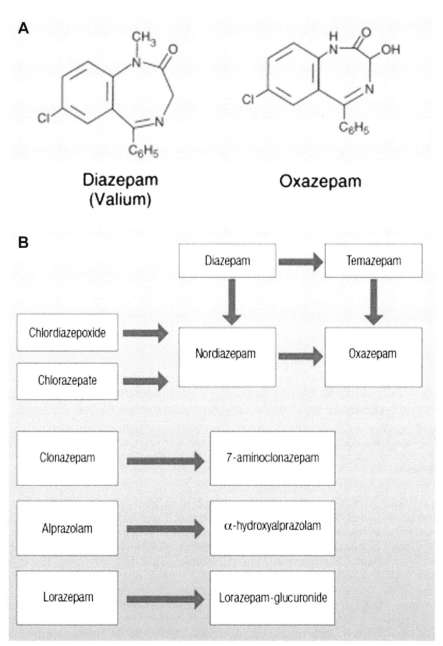

Fig. 8. (*A*) Chemical structures of benzodiazepines. (*B*) Benzodiazepine metabolic pathways. (*From* [*A*] *From* Pincus MR, Bluth MH, Abraham NZ. Toxicology and therapeutic drug monitoring. In: Pincus MR, McPherson RA, editors. Henry's clinical diagnosis and management by laboratory methods. 23rd edition. Elsevier; 2017. p. 331.e2, with permission; and [*B*] *Reprinted with* permission from Pract Pain Manage 2014;14(1):38–41. © 2016 Vertical Health Media, LLC.)

HALLUCINOGENS

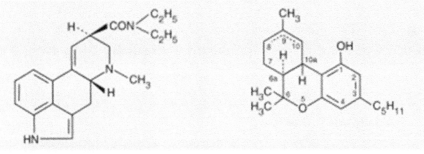

Phencyclidine   Methaquaalone

Lysergic acid   Tetrahydro
diethylamide   cannabinol
(LSD)

Fig. 9. Chemical structures of hallucinogens. (*From* Pincus MR, Bluth MH, Abraham NZ. Toxicology and therapeutic drug monitoring. In: Pincus MR, McPherson RA, editors. Henry's clinical diagnosis and management by laboratory methods. 23rd edition. Elsevier; 2017. p. 332.e2; with permission.)

drug is traded on the streets under the name of *angel dust* or *angel hair*. It is peculiar that the use of this drug seems to be periodic. The physiologic effects of PCP seem to be analgesic and anesthetic and, paradoxically, stimulatory. This drug has been found to interact with cholinergic, adrenergic, GABA-secreting, serotonergic, and opiate neuronal receptors. As with ketamine, PCP has also been found to block NMDA receptors with slight variations.[39] Thus, a wide variety of bizarre and apparently paradoxic symptoms can be seen in the same patient. This drug has been shown to bind to specific regions of the inner chloride channels of neurons, apparently profoundly affecting chloride transport. It has also been found to bind strongly to a class of neural receptors referred to as sigma-receptors.[40] This type of receptor binds strongly to the neuroleptic, antipsychotic drug haloperidol (Haldol)—a finding that may implicate the sigma-receptor in some of the clinical findings of severe psychosis in patients suffering from overdose with PCP.

Because of its varied actions, clinically acute manifestations vary from depression to euphoria and can involve catatonia, violence, rage, and auditory and visual hallucinations. Vomiting, hyperventilation, tachycardia, shivering, seizures, coma, and death are among the common occurrences that result from abuse of this drug. Most fatalities occur from the hypertensive effects of the drug, especially on the large cerebral arteries. As can be inferred from this spectrum of possible symptoms, diagnosis based on clinical findings alone can be quite challenging. Only the results of a drug screen and/or urine drug confirmation studies can be diagnostic. The general detection window in urine can be 5 to 7 days after ingestion and even longer (approximately 30 days) with heavy use. Treatment of drug abuse with PCP is supportive, with the patient kept in isolation in a darkened, quiet room. Acidification of the urine increases the rate of PCP excretion. As might be expected from findings regarding the sigma-receptor, treatment with haloperidol results in sedation of the violent, hallucinating patient.

BARBITURATES

An almost bewildering variety of these major sedative drugs is available. However, all are derivatives of barbituric acid, which may be regarded as the condensation product of urea and malonic acid, as indicated in **Fig. 10**. Depending on the substituents of the –CH$_2$ group of the malonic acid portion, the particular drug may be long acting, as is phenobarbital, with a benzene ring and ethyl group substituents on this carbon; short acting, as is pentobarbital, with neopentyl and ethyl groups at this position; or ultrashort acting, as is the case with thiopental. The long-acting barbiturate phenobarbital is a therapeutic drug that is used as an anticonvulsant, unlike the

BARBITUATES; SEDATIVE - HYPNOTICS

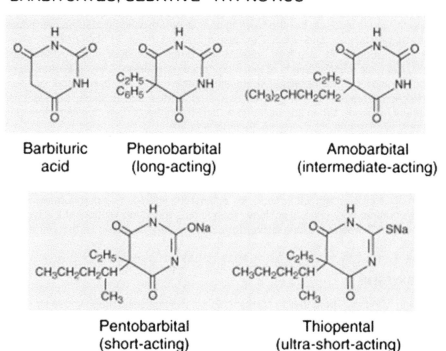

Fig. 10. Chemical structures of barbiturates and sedative–hypnotics. (*From* Pincus MR, Bluth MH, Abraham NZ. Toxicology and therapeutic drug monitoring. In: Pincus MR, McPherson RA, editors. Henry's clinical diagnosis and management by laboratory methods. 23rd edition. Elsevier; 2017. p. 331.e2; with permission.)

short- and ultrashort-acting drugs. All of the barbiturates are fat soluble and therefore pass easily across the blood–brain barrier. All of them seem to stabilize membranes such that depolarization of the membranes becomes more difficult.

As with the benzodiazepines, the barbiturates are known to interact with GABA receptors. In particular, they bind to the α subunit of the GABA$_A$ receptor at a site that is distinct both from the GABA binding site and from the benzodiazepine binding site. Their effect is to increase the duration of chloride ion channel opening at the GABA$_A$ receptor, potentiating the GABA effect (ie, inhibition of dopamine-dependent nerve conduction). It is thought that this action of chloride channel opening, called direct gating of the chloride channel, is the basis for barbiturate toxicity, which is greater than for the benzodiazepines, which do not increase the duration of chloride channel opening but rather increase the frequency of channel opening. In addition, at higher doses, barbiturates have been found to inhibit a subtype of glutamate receptors, called AMPA receptors. Glutamate is a major excitatory neurotransmitter. More generally, barbiturates have been found to block calcium ion–induced release of neurotransmitters.[41]

For unknown reasons, the short-acting and ultrashort-acting barbiturates seem to inhibit selectively the reticular activating system, involved with arousal—hence their sedative and hypnotic effects. The ultrashort-acting barbiturates rapidly diffuse out of the CNS, accounting for their rapid action. Phenobarbital, however, selectively reduces the excitability of rapidly firing neurons and is therefore a highly effective anticonvulsant. It may be more than coincidence that phenobarbital and the equally effective anticonvulsant phenytoin (Dilantin) bear structural resemblance to one another and may exert similar effects on rapidly firing neurons.

Clinically, at low doses, the short-acting and ultrashort-acting barbiturates produce sedation, drowsiness, and sleep. They also impair judgment. At higher doses, anesthesia is produced. At very high doses, these drugs can cause stupor, coma, and death. The toxic manifestations of these drugs are depression, Cheyne-Stokes respiration, cyanosis, hypothermia, hypotension, tachycardia, areflexia, and pupillary constriction. Treatment of drug overdose is supportive and includes the standard treatment for shock. When administered within 30 minutes of drug ingestion, activated charcoal is an effective barbiturate chemoadsorbent.

Diagnosis of drug abuse with short- and ultrashort-acting barbiturates is done by immunoassay and TLC screening procedures. High-performance liquid chromatography has found some use in this regard, but is not a standard method. Immunoassays for those drugs are also excellent, the one caveat being that high levels of phenobarbital in urine cross-react with antibodies against the short-acting barbiturates. Additionally, confirmatory urine toxicology testing has a detection window of 2 days and greater than 3 weeks for long-acting formulations after ingestion of barbiturates in general.

PROPOXYPHENE

Although withdrawn from the US market in 2010, this analgesic drug, whose structure is shown in **Fig. 3**, has pharmacologic properties very similar to those of the opiates, like morphine. As can be seen in the figure, the structure of propoxyphene (Darvon) is quite similar to that of methadone. This drug can be taken orally, so that the sedated, good feelings induced by opiates can be induced without the need to have recourse to the intravenous apparatus needed for infusion of heroin. A major cause of drug-related death is propoxyphene overdose alone or in combination with CNS depressants like barbiturates and alcohol. Toxic symptoms are similar to those seen with overdoses of opiates (namely, respiratory depression, cardiac arrhythmias, seizures, pulmonary edema, and coma). Nephrogenic diabetes insipidus may also occur. In addition, propoxyphene has been found to cause cardiac arrhythmias.[42] Treatment for propoxyphene overdose is mainly supportive. Administration of naloxone reverses the toxic effect of the drug. Urine confirmatory testing (ie, LC/MS) has a detection window of 2 to 3 days after ingestion and can be used to differentiate propoxyphene from other opiates.

METHAQUALONE (QUAALUDE)

Methaqualone is a 2,3-disubstituted quinazoline (see **Fig. 9**). Although not structurally similar to the barbiturates, it has many of the same sedative–hypnotic properties as the barbiturates. This compound also possesses anticonvulsant, antispasmodic, local anesthetic, antitussive, and weak antihistamine actions. Oral administration leads to rapid and complete absorption of the drug, with approximately 80% bound to plasma protein. Peak plasma concentrations are reached in approximately 2 to 3 hours, and almost all of the drug seems to be metabolized by the hepatic cytochrome P450 microsomal enzyme system, with only a small percentage (<5%) excreted unchanged in the urine. The serum half-life ranges from 20 to 60 hours. The dosages used for its hypnotic–sedative actions range from 150 to 300 mg daily. Toxic serum concentrations are generally reached at 10 μg/mL. Tolerance to some of its actions, as well as dependence, occurs, such that abusive dosages can be up to 6 to 7 times greater than those used therapeutically. Symptoms of overdose can be similar to barbiturate toxicity and produce CNS depression with lethargy, respiratory depression, coma, and death. However, unlike barbiturate overdose, muscle spasms, convulsions, and pyramidal signs (hypertonicity, hyperreflexia, and myoclonus) can result from severe methaqualone intoxication. Treatment for overdose includes supportive therapy, as well as delaying absorption of remaining drug with activated charcoal and drug removal by gastric lavage.

MARIJUANA (CANNABIS)

This is one of the oldest and most widely used of the mind-altering drugs. Marijuana is a mixture of cut, dried, and ground portions of the hemp plant *Cannabis sativa*. Hashish refers to a more potent product produced by extraction of the resin from the plant. The principal psychoactive agent in marijuana is considered to be δ-9-tetrahydrocannabinol (δ-9-THC; see **Fig. 9**), a lipid-soluble compound that readily enters the brain and may act by producing cell membrane changes. δ-9-THC binds to the presynaptic neural cannabinoid receptor CB1, which releases the inhibitory neurotransmitter GABA in the hippocampus, amygdala, and cerebral cortex. Different forms of THC have been found to cause distinctly different physiologic effects.[43] δ-9-THC induces an increase in anxiogenic effects, and cannabidiol produces a diminution in anxiety. The latter derivative was found to attenuate blood oxygenation levels in the amygdala and the anterior and posterior cingulate cortex; δ-9-THC was found to modulate activation in frontal and parietal regions of the brain.

Marijuana may be introduced through the lungs by smoking or through the GI tract by oral ingestion in food. Once THC enters the body, it is readily stored in body fat and has a half-life of approximately 1 week. Biotransformation is complex and extensive, and less than 1% of a dose is excreted unchanged. About one-third is excreted in the urine, primarily as δ-9-carboxy-THC and 11-hydroxy-δ-9-THC. These metabolites may be detected in the urine from 1 to 4 weeks after the last ingestion, depending on both dosage and frequency of ingestion.

Marijuana does not seem, in general, to cause physiologic dependence, but tolerance and psychological dependence do seem to occur, and a proportion of chronic users of this drug can develop physiologic dependence. Two major physiologic effects of marijuana are reddening of the conjunctivae and increased pulse rate. Muscle weakness and deterioration in motor coordination can also occur. The preponderant changes seen with cannabis intoxication are perceptual and psychic changes. These range from euphoria, relaxation, passiveness, and altered time perception, seen at low doses, to adverse reactions such as paranoia, delusions, and disorientation, which can be seen at high doses in psychologically susceptible individuals.

The dosage, the route of administration, the individual's psychological makeup, and the setting are important determinants in each individual's reaction to cannabis intoxication. Thus, high doses in an individual unprepared or unaware of drug consumption may produce a disturbing experience. More commonly, experienced users report mild euphoria, enhancement or alteration of the physical senses, introspection with altered emphasis or importance of ideas, and heightening of subjective experiences. Heavy chronic use may produce bronchopulmonary disorders; although the relative safety of chronic use is controversial, acute panic reactions, delirium, and psychoses occur rarely. Few users seek treatment, and when this occurs in a distressed patient, medical intervention is generally conservative. However, after an acute episode, psychological evaluation may be necessary in an individual with an underlying psychiatric disturbance. Rarely, marijuana may be ingested by intravenous infusion of a boiled concentrate. Severe multisystem toxicity may be produced by this route of administration. Symptoms may include acute renal failure, gastroenteritis, hepatitis, anemia, and thrombocytopenia.

LYSERGIC ACID DIETHYLAMIDE (LYSERGIDE)

Lysergic acid diethylamide (LSD; see **Fig. 9**) is a semisynthetic indolalkylamine and a hallucinogen. It is one of the most potent pharmacologic materials known, producing effects at doses as low as 20 μg, and is equally effective by injection or oral administration. Comparison of the structure of LSD with that of 5-hydroxytryptamine (serotonin), as shown in the group 6 drugs in **Fig. 9**, reveals that LSD has a tryptaminelike nucleus, but it lacks the 5-hydroxyl group of serotonin. LSD has multiple complex effects in the CNS. In the locus coeruleus and the median raphe of the midbrain, which use serotonergic pathways, it has the paradoxic effect of inhibiting both the firing of neurons in these structures and the release of serotonin at the axonal sides of synapses.[44] This process, in turn, may produce a state of CNS hyperarousal. In contrast, it actually acts as a serotonin agonist on postsynaptic HT_{1A} receptors. It is a pure agonist on $5\text{-}HT_2$ receptors in other serotonergic pathways. Recently, it has been found that the hallucinogenic effect of LSD is owing to its agonistic effect on $5\text{-}HT_2$ receptors, and that it behaves very much like the tryptamines (see **Fig. 6**) and phenylethylamines (see **Fig. 5**), discussed previously, in producing this effect. In addition, it has been found to have both agonistic and antagonistic effects on dopaminergic pathways. Thus, it acts at multiple sites in the CNS in complex ways. LSD further affects both the sympathetic and parasympathetic nervous systems. However, the sympathetic effect seems to be greater, and initial symptoms include hypertension, tachycardia, mydriasis, and piloerection.

The usual dosage of LSD is 1 to 2 μg/kg; LSD produces an experience that begins within an hour of ingestion, usually peaks at 2 to 3 hours, and generally lasts 8 to

12 hours, after ingestion. Metabolism occurs in the liver, whereas excretion occurs mainly in the bile. The detection window in urine is 1 to 2 days after ingestion.

LSD is the most commonly abused drug in its class and is believed by its users to provide insights and new ways of solving problems. The psychological effects are usually intense and vary, depending on the user's personality, expectations, and circumstances. LSD acts on all body senses, but visual effects are most intense. Common perceptual abnormalities include changes in the sense of time, organized visual illusions or hallucinations, blurred or undulating vision, and synesthesias. Mood may become very labile, and dissolution and detachment of ego may occur. LSD toxicity levels are low, and deaths are generally owing to trauma secondary to errors in the user's judgment. Panic reactions—a bad trip—are the most common adverse reactions. These may occur in any user and cannot be reliably predicted or prevented. Borderline psychotic and depressed individuals are at risk for the precipitation of suicide or a prolonged psychotic episode by the usage of LSD. Flashbacks, which are poorly understood, occur days to months after ingestion. This occurs when the user experiences recurrences of a previous hallucinogenic experience in the absence of drug ingestion. Acute panic reactions may be treated by frequent reassurance and a quiet and calm environment; diazepam may also be effective. However, except for treating specific complications, LSD abuse has no systematic program of treatment.

CATHINONES (BATH SALTS)

Synthetic cathinones (ie, "bath salts"; **Fig. 11**) are a type of psychoactive designer drug that produce amphetaminelike or cocainelike subjective effects by activating monoamine systems in the brain and periphery.[45] Bath salts produce the expected desirable effects at lower doses. However, high doses as well as chronic exposure can foster psychosis, violent behaviors, tachycardia, hyperthermia, and even death. There are 3 main synthetic cathinones: 4-methyl-*N*-methylcathinone (mephedrone),

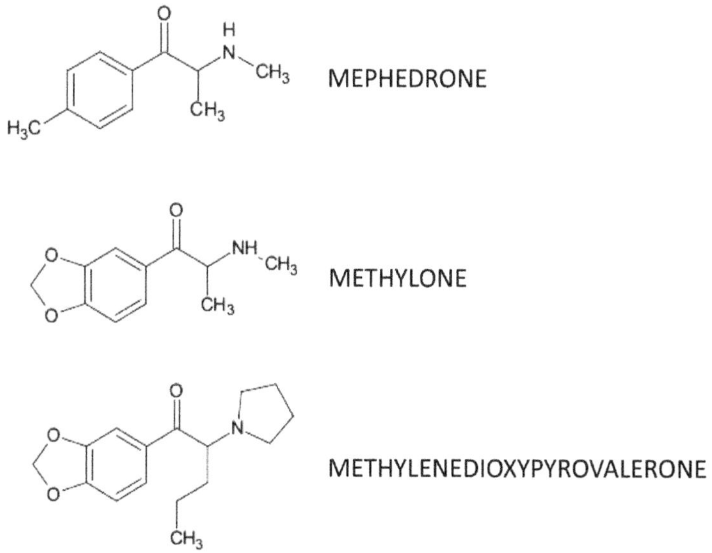

Fig. 11. Chemical structures of bath salts.

3,4-methylenedioxy-*N*-methylcathinone (methylone), and 3,4-methylenedioxypyro-valerone. These compounds are structurally related to the parent compound cathinone, which is a naturally occurring β-keto amphetamine with known psychos-timulant properties. Bath salts enhance sympathetic nervous system activity and are thought to act by increasing the concentration of dopamine in the synaptic cleft that results in increased activation of postsynaptic dopamine receptors (see **Fig. 1**). Furthermore bath salts such as methcathinone is a substrate for the dopamine transporter, thereby blocking the ability of dopamine to bind to the transporter and subsequently reducing one of the main mechanisms of dopaminergic neuro-transmission termination.

The diagnosis of bath salt ingestion requires a high index of suspicion when evalu-ating a patient presenting with intoxication or overdose, because there are no commonly available laboratory drug screening testing approaches that can be used at a point of care or office setting at the time of presentation. They may precipitate a false-positive methamphetamine drug screening result. Laboratory detection of syn-thetic cathinones requires high complexity GC/MS or LC/MS confirmatory testing with a detection window for urine sample of 2 to 3 days after ingestion. Serum and urine toxicologic studies can also identify potential coingestion of other toxic agents. Treat-ment of synthetic cathinone overdose is primarily supportive care as a specific anti-dote does not exist. The most common treatments used in emergency departments are intravenous fluids, benzodiazepines, oxygen, and sedatives. Specific metabolic sequelae (hyponatremia, myocarditis, and necrotizing fasciitis) should be treated by medical and/or surgical interventions as required.[46]

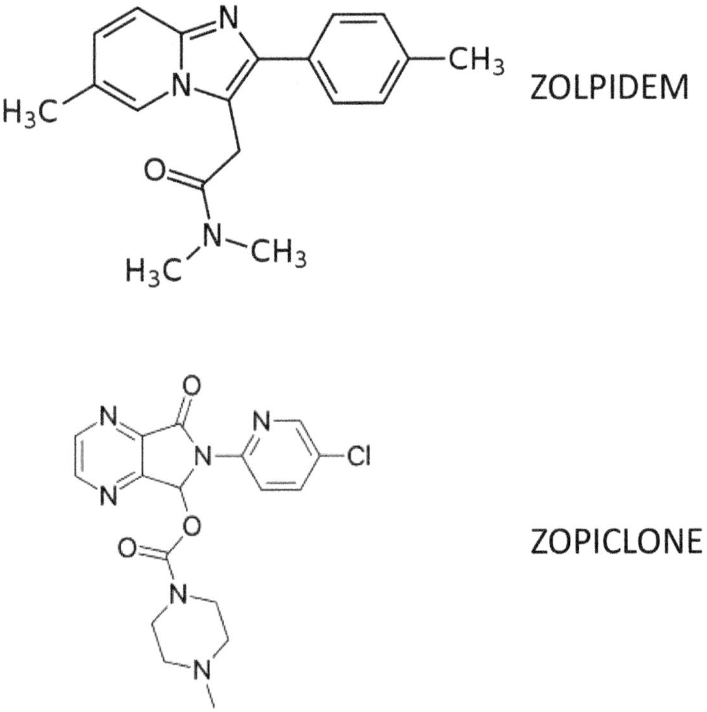

Fig. 12. Chemical structures of sleep aids.

SLEEP AIDS

It is estimated that 1 in 6 adults with a diagnosed sleep disorder and 1 in 8 adults with trouble sleeping reported using sleep aids, that 50 to 70 million Americans suffer from sleep disorders or deprivation and that 4% of adults aged 20 and over reported using a prescription sleep aid in the past month, with greater use in the elderly.[47] Furthermore, sleep aids include sedative/hypnotic agents and are also subject to dependency and abuse. Prescription sleep aids include barbiturates and benzodiazepine in addition to other agents. The imidazopyridine zolpidem (Ambien), represents a chemically novel nonbenzodiazepine hypnotic agent (**Fig. 12**), which binds to the ω-1 receptor in the brain. Unlike benzodiazepines, zolpidem does not contain myorelaxant or anticonvulsant effects and its effects on anxiety seem to be minor. It does not seem to affect sleep stages, but does seem to reduce the latency to and prolongs the duration of sleep in patients with insomnia owing to its rapid onset of action and short elimination half-life.[48] In contrast, the cyclopyrrolone zopiclone/eszopiclone (Lunesta), another nonbenzodiazepine hypnotic agent (see **Fig. 12**), modulates the $GABA_A$ receptor through allosteric mechanisms.[49] Although its receptor binding is not facilitated directly by GABA, its interaction with the $GABA_A$ receptor can potentiate responses to GABA. As such, coadministration of benzodiazepines, which is not uncommon in those with sleep disorders, can have deleterious potentiating effects. The detection window for these sleep aids are generally 1 to 7 days after ingestion when conventionally assessed via GC/MS or LC/MS confirmatory testing approaches.

MUSCLE RELAXANTS

Pain management of musculoskeletal conditions include carisoprodol (ie, Soma; **Fig. 13**), a CNS depressant with an unknown mechanism of pharmacologic action. Its sedative effects are generally attributed to the actions of its primary metabolite, meprobamate, at $GABA_A$ receptors. Interestingly, although its primary metabolite meprobamate (ie, Miltown, Equanil; see **Fig. 13**) is classified as a controlled substance at the federal level, carisoprodol is not.[50] These agents are available in varying doses and ingestion recommendations and the general detection window in a urine sample after ingestion is 1 to 3 days. There have been reports of carisoprodol-related abuse,

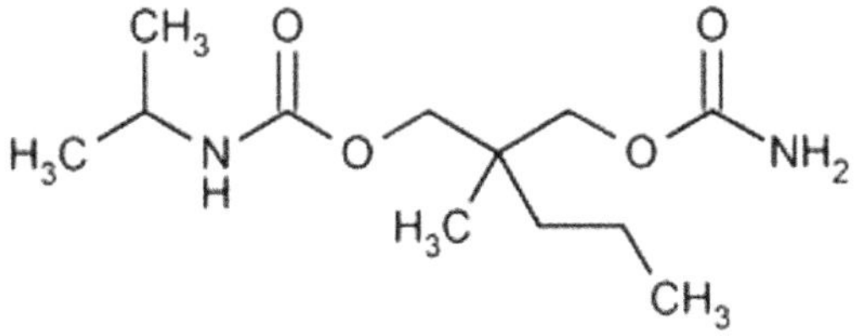

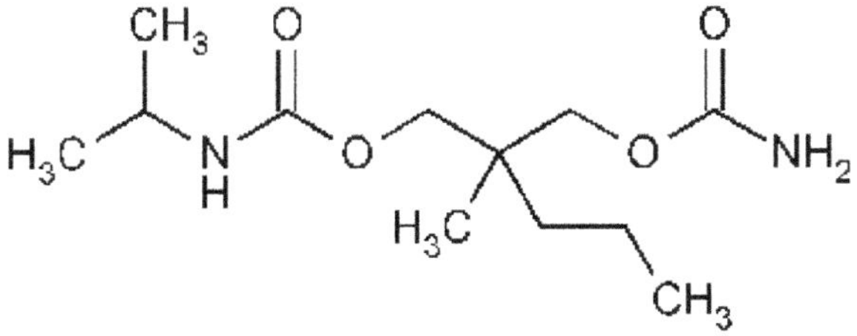

Fig. 13. Chemical structures of muscle relaxants: carisoprodol and meprobamate.

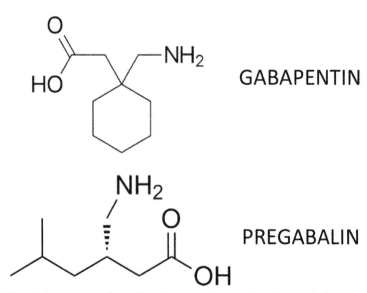

Fig. 14. Chemical structures of muscle relaxants: gabapentin and pregabalin.

diversion, and death thus deeming it a drug of concern for the US Department of Justice Drug Enforcement Agency Office of Diversion Control. In Florida, the number of carisoprodol/meprobamate–related deaths in 2005 exceeded those attributed to opioids, including heroin and fentanyl. Thus, abuse of carisoprodol has become an international problem. Recently, the Committee for Medicinal Products for Human Use concluded the abuse potential associated with carisoprodol outweighs its benefits as a therapeutic drug.

ANTIEPILEPTICS

Gabapentin (ie, Neurontin), a 3-alkylated analog of GABA, and pregabalin (Lyrica; **Fig. 14**) are commonly prescribed agents used to treat epilepsy. Other applications of these drugs include neuropathic pain, fibromyalgia, and possibly for treating postoperative pain. In addition gabapentin has been considered effective for the treatment of restless leg syndrome, Guillain–Barré syndrome, uremic pruritus, and phantom limb pain, whereas pregabalin has also been considered effective for the treatment of generalized anxiety disorder.[51] The mechanism of action is thought to include the activity as a ligand at the alpha2-delta subunit of voltage-gated calcium channels by calcium influx at nerve terminals. This interaction reduces the release of neurotransmitters, such as glutamate norepinephrine and substance P. To this end, gabapentin has recently been reported to facilitate cannabis abstinence by producing effects that overlap with those of cannabinoids[52] and recent animal studies show synergistic pain reduction effects when coadministered with morphine and its metabolites.[53] This has propagated abuse potential both in synergy with other agents to potentiate their effects as well as for this drug class in its own right.[54] The general detection window (urine) for gabapentin and pregabalin is 1 to 4 days after ingestion.

OTHER DRUGS

There is no lack of ingenuity when it comes to conjuring up new synthetics. There have been a number of new synthetic cannabinoids available to the clinical marketplace, many of which have deleterious health effects that are more severe than that of marijuana. These have brand names like "Spice" or "K2," among other, and their effects can be physical and affect cardiovascular, neurologic, renal, pulmonary, metabolic, or psychological and can also affect cognitive and behavioral functions, among others.[55] These synthetic cannabinoids, propagated by "street" chemists, can be of the benzoyl, naphthoyl, alkoyl, and phenylacetyl derivatives among others and comprise greater than 50 different types.[56] For example, the aminoalkylindole cannababinoid derivative JWH-018 (1-penthyl-3-(1-napthoyl)indole), one of the first derivatives detected in K2 preparations seized in the United States, is thought to exert its effects via G protein coupled cannabanoid type 1 (CB-1) receptors. The affinity of JWH-018 for the CB-1 receptor is about 15 times greater than conventional Δ^9-THC. Although the general detection window for urine testing is about 3 to 5 days after ingestion of JWH-018 and similar analogs, there are no quality control and manufacturing standards for such illicit substances.

SUMMARY

The management of pain is an ever evolving discipline. New formulations of narcotic analgesics mature to the marketplace in a timely fashion with the promises of availing improved pain control, better dosing, fewer side effects, and the like. These agents also avail an equal risk for abuse, which may mature as a result of physiologic tolerance, polypharmacy, metabolic factors, phramacogenomics, and economic concerns among others. Street chemists are equally adept at both manipulating current and evolving drugs to more potent versions in addition to creating new compositions of matter for consumption in the medical and illicit marketplaces. Although the clinical assessment of the patient is paramount to developing an index of suspicion of overdose, toxicity or illicit drug use, the clinical laboratory can provide a unique and valuable resource to support such investigations and guide appropriate therapy. As new agents pervade the health care system so too does the clinical toxicology laboratory keep in step with adapting its technology and methodology to facilitate detection of such substances.

REFERENCES

1. Substance Abuse and Mental Health Services Administration (SAMHSA), Center for Behavioral Health Statistics and Quality. Results from the 2014 national survey on drug use and health: detailed tables. Rockville (MD): SAMHSA. Available at: http://www.samhsa.gov/data/sites/default/files/NSDUH-DetTabs2014/NSDUH-DetTabs2014.pdf. Accessed April 15, 2016.
2. Meyer MR, Maurer HH. Absorption, distribution, metabolism and excretion pharmacogenomics of drugs of abuse. Pharmacogenomics 2011;12:215–33.
3. Smith ML, Hughes RO, Levine B, et al. Forensic drug testing for opiates. VI. Urine testing for hydromorphone, hydrocodone, oxymorphone, and oxycodone with commercial opiate immunoassays and gas chromatography-mass spectrometry. J Anal Toxicol 1995;19:18–26.
4. Vadivelu N, Lumermann L, Zhu R, et al. Pain control in the presence of drug addiction. Curr Pain Headache Rep 2016;20:35.
5. Knittel JL, Holler JM, Chmiel JD, et al. Analysis of parent synthetic cannabinoids in blood and urinary metabolites by liquid chromatography tandem mass spectrometry. J Anal Toxicol 2016;40:173–86.
6. Tsai IL, Weng TI, Tseng YJ, et al. Screening and confirmation of 62 drugs of abuse and metabolites in urine by ultra-high-performance liquid chromatography-quadrupole time-of-flight mass spectrometry. J Anal Toxicol 2013;37:642–51.

7. Manchikanti L, Malla Y, Wargo BW, et al. Comparative evaluation of the accuracy of benzodiazepine testing in chronic pain patients utilizing immunoassay with liquid chromatography tandem mass spectrometry (LC/MS/MS) of urine drug testing. Pain Physician 2011;14:259–70.
8. Blum K, Chen AL, Giordano J, et al. The addictive brain: all roads lead to dopamine. J Psychoactive Drugs 2012;44:134–43.
9. Hurd YL, Kehr J, Ungerstedt U. In vivo microdialysis as a technique to monitor drug transport: correlation of extracellular cocaine levels and dopamine outflow in the rat brain. J Neurochem 1988;51:1314–6.
10. Baldessarini RJ. Drug therapy of depression and anxiety disorders. In: Brunton LL, Lazo JS, Parker KL, editors. Goodman and Gilman's the pharmacological basis of therapeutics. 11th edition. New York: McGraw-Hill; 2006. p. 429–59.
11. Kablinger AS, Lindner MA, Casso S, et al. Effects of the combination of metyrapone and oxazepam on cocaine craving and cocaine taking: a double-blind, randomized, placebo-controlled pilot study. J Psychopharmacol 2012;26: 973–81.
12. Li P, Eaton MM, Steinbach JH, et al. The benzodiazepine diazepam potentiates responses of $\alpha1\beta2\gamma2L$ γ-aminobutyric acid type A receptors activated by either γ-aminobutyric acid or allosteric agonists. Anesthesiology 2013;118:1417–25.
13. Fujii H, Narita M, Mizoguchi M, et al. Drug design and synthesis of epsilon opioid receptor agonist: 17-(cyclopropylmethyl)-4,5alpha-epoxy-3,6beta-dihydroxy-6,14-endoethenomorphinan-7alpha-(N-methyl-N-phenethyl)carboxamide (TAN-821) inducing antinociception mediated by putative epsilon opioid receptor. Bioorg Med Chem 2004;12:4133–45.
14. Zhuo M. Plasticity of NMDA receptor NR2B subunit in memory and chronic pain. Mol Brain 2009;2:1–11.
15. Gonzalez J, Tukey RH. Drug metabolism. In: Brunton LL, Lazo JS, Parker KL, editors. Goodman and Gilman's the pharmacological basis of therapeutics. 11th edition. New York: McGraw-Hill; 2006. p. 71–91.
16. Smith HS. Opioid metabolism. Mayo Clin Proc 2009;84:613–24.
17. Dwyer JP, Jayasekera C, Nicoll A. Analgesia for the cirrhotic patient: a literature review and recommendations. J Gastroenterol Hepatol 2014;29:1356–60.
18. Jones JH, Wie WB. Cocaine-induced chest pain. Clin Lab Med 2006;26:127–46.
19. Hoffman RS. Cocaine. In: Flomenbaum NE, Goldfrank LR, Hoffman RF, et al, editors. Goldfrank's toxicologic emergencies. 8th edition. New York: McGraw-Hill; 2006. p. 1133–47.
20. Azmitia EC, Murphy RB, Whitaker-Azmitia PM. MDMA (ecstasy) effects on cultured serotonergic neurons: evidence for Ca2+-dependent toxicity linked to release. Brain Res 1990;510:97–103.
21. Cami J, Farre M. Drug addiction. N Engl J Med 2003;349:975–86.
22. Forray A, Foster D. Substance use in the perinatal period. Curr Psychiatry Rep 2015;17:91.
23. Tso PH, Wong YH. Molecular basis of opioid dependence: role of signal regulation by G-proteins. Clin Exp Pharmacol Physiol 2003;30:307–16.
24. von Euler M, Villén T, Svensson JO, et al. Interpretation of the presence of 6-monoacetylmorphine in the absence of morphine-3-glucuronide in urine samples: evidence of heroin abuse. Ther Drug Monit 2003;25:645–8.
25. Smith ML, Nichols DC, Underwood P, et al. Morphine and codeine concentrations in human urine following controlled poppy seeds administration of known opiate content. Forensic Sci Int 2014;241:87–90.

26. Chen P, Braithwarte RA, George C, et al. The poppy seed defense: a novel solution. Drug Test Anal 2014;6:194–201.
27. Bell J, Seres V, Bowron P, et al. The use of serum methadone levels in patients receiving methadone maintenance. Clin Pharmacol Ther 1988;43:623–9.
28. Diong SH, Mohd Yusoff NS, Sim MS, et al. Quantitation of methadone and metabolite in patients under maintenance treatment. J Anal Toxicol 2014;38:660–6.
29. Haroz R, Greenberg MI. New drugs of abuse in North America. Clin Lab Med 2006;26:147–64.
30. Schier J. Avoid unfavorable consequences: dextromethorphan can bring about a false-positive phencyclidine urine drug screen. J Emerg Med 2000;18:379–81.
31. Smith MT. Differences between and combinations of opioids re-visited. Curr Opin Anaesthesiol 2008;21:596–601.
32. Gerra G, Borella F, Zaimovic A, et al. Buprenorphine versus methadone for opioid dependence: predictor variables for treatment outcome. Drug Alcohol Depend 2004;75:37–45.
33. Smith ML, Nichols DC, Underwood P, et al. Methamphetamine and amphetamine isomer concentrations in human urine following controlled Vicks Vapolnhaler administration. J Anal Toxicol 2014;38:524–7.
34. Haslam D. Weight management in obesity - past and present. Int J Clin Pract 2016;70:206–17.
35. Montesano C, Sergi M, Moro M, et al. Screening of methylenedioxyamphetamine- and piperazine-derived designer drugs in urine by LC-MS/MS using neutral loss and precursor ion scan. J Mass Spectrom 2013;48:49–59.
36. Campo-Soria C, Chang Y, Weiss DS. Mechanism of action of benzodiazepines on $GABA_A$ receptors. Br J Pharmacol 2006;148:984–90.
37. Fraser AD. Use and abuse of the benzodiazepines. Ther Drug Monit 1998;20: 481–9.
38. Perez ER, Knapp JA, Horn CK, et al. Comparison of LC-MS-MS and GC-MS analysis of benzodiazepine compounds included in the drug demand reduction urinalysis program. J Anal Toxicol 2016;40:201–7.
39. Hevers W, Hadley SH, Luddens H, et al. Ketamine, but not phencyclidine, selectively modulates cerebellar $GABA_A$ receptors containing $\alpha6$ and δ subunits. J Neurosci 2008;28:5383–93.
40. Skuza G. Pharmacology of sigma (σ) receptor ligands from a behavioral perspective. Curr Pharm Des 2012;18:863–74.
41. Löscher W, Rogawski MA. How theories evolved concerning the mechanism of action of barbiturates. Epilepsia 2012;53:12–25.
42. Barkin RL, Barkin SJ, Barkin DS. Propoxyphene (dextropropoxyphene): a critical review of a weak opioid analgesic that should remain in antiquity. Am J Ther 2006; 13:534–42.
43. Fusar-Poli P, Crippa JA, Bhattacharyya S, et al. Distinct effects of $\Delta9$-tetrahydrocannabinol and cannabidiol on neural activation during emotional processing. Arch Gen Psychiatry 2009;66:95–105.
44. Passie T, Halpern JH, Stichtinoth DO, et al. The pharmacology of lysergic acid diethylamide: a review. CNS Neurosci Ther 2008;14:295–314.
45. Banks ML, Worst TJ, Rusyniak DE, et al. Synthetic cathinones ("bath salts"). J Emerg Med 2014;46:632–42.
46. Thornton MD, Baum CR. Bath salts and other emerging toxins. Pediatr Emerg Care 2014;30:47–52.
47. Centers for Disease Control and Prevention (CDC), National Center for Health Statistics. Prescription sleep aid use among adults: United States 2005-2010.

Atlanta (GA): CDC; 2013. Available at: http://www.cdc.gov/nchs/products/databriefs/db127.htm.

48. Langtry HD, Benfield P. Zolpidem. A review of its pharmacodynamic and pharmacokinetic properties and therapeutic potential. Drugs 1990;40:291–313.

49. Döble A, Canton T, Malgouris C, et al. The mechanism of action of zopiclone. Eur Psychiatry 1995;10:117s–28s.

50. Gonzalez LA, Gatch MB, Forster MJ, et al. Abuse potential of soma: the GABA(A) receptor as a target. Mol Cell Pharmacol 2009;1:180–6.

51. Calandre EP, Rico-Villademoros F, Slim M. Alpha2delta ligands, gabapentin, PGB and MGB: a review of their clinical pharmacology and therapeutic use. Expert Rev Neurother 2016. [Epub ahead of print].

52. Lile JA, Wesley MJ, Kelly TH, et al. Separate and combined effects of gabapentin and [INCREMENT]9-tetrahydrocannabinol in humans discriminating [INCREMENT]9-tetrahydrocannabinol. Behav Pharmacol 2016;27:215–24.

53. Papathanasiou T, Juul RV, Gabel-Jensen C, et al. Population pharmacokinetic modelling of morphine, gabapentin and their combination in the rat. Pharm Res 2016. [Epub ahead of print].

54. Bossard JB, Ponté C, Dupouy J, et al. Disproportionality analysis for the assessment of abuse and dependence potential of pregabalin in the French Pharmacovigilance Database. Clin Drug Investig 2016;36(9):735–42.

55. Castellanos D, Gralnik LM. Synthetic cannabinoids 2015: an update for pediatricians in clinical practice. World J Clin Pediatr 2016;5:16–24.

56. Debruyne D, Le Boisselier R. Emerging drugs of abuse: current perspectives on synthetic cannabinoids. Subst Abuse Rehabil 2015;6:113–29.

Liquid Chromatography–Tandem Mass Spectrometry

An Emerging Technology in the Toxicology Laboratory

Yan Victoria Zhang, PhD, DABCC[a], Bin Wei, PhD[b], Yu Zhu, PhD[c],*,
Yanhua Zhang, PhD[d], Martin H. Bluth, MD, PhD[c,e]

KEYWORDS

- LC-MS/MS • Toxicology application • Quadrupole mass spectrometer • MRM • ESI
- APCI • APPI • Immunoassay

KEY POINTS

- Both licit and illicit opiates have effects on the immune and neurologic components of asthma inflammation and clinical disease as well as associated allergic responses.
- The end product of these interactions determines the clinical output of this complex interplay, with either worsening or improvement of asthma, and possible increase in allergic responses.
- In the last decade, Liquid Chromatography - Tandem Mass Spectrometry (LC-MS/MS) has seen enormous growth in routine toxicology laboratories.
- Major strengths of LC-MS/MS are improved specificity, flexibility and sample high throughput compared with other techniques.
- Technology advances in LC-MS/MS are taken place, such as automation, miniaturization, detector and LC improvements. Efforts in standardizing method development and forthcoming regulation will greatly impact the role of LC-MS/MS in toxicology laboratories.

INTRODUCTION

History of Liquid Chromatography–Tandem Mass Spectrometry

With roots stretching back more than 100 years, mass spectrometry (MS) is an analytical technique with both an interesting history and a promising future. MS was born from early studies of electromagnetism. It first gained importance in physics, where

[a] University of Rochester Medical Center, 601 Elmwood Avenue, Box 608, Rochester, NY 14642, USA; [b] Toxicology Laboratory, Michigan Surgical Hospital, 21230 Dequindre Road, Warren, MI 48091, USA; [c] Consolidated Laboratory Management Systems, LLC, 24555 Southfield Road, Southfield, MI 48075, USA; [d] Total Toxicology Labs, LLC, 24525 Southfield Road Suite 100, Southfield, MI 48075, USA; [e] Department of Pathology, Wayne State University School of Medicine, 540 East Canfield, Detroit, MI 48201, USA
* Correspondence author.
E-mail address: yu.zhu@consolidatedlabsmgt.com

Clin Lab Med 36 (2016) 635–661
http://dx.doi.org/10.1016/j.cll.2016.07.001
0272-2712/16/© 2016 Elsevier Inc. All rights reserved.
labmed.theclinics.com

it was used to determine the existence of isotopes and the atomic weights of the elements.[1–4] Subsequently, MS was used on a massive scale for the separation of the isotopes of uranium as part of the Manhattan Project.[5] During the 1950s, MS became part of chemistry, being used to study small molecules, particularly by the petrochemical industry.[6] During that era, gas chromatography (GC)–MS was born,[7] and forecasted the path toward liquid chromatography–tandem mass spectrometry (LC-MS/MS) (or LC–mass spectrometry/mass spectrometry).

Instrumental developments in the field of MS accelerated throughout the latter half of the twentieth century. These developments included quadrupole, time-of-flight (TOF), and Fourier-transform MS.[8] The development and commercialization of thermospray,[9] atmospheric pressure chemical ionization (APCI),[10] and electrospray ionization (ESI)[11] in the 1980s enabled the successful interface of LC to mass spectrometers. The performance, sensitivity, and reliability of the instruments have been areas of active development. New mass analyzers continue to improve performance across the field, as have developments in ionization sources.

Although LC-MS is now commonly used in many clinical applications, the difficulties faced in interfacing a liquid chromatograph to a mass spectrometer were enormous. At the time of the first experiments in interfacing those techniques, most mass spectrometers operated at high vacuum, in the magnitude of 10 to 6 mm Hg ($\sim$ 10–4 Pa, 1 mm Hg = 133.3 Pa). Similarly, most liquid chromatographs were operated at flow rates near 1 mL/min. Because 1 mL of liquid water produces more than 1 L of gas at atmospheric pressure and the volume expands as pressure is reduced, vacuum systems were greatly challenged to deal with the volume of gas present at an LC/MS interface. A further challenge was that many mass spectrometers at the time operated at high voltage (kV), which is incompatible with high pressures.

A confluence of developments enabled the coupling of LC with MS. First, improvements in quadrupole mass spectrometers, which operate at lower voltages (hundreds of volts lower), made them viable candidates toward the maturation of LC-MS instruments. Next, improvements in vacuum systems made it possible to deal with the volume of gas generated in an LC-MS interface. Improvements in chromatography made the use of lower flow rates possible. In addition, improvements in interfaces reduced the volume of gas presented to the vacuum system. Simultaneously, Yost and Enke[12] introduced the triple quadrupole mass spectrometer. Another critical component was the use of computers to control mass spectrometers and chromatography systems, which also happened during this timeframe, making complex MS/MS scans possible.

These developments culminated in the introduction of the first commercial, dedicated LC-MS/MS instrument in 1989. The next year saw the publication of the first LC-MS/MS publication in the field of clinical chemistry.[13] From there, the field has grown enormously, as shown in **Fig. 1**.

Along the way, the field has been well-recognized. Nobel Prizes have been awarded to 6 practitioners in the field, starting with the 1906 Prize in Physics awarded to J.J. Thomson of Cambridge University, "In recognition of the great merits of his theoretical and experimental investigations on the conduction of electricity by gases," which allowed him to invent the first mass spectrometer. His student, F.W. Aston, was awarded the 1922 Nobel Prize in Chemistry for the discovery of isotopes. In 1989, Hans Dehmelt and Wolfgang Paul shared half of the Nobel Prize in Physics for their development of the ion trap, which was fundamental in the development of quadrupole mass spectrometers. Most recently, John Fenn and Koichi Tanaka shared half of the 2002 Prize in Chemistry for "their development of soft desorption ionization methods for mass spectrometric analyses of biological macromolecules," which meant electrospray for John Fenn and soft laser desorption for Koichi Tanaka.

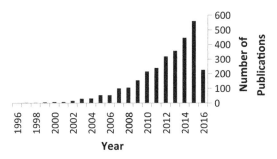

Fig. 1. Number of publications in the past decades in the field of clinical MS. The search was done on April 8, 2016 on PubMed, based on searching terms of "LC-MS MS" and "clinical."

Basic Principles of Tandem Mass Spectrometry

Fundamentally, mass spectrometers can be thought of as devices for weighing molecules. Tandem mass spectrometers, or MS/MS instruments, can be thought of as devices to perform chemistry on molecules, followed by weighing the results.[14] To accomplish these measurements, mass spectrometers work with charged molecules (ions) in vacuum. LC, on the other hand, works with molecules in solution. The transition of the sample into a charged, gas phase ion is the first step in MS followed by measurement.

Modern mass spectrometers consist of several discrete components: the ion source, mass analyzer, and detector, as shown in **Fig. 2**. The ion source often combines the interface between a chromatography system and the ionization process, as presented in later discussion. The mass analyzer separates the resulting ions. There are a variety of types of mass analyzers, including analyzers that separate different masses in space, like quadrupole and orbitrap analyzers, and analyzers that separate different masses in time, like the TOF analyzer. Multiple mass analyzers can be linked together with a collision cell to provide structural information from ions, as shown in **Fig. 2**, or, for analyzers that separate different mass in time, collisions can take place as part of a sequential experiment. Last, the ions must be detected. Two common detection methods are currently in use: one based on discrete particle impacts on an electron- or photomultiplier and the other based the detection of an image current.

There are 3 methods currently in wide use for transitioning molecules from the LC to the mass spectrometer: ESI, APCI, and atmospheric pressure photoionization (APPI). ESI and APCI are the most commonly used ionization methods, whereas APPI is a relative newcomer and has become a method of choice for many applications.

ESI uses a high voltage to create a fine aerosol of charged particles (**Fig. 3**A).[15] For larger chromatographic flow rates (above nanoliters per minute), aerosol production

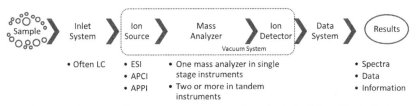

Fig. 2. Schematic diagram of a mass spectrometer. The 3 basic building blocks (inlet, mass spectroscopy, data system) of all mass spectrometers are shown. The ion source used depends on the inlet system and the analyte; other ion sources are used for non-LC inlet systems.

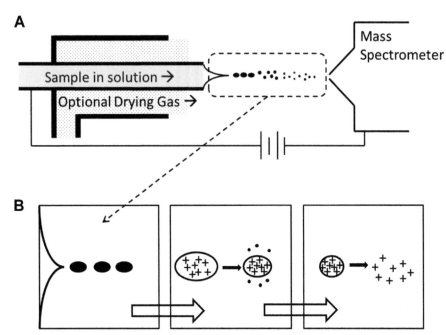

Fig. 3. ESI process. (*A*) Aerosol production. (*B*) Solvent evaporation/ion declustering. Electrospray produces ions through the application of a voltage to a liquid. The liquid disperses into charged droplets, which then decluster. A drying gas can be used to enhance the process, depending on the flow rate.

can be assisted by nebulization with a heated inert gas. Solvent molecules evaporate from the charged droplet until the Rayleigh limit (criterion for the minimum resolvable detail) is reached, after which the droplet undergoes Coulomb fission, essentially exploding and creating smaller charged droplets (**Fig. 3**B). This process continues until the droplets are small enough that, for small molecules, charged analyte ions evaporate from the droplet. For large molecules, the fission cycle continues until the droplet contains one charged analyte ion, which is then transferred into the mass spectrometer, resulting in multiple charges being associated with larger molecules.

APCI (**Fig. 4**) takes place in a heated nebulizer, with a corona discharge providing ionization.[16] The effluent from an LC flows into the ion source region. A concentric flow of gas assists with nebulization and the effluent flows through a region of high heat at the end of the APCI probe. This ionization procedure produces a thin "fog" of gas, which reacts with a corona discharge. Because most of the fog is the high-performance liquid chromatography (HPLC) solvent, an excess of reactant ions is formed from the solvent molecules, which then interact with the analyte molecules and ionize them. In positive ion mode, analyte molecules are ionized primarily by proton transfer from the reactant or by charge transfer. For proton transfer, the gas phase basicity of the analyte must be sufficient to abstract a proton from the reactant gas. For charge transfer, the ionization potential (IP) of the analyte must be sufficiently low for the analyte to lose an electron to the ionized solvent cloud. A third reaction pathway is via adduct formation, in which a positively charged species in the solvent cloud "sticks" to the analyte, forming a charged complex. In negative ion mode, the opposite reactions take place. Protons are abstracted from the analyte molecules to

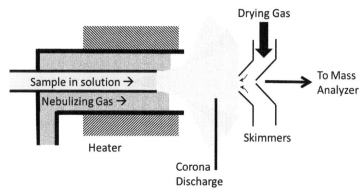

Fig. 4. APCI. APCI uses gas-phase ion-molecule reactions to produce charged analyte species. The effluent from an LC is converted to an aerosol, which is exposed to a corona discharge. Species produced by the discharge interact with the sample, producing ions that are detected by the mass spectrometer.

form negatively charged species, and electrons are transferred or negatively charged adducts are formed.

A variant of APCI uses short wavelength (UV) photons to ionize the analyte molecules in place of the corona discharge. This technique, known as APPI,[17] is most useful for analytes incorporating aromatic chemistry and has found utility in the field of clinical chemistry in the analysis of steroids. A krypton discharge UV lamp produces 10.6-eV photons that excite analyte molecules that undergo electron ejection to form cations. Ionization of analytes depends on the IP of the analyte; the IP of the analyte must be less than 10.6 eV. Most HPLC solvents have IPs greater than 10.6 eV and are not ionized. Deliberate addition of an ionizable species such as toluene or acetone can enhance the ionization by providing additional ionization pathways involving charge transfer or proton exchange. There is evidence to suggest that APPI is the least susceptible to ion suppression of the 3 atmospheric pressure ionization techniques, at least at low flow rates.[18] This phenomenon of reduced ion suppression is thought to be due to the lack of competition for charge in the ionization, because the photon flux is sufficient to promote ionization of all molecules present. The 3 ionization techniques are compared in **Table 1**, and the applicability of the techniques to different regions of chemical space is shown in **Fig. 5**.

APCI, APPI, and ESI take place at atmospheric pressure, which removes a great deal of the burden on the vacuum systems of the mass spectrometer. Because the analyte is charged at the end of the process, the ions can be focused through a small orifice into the mass spectrometer, which is operated at a higher vacuum. APCI is somewhat more robust and more energetic than ESI and works particularly well for less polar species. ESI works particularly well for more polar species. Because both techniques work predominantly by protonation/deprotonation, neither will work for species that do not exhibit some degree of gas-phase basicity (for the formation of positive ions by proton transfer) or gas-phase acidity (for the formation of negative ions by proton abstraction). In practice, that means that the analyte molecules must contain heteroatoms like nitrogen, oxygen, or sulfur to be successfully analyzed.

Mass spectrometers operate on charged species and measure the mass-to-charge ratio (m/Q or m/z) of analytes. Once molecules are charged, they can be influenced by electrostatic and magnetic fields. Because there are many ways to generate electrostatic and magnetic fields, there are many ways to manipulate ions and many different

Table 1
The advantages and disadvantages of electrospray ionization, atmospheric pressure chemical ionization, and atmospheric pressure photoionization ionization methods for clinical analysis

ESI	APCI	APPI
Softest ionization	More robust than ESI	Excellent for PAH
Capable of multiple charging (higher molecular weights)	More energetic ionization	Used for steroids
Most susceptible to ion suppression	Ionizes smaller, less polar molecules than ESI: steroids, benzodiazepines, carbamates	May require use of a dopant for ionization
Greatest coverage	Forms only singly charged ions	Can provide superior signal/ noise ratio
Best compatibility with thermally labile species	Moderate susceptibility to ion suppression	Least susceptible to ion suppression
Most susceptible to ion suppression		

configurations for mass spectrometers. Subsequent focus is on triple quadrupole mass spectrometers. As suggested by the name, a triple quadrupole mass spectrometer consists of 3 quadrupole mass spectrometers joined together, usually inside one vacuum system. The first and third quadrupoles, typically called Q1 and Q3, respectively, are used to scan masses, while the middle quadrupole is used as a collision chamber. This arrangement is very versatile, and there are many different scan modes available, as shown in **Fig. 6**.[19,20] In the most basic mode, Q1 is scanned; there is no collision gas present in the collision chamber, and Q3 is set to pass all masses (or scans in sequence with Q1) (see **Fig. 6A**). This scanning mode results in a full scan mass spectrum, where all ions of the correct polarity that are produced in the source

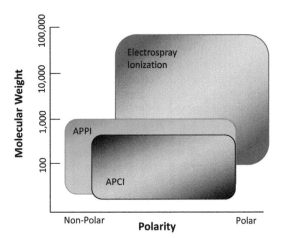

Fig. 5. Coverage map of ESI, APPI, and APCI in chemical space. APPI and APCI are more applicable to lower-polarity analytes of lower molecular weight, whereas ESI performs better for analytes with greater polarity. For ESI, a less-energetic ionization method is able to ionize higher molecular weight species than either APPI or APCI. There is considerable overlap between the techniques.

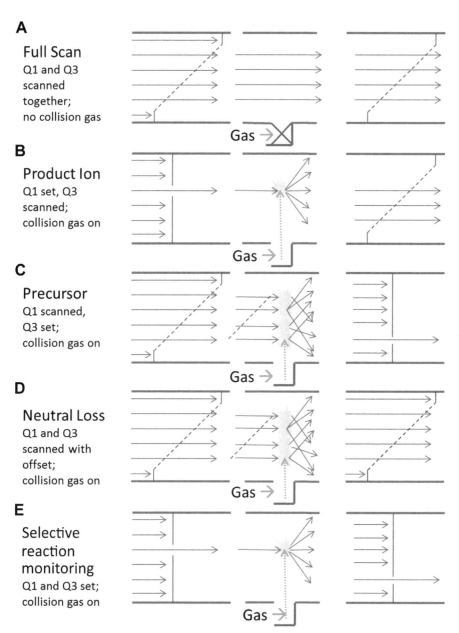

A

Full Scan

Q1 and Q3 scanned together; no collision gas

Gas →

B

Product Ion

Q1 set, Q3 scanned; collision gas on

Gas →

C

Precursor

Q1 scanned, Q3 set; collision gas on

Gas →

D

Neutral Loss

Q1 and Q3 scanned with offset; collision gas on

Gas →

E

Selective reaction monitoring

Q1 and Q3 set; collision gas on

Gas →

Fig. 6. The 5 main experiments performed with triple quadrupole mass spectrometers. (*A*) Full scan. (*B*) Product ion scan. (*C*) Precursor ion scan. (*D*) Neutral loss scan. (*E*) SRM. Note that collision gas is used for all experiments except full scan.

are observed in the mass spectrum, within the defined upper and lower limits of the scan. This scan mode is a useful scan mode, for example, for determining the molecular weights of species in a chromatogram. A second common scan mode is the product ion scan (see **Fig. 6**B). In this scan mode, one mass (actually a selected m/z ratio with a defined mass window) is selected in Q1 and allowed to collide with gas in the collision quadrupole, and the resulting charged fragments are observed by scanning Q3. This scan mode is useful for determining the structure of an unknown species or for determining the product ions that are potential candidates for monitoring in other types of MS/MS scans. **Fig. 6**C shows the reverse of a product ion scan, the precursor ion scan. In this scan mode, ions are scanned in Q1 and allowed to fragment in the collision quadrupole, and only one fragment ion mass is allowed through by Q3. This scan is useful for determining all of the species in a sample that contain a common structural element and is used for determining, for example, the metabolites of a drug. The neutral loss scan is depicted in **Fig. 6**D and shows a scan mode that is complementary to the precursor ion scan. In this mode, Q1 and Q3 are offset, and the difference between the masses is set to determine the mass of a substructural group that is being observed. This scan mode is used to show, for example, all of the species in a sample that might contain a hydroxyl group, which would lead to loss of H_2O and which is observed by setting an offset of 18 Da between Q1 and Q3. The final common scan mode is selective reaction monitoring (SRM), shown in **Fig. 6**E. This method of scanning is the one typically used for quantitation. Q1 and Q3 are set to observe a preselected transition, and collision gas is present, resulting in a stable transition indicative of a particular species. An even more common variant of SRM is multiple reaction monitoring (MRM). In this mode, multiple selected product ions from a common precursor are observed to provide additional confirmation in the quantitation process. This scanning mode is the most popular method used in the toxicology laboratory for monitoring small molecule drugs. In all scan modes where collisions are used, the energy of collision is a variable that must be optimized and set.

APPLICATION OF LIQUID CHROMATOGRAPHY–TANDEM MASS SPECTROMETRY IN THE TOXICOLOGY LABORATORY
Traditional Toxicology Techniques

Before going to the in-depth discussion about the applications of LC-MS/MS in toxicology laboratories, an initial introduction to the traditional techniques that were popular in toxicology testing is warranted. Technology limitations of traditional techniques lead to the transition of using LC-MS/MS as the method of choice in clinical testing. The advantages and disadvantages of each technique are summarized in **Tables 2** and **3**.

Immunoassay
History and introduction Immunoassay (IA) was first developed to identify antigen-antibody complex formation. One example of the older IA method is the Ouchterlony double immunodiffusion assay developed in the 1940s, whereby both antigen and antibody diffuse through a semisolid gel independently to identify if the specific

Table 2 Comparison of the advantages of different toxicology techniques			
	IA	GC-MS	LC-MS/MS
Fast turnaround	√	—	—
Specificity	—	√	√
Sensitivity	√	√	√
Ease of sample preparation	√	—	√
Ease of developing new test	—	√	√
High throughput	—	—	√

Table 3 Disadvantages of different techniques for clinical analysis		
IA	**GC-MS**	**LC-MS/MS**
Lack of analytical specificity	Longer run times	More expensive instrumentation
Not suitable for testing large panel of analytes in one run	More complex sample preparation for larger molecules	Higher maintenance
Low requirement for qualified staff raises the concern of human error	Limited utility for large, polar, or thermally labile analytes	Ion suppression/matrix effect concerns
Not flexible for developing new assays		

antigen/antibody complex is formed.[21,22] In late 1950s, Yalow and Berson[23] first reported the development of a radioimmunoassay (RIA) for insulin that used radioactive isotopes. The radioactive labels used in this method emit gamma rays, which allow the quantitative detection of trace levels of insulin using a gamma counter. Since then, IAs have evolved considerably in the area of both research and clinical diagnostics. Depending on the detection methods, IA can be defined as RIA, enzyme immunoassay (EIA), fluorescent immunoassays, and chemiluminescent IAs.[24] The IAs most frequently used in clinical laboratories are quantitative or semiquantitative automatic IA analyzers with methods such as enzyme multiplied immunoassay technique (EMIT), fluorescent polarization immunoassay (FPIA), and chemiluminescent EIA.[25]

Primary use IA is widely used in the field of clinical toxicology primarily because of its ease of performance, minimal sample preparation requirement, and rapid turnaround time. IA is the dominant screening method at the point of care. The IA screening method is typically followed by the confirmation of individuals who test positive for drug use by other more specific assays such as MS.[26] According to the product guide 2015 from the College of American Pathologist, there are more than 20 manufacturers and 60 analyzers on the market serving the needs of clinical laboratories. Assays are available for blood, serum, or urine samples for the determination of ethanol, drugs of abuse, and therapeutic drug monitoring (eg, benzodiazepines, amphetamine and methamphetamine, cannabinoids). For example, Abbott Laboratories (Chicago, IL, USA) with its ARCHITECT analyzer and AXSYM analyzer, and Roche Diagnostic Laboratories (Nutley, NJ, USA) with its COBAS and INTEGRA analyzers, are 2 of the pioneers using this technique for monitoring a large variety of analytes.[24]

There are also IA test devices for point-of-care testing (POCT), which do not need large-scale instruments. These "devices" may be dipstick, cup, card, or cassette based.[27] The simple-to-use POCT device combines the sample collection and testing, thereby facilitating a fast turnaround time. However, the operator for this kind of assay needs to perform multiple steps, including sample collection, timing for the reaction end point, result interpretation, and data recording. One often-cited issue for these devices is that the resolution/interpretation of the result varies between different operators, because the positive readings are often solely dependent on visual signs, for example, change of color or absence of a line. On the other hand, laboratory IA instruments have the advantage of automation to capture data on a computer system, reducing the chance of human error.

Advantages The attributes of toxicology diagnostics consist of the following aspects: specificity, sensitivity, fast turnaround time, high throughput, ease of sample preparation, and the flexibility to develop laboratory-based tests.[28] The major advantage of IA in the clinical testing is its rapid turnaround time. Since the 1980s, many companies have been devoted to developing fully automated IA systems for rapid and sensitive testing. It has been reported that, with an automated IA system, the analysis time of a total of 11 drugs (cyclosporine, tacrolimus, mycophenolic acid, valproic acid, digoxin, theophylline, carbamazepine, phenytoin, phenobarbital, vancomycin, and gentamicin) was 1.1 minutes and the time for reporting was 11 minutes, using the Viva-E Drug Testing System (Siemens, Palo Alto, CA, USA).[29] Moreover, most of the testing is performed using the homogeneous IA, which means that the assays are performed in solution without the need of excess sample preparation (phase separation, sample extraction, and so forth). Another advantage of IA is its sensitivity or limits of detection. With the development of this technique, nowadays both EMIT and FPIA assays can detect analyte levels in the nanomolar range, which fulfill the needs of most clinical diagnostics.

Disadvantages Analytical specificity is a major concern for the IA techniques. It is almost impossible to raise antibodies toward a single molecular structure, but rather, most antibodies are used to detect a family of compounds with the same chemical backbone, which may lead to false positive or false negative results. For example, cross-reactivity has been identified using IA for the detection of tricyclic antidepressants (TCA; eg, amitriptyline, imipramine, desipramine, and nortriptyline).[30] Positive results can be observed due to TCA, or a non-antidepressant drug cyclobenzaprine, due to the similarity of the 3-ring structure. When blood samples are tested, the monoclonal antibodies used in IA may bind nonspecifically with the proteins present in patient's serum and plasma, thereby producing false positive results.[31] IAs are limited to the assays for which the manufacturers can develop suitable antibodies. The average time for developing commercial IAs takes 2 to 5 years. Large discrepancies can be found in terms of sensitivity, result interpretation, cutoff values, and reference ranges from the kits and instruments designed by different manufacturers.[32–34] In addition, the throughput of IA is dependent on the manufacturer's assay kit; most of the time, individual IAs are necessary for the detection of each group of drugs, thus rendering it impractical to measure all the analytes of interest simultaneously. It is also worth noting that immunoanalyzers and assay kits are designed specifically for use with a certain matrix (urine or plasma). When modification is made for using a kit with a different matrix, the laboratory needs to thoroughly validate the method.[35] Ideally, clinical and laboratory staff need to be trained to know the limitations of IA and be aware of false positive/negative results related to this methodology. Both automated immunoanalyzers and POCT devices are easy to use, which leads to minimal technical requirements for the staff performing the test. When no specialist is present in the laboratory, results may not be interpreted properly.

Gas chromatography-mass spectrometry

Technology advancement of MS offers robust solutions that can be applied to clinical testing toward obtaining better specificity, accuracy, and sensitivity. Modern MS would not exist without the chromatographic systems used to provide separation of analytes. The 2 major chromatographies currently in use are GC and LC. Both use a stationary phase and a mobile phase, and they are distinguished by their mobile phases. GC uses an inert gas, typically helium, hydrogen, or nitrogen, as a mobile phase, whereas LC uses a liquid solvent system. The separation is affected by the analytes moving between the stationary phase and the mobile phase, in a process known as partitioning. LC and GC are used for different types of compounds and situations, and the 2 techniques are now very complementary. GC is used for smaller, less polar molecules, and LC is used for larger or more polar molecules that are not amenable to GC (**Fig. 7**).

History and introduction GC is a robust technique that offers the ability to resolve volatile analytes from a complex biological matrix. MS provides the unambiguous identification of a compound based on its mass-to-charge ratio. In combination, GC and MS serve as a powerful and versatile analytical tool for both qualitative and quantitative purposes.[36] It was first reported in early 1950s that GC technology can be used for the separation of volatile compounds in a mixture.[37] In the mid 1950s, Roland S. Gohlke and Fred W. McLafferty at Spectroscopy Lab at Dow Chemical Co. worked in collaboration with Bill Wiley, Ian McLaren, and Dan Harrington at Bendix Labs, where they successfully produced the first direct-coupling GC-MS. Later, the technology of GC-MS started to quickly evolve with the introduction of capillary chromatographic columns and the advance of carrier gas separators to remove the GC carrier gas before introduction of a sample into the high-vacuum mass spectrometer. Nowadays, the modern GC-MS instrumentation is widely used as a high-resolution technique for analyte separation and identification. Applications of modern GC-MS include environmental analysis, forensics, clinical laboratory drug testing, and pharmacologic studies.

Advances in the ionization techniques promoted the variety of applications of GC-MS in the clinical testing. The electron ionization (EI) full-scan mode is the gold standard for comprehensive screening and systematic toxicologic analysis of drugs and metabolites.[38,39] Positive ion chemical ionization (PCI) is suitable for the identification of drug metabolites in biosamples.[40] PCI can give the molecular mass information of analytes when EI fails to produce a corresponding molecular ion.[41] Negative ion chemical ionization (NICI) can improve the sensitivity of analytes with electronegative moieties (eg, benzodiazepines) by several thousand-fold.[42]

Primary usage GC-MS has been used for drug monitoring for several decades, and it continues to be the definitive standard for toxicology laboratory confirmation analysis.[30] Because the detection of therapeutic drugs and drug of abuse can have serious consequences in patients' professional, social, and financial situations, it is generally accepted that positive results of certain drugs from screening procedures (eg, IA) need to be confirmed by a second method. GC-MS is one of the gold-reference methods for confirmation.

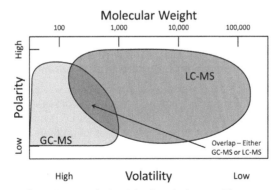

Fig. 7. Coverage map for GC-MS and LC-MS in chemical space. The coverage was illustrated based on volatility (lower x-axis), polarity (y-axis), and molecular weight (higher x-axis). GC-MS is useful for higher-volatility, lower-molecular-weight analytes, whereas LC-MS is useful for lower-volatility, higher-polarity analytes.

Another merit of this technique is that GC-MS can also be used for screening procedures for simultaneous detection of several drug classes.[43] Reliable screening methods have been developed for the detection of drugs of abuse[44,45]; therapeutic drug monitoring, including barbiturates, benzodiazapines, antidepressants, and morphine[46]; and pesticides.[47,48] There are several commercially available libraries for drugs, drug metabolites, poisons, and pesticides, providing universal spectra that can be applied on different GC-MS instruments from various manufacturers.[49]

Advantages Advances in technology have allowed the introduction of bench-top GC/MS instrumentation into clinical laboratories. GC/MS has been widely recognized for its reproducibility, specificity, and sensitivity to detect trace amounts of analytes. The long GC capillaries ($\sim$30 m) lead to better analyte separation from matrix and interferences compared with other chromatography techniques, which increases the specificity of targeted compounds. Sensitivity of GC-MS is significantly higher than IA for the detection of drugs and metabolites in relation to clinical toxicology testing. It is reported that the limit of detection (LOD) for opioids, tetrahydrocannabinol, and benzodiazepines ranges from 1 pg/mL to 0.1 ng/mL in biosamples using the GC-MS-NICI technique.[41] In addition, GC-MS offers improvement in specificity compared with the IA method, by combining high chromatographic resolution with full spectra information.

Similar to the IA screening method, GC-MS can also be configured for screening large panels of drugs in the same run, which is beneficial because IAs typically only screen one class of drug in one assay. In addition, toxicology laboratories can develop their own GC-MS applications for the less commonly tested drugs (eg, lysergic acid diethylamide [LSD]), for which IA methods are not available.

Disadvantages A major drawback for the GC-MS technology is its labor-intensive sample preparation procedures. Because of the nature of GC, GC-MS analysis is limited to small nonpolar analytes that are sufficiently volatile as well as thermally stable to vaporize at practical temperatures (the temperature in the GC injector and oven often do not exceed 300°C). For polar and thermally labile analytes, sample derivatization is the prerequisite to convert the analytes to volatile products before injecting into the gas chromatograph. The sample preparation steps may also include the cleavage of conjugates, extraction, and cleanup procedures; these factors contribute to the prolonged turnaround time and reduced throughput. In addition, GC-MS instruments are not available at most hospital laboratories; thus, positive IA samples need to be sent out to comprehensive or reference toxicology laboratories for GC-MS confirmation. In this case, the turnaround time can be delayed for days.

Liquid Chromatography–Tandem Mass Spectrometry Application in the Toxicology Laboratory

Although GC provides higher resolution separations, it comes with the cost of longer run times and only for thermally stable, volatile species. LC is more amenable to rapid separations and is optimized for larger analytes. Although there is much overlap, analyses are moving toward LC-MS/MS for speed, and in many cases, sensitivity. Many clinical methods were developed for GC and GC-MS before reliable LC-MS interfaces were available. LC, being more compatible with most clinical matrices and analytes and also using shorter run times with often-simpler sample preparation, is commanding an ever-growing share of the clinical laboratory landscape. Today, with its well-known merits of sensitivity, selectivity, and robustness, LC-MS/MS is serving the toxicology laboratories with fast, accurate, and comprehensive testing for nearly all the analytes of interest in the field of drug-of-abuse and therapeutic drug monitoring. With proper sample preparation, LC-MS/MS can provide the solution for testing nearly all common biological fluids.

Common sample matrix and sample preparation methods

Urine, blood plasma, and oral fluid are the most commonly used matrices for clinical applications of LC-MS/MS. Because of the presence of endogenous components in different biomatrix fluids, especially in oral fluid and blood samples, ionization suppression or enhancement can occur, which is known as the "matrix effect." The precision as well as accuracy will be affected if the compounds of interest coelute with the matrix fluid. Sample cleaning also helps improve the sensitivity of the assay by achieving lower limits of detection. Therefore, the sample preparation is a very important step to ensure the quality of instrument performance for every assay.

The purpose of the sample preparation is to remove the interferences that can affect the detection of the target analytes and the lifetime of the column and the instrument. Also, the preparation steps serve to enrich the analytes of interests to be categorized within the method detectable range. **Table 4** shows the sample preparation options with their strength and shortcomings.

Workflow and high throughput are of key importance in the clinical laboratory, whereas the sample preparation is usually the "rate-limiting" step. The "dilute-and-shoot" method is gaining popularity in clinical applications by offering the quickest preparation, while reducing the matrix effect to a certain extent with simply diluting urine samples with mobile phases. When it comes to blood samples, cleanup is a prerequisite before the sample can be loaded for LC-MS/MS analysis. Simple methods like liquid-liquid extraction (LLE) and protein precipitation (PPT) are the 2 commonly used methods for sample cleanup. However, because LLE cannot remove phospholipids, which can cause formation of an emulsion during the extraction procedure, the recovery rate of analytes can be significantly affected. In addition, extraction solvents are typically nonpolar organics; therefore, it is expected that the recovery of polar drugs would be minimal. PPT is less selective than LLE, and it does not remove most of the interference component. An improvement to PPT is the commercially available protein removal plates, which removes the phospholipids and other interference components. The solid-phase extraction method (SPE) is perhaps the most

Table 4
Advantages and disadvantages of different sample preparation methods

Method	Advantages	Disadvantages	Suitable Matrices
Dilution-and-shoot	Simple, quick, and low cost	No cleanup and no selectivity	Urine
LLE	Simple, better cleanup than PPT	Difficult to automate, not suitable for highly polar analytes, solvent evaporation needed	Urine, plasma, serum, oral fluid
PPT	Simple, quick	No matrix interference removal, minimal selectivity, solvent evaporation needed	Whole blood, plasma, serum
SPE	Can be automated, best cleanup option, high reproducibility	Costly and method development can be difficult	Urine, whole blood, plasma, serum, oral fluid

powerful technique for sample preparation for clinical applications. SPE columns and kits are available for various analytes with selectivity in size or polarity. It is currently the best option for sample cleanup, because of its high recovery rate and reproducibility. SPE is particularly suitable for oral fluid sample preparation. Oral fluid contains extraction buffers, proteins, enzymes, and even oral swab tissues, and the analyte concentrations are 5 to 10 times lower in oral fluid than in a urine sample. Enrichment through SPE is essential to detect low concentration of drugs in oral fluid samples.

Drug monitoring for pain management drugs and drugs of abuse

MRM with ESI mode has been widely used in toxicology laboratories for developing in-house drug testing panels. MRM methods are commonly established on triple quadrupole mass spectrometers, where the first and third quadrupoles (Q1 and Q3) function as mass analyzers; the second quadrupole (Q2 or q) functions as a collision cell to introduce fragmentation of targeted ions through collision-induced dissociation. In order to develop an MRM method for a given analyte panel, each analyte needs to be "tuned" by direct infusion into the mass spectrometer to gain the best intensity, sensitivity, and selectivity. Although parameters vary from different mass spectroscopy manufacturers, the universally important parameters include the m/z for precursor ions (Q1) and transition ions (Q3), declustering potential (DP), and collision energy (CE). One or more Q3 masses could be chosen as both quantifier and qualifier to ensure a better identification of certain drug analytes. DP refers to the voltage applied to the orifice to prevent the target ions from being clustered with other ions in the matrix or solvent. CE is the voltage applied at the collision cell and determines the rate of acceleration when the drug ions enter Q2. The first step in method development is to optimize the values for each of these parameters because these values can be compounded as well as instrument dependent.

Two working examples for analysis of 72 pain management drugs and 52 psychiatric drugs are presented using MRM methods developed on a Sciex 4500 Q-Trap Mass Spectrometer (Sciex, Framingham, MA, USA) equipped with ESI. Drugs in the pain management panel and psychiatric panel were both separated through Shimadzu Nexera XR HPLC system (Shimadzu, Kyoto, Japan) and Restek Raptor Bi-phenol analytical column. For each drug panel, the methods were validated for accuracy, linearity, precision, LOD, limit of quantitation (LOQ), and carryover limits, which are all important aspects of clinical MS. Methods for both pain management and psychiatric drug panels were developed and validated according to standard procedures.

Chronic pain was defined by the International Association for the Study of Pain as "… an unpleasant sensory and emotional experience associated with actual or potential tissue damage…."[50] Currently, chronic pain has affected more than a quarter of million American lives leading to a cost of about $600 billion per year.[51–53] Pharmacologic therapies with pain-relieving medications (analgesics) are frequently recommended by physicians for pain management. There are 2 major categories of analgesics commonly available for a pain management program: opioid drugs and non-opioid drugs. Non-opioid drugs, such as aspirin and paracetamol, are mainly used for treatment of moderate levels of pain. Opioid drugs, such as codeine, morphine, and oxycodone, are usually recommended for treatment of severe pain. However, addiction to opioid analgesics, such as oxycodone or heroin, which share chemical similarities, has been frequently identified at various stages of a prescribed pain management program. Therefore, effective pain management drug monitoring via urine specimen assessment is essential to build the confidence for both physicians and pain patients alike, to affirm that patients are being compliant with the prescribed medications as well as to detect abused substances or illicit drugs. However, if the expected drugs or metabolites are not present, this may be indicative of noncompliance, sample adulteration, or poor drug absorption, in addition to limitations of methodology, instrumentation, or detection sensitivities. An MRM method for pain management drug monitoring is presented in **Table 5**, which covers 32 drug categories that are widely prescribed to chronic pain patients as well as some of the commonly identified illicit drugs and abused substances. A comprehensive list of the drug category (see **Table 5**) includes amphetamine, benzodiazapines, opiates, opiate analogues, opioid, synthetic opioid, oxycodone, buprenorphine, fentanyl, methadone, gabapentin, heroin metabolite, methylphenidate, ketamine and norketamine, methylenedioxyamphetamines (MDA), muscle relaxant, phencyclidine (PCP), pregabalin, propoxyphene, sedative hypnotics, synthetic cannibinoids, tapentadol, tramadol, TCA, stimulant, cocaine metabolite, and bath salts, among others.

Psychiatric medication represents another category of prescription medications where drug monitoring has become of recent interest. There are 6 major psychiatric medication categories: antidepressants, antipsychotics, anxiolytics, depressants, mood stabilizers, and stimulants. Because of the high rates of poor compliance by the patients with mental health issues and the considerable genetic variability of metabolism of the psychiatric drugs, therapeutic monitoring of the psychiatric medication for many patients with psychiatric disorders has been proven valuable for improving the patients' compliance with the medication, avoiding toxicity, optimizing psychopharmacotherapy strategy, and discovering genetic polymorphism and pharmacokinetic mechanisms.[54,55] An LC-MS/MS method for monitoring of 52 psychoactive drugs using positive MRM mode is presented in **Table 6**. The present method covers 12 drug categories focusing on antidepressants (serotonergic), antidepressants (tricyclic), antidepressants (other), antiepileptics, antipsychotics, stimulants, muscle relaxants, alkaloids, ketamine, and methylphenidates.

Methodologies have been developed for the determination of analyte concentrations in urine using a dilute-and-shoot method. Urine aliquots were first separated by centrifugation, followed by hydrolysis with β-glucuronidase to remove β-D-glucuronic acid conjugates that were formed by human metabolism. The mixed urine samples were then diluted with a mobile phase gradient by a dilution factor of 4, followed by vortex and further centrifugation. The supernatant from the resulted urine sample was transferred into HPLC vials and loaded onto the column for MRM analysis. Total run time for this assay is 7 minutes using a gradient elution of mobile phase A (0.1% formic acid and 2 mM ammonium acetate in water) and mobile phase B (0.1% formic acid and 2 mM ammonium acetate in methanol). The gradient was increased from 5% to 95% mobile phase B over 5 minutes at a flow rate of 0.7 mL/min.

The precursor (Q1) and transition (Q3) ions for each of the 72 pain management drug and 52 psychiatric drug analytes, as well as their retention time, LOQ, and LOD, are listed in **Tables 5** and **6**, respectively. Calibration curves for each analyte covers the range from below the cutoff to above the commonly detected confirmation levels. Accuracy was achieved for all drug analytes within the entire calibration range. Coefficients of variation were less than 15% (data not shown). For all the drug analytes, the quantitation method showed linearity in the calibration range of r >0.99. A representative chromatogram of all 72 pain management drug analytes identified using the ESI + mode MRM method is provided in **Fig. 8**. The total MRM detection window was 3 minutes. An overlay of MRM ion traces for both quantifier and qualifier transition ions of each drug is shown in different colors. The scheduled MRM algorithm provided by AB Sciex Analyst software allowed the monitoring of the MRM for each drug transition being triggered only within an appropriate time window flanking the retention

Table 5
List of 72 pain management drugs and their categories, precursor and transition ions, retention time, cutoff concentration, as well as method validation results for limit of detection and limit of quantitation

Group	Analyte	Q1 Mass (Da)	Q3 Mass (Da)	RT (min)	Cutoff (ng/mL)	LOD (ng/mL)	LOQ (ng/mL)
Adrenergic agonist	Ephedrine	166.115	91.1/115	1.35	25	0.35	1.07
Amphetamine	Amphetamine	136.1	91/119	1.49	100	1.02	3.08
	Methamphetamine	150.1	91.2/119.2	1.67	100	2.63	7.96
Bath salts	Mephedrone	178.3	145/144	1.91	3	0.15	0.47
	Methylone	208.1	160.1/132.1	1.74	3	0.13	0.39
	Methylenedioxypyrovalerone	276.2	126.1/135	2.41	3	0.17	0.50
Benzodiazepines	Diazepam	285.1	193.1/154	3.57	25	1.78	5.41
	Midazolam	326.1	291.1/222	2.96	25	0.35	1.08
	α-Hydroxyalprazolam	325.1	297/216.1	3.25	25	0.03	0.09
	Alprazolam	309.1	281/205.1	3.43	25	0.85	2.57
	7-Aminoclonazepam	286.1	222.1/121.1	2.39	25	0.51	1.55
	Flunitrazepam	314.1	268.2/239.2	3.38	25	0.56	1.70
	Flurazepam	388.2	315.1/134.1	2.76	25	0.40	1.22
	Lorazepam	321	275/229.1	3.06	25	0.61	1.84
	Nordiazepam	271.1	140/165.1	3.3	25	0.59	1.79
	Oxazepam	287.1	241/269.1	3.13	25	0.83	2.52
	Temazepam	301.1	255.1/177.1	3.39	25	0.83	2.50
	Triazolam	343	239/314.9	3.36	25	0.14	0.41
Buprenorphine	Buprenorphine	468.4	396.3/414.3	2.7	25	0.81	2.45
	Norbuprenorphine	414.3	101.1/165.1	2.42	25	3.51	10.64
Cocaine	Benzoylecgonine	290.2	168.1/105	2.27	25	0.46	1.40
Fentanyl	Fentanyl	337.2	105.1/188.1	2.69	3	0.14	0.42
	Norfentanyl	233.3	84.3/150.2	2.1	10	0.36	1.09
Gabapentin	Gabapentin	172.1	154.2/95.2	1.5	200	5.25	15.90
Heroin metabolite	6-MAM	328.1	165.2/211.2	1.7	10	0.70	2.12

		238.1	125/220.2	2.23	25	0.61	1.84
Ketamine & norketamine	Ketamine	238.1	125/220.2	2.23	25	0.61	1.84
Methadone	EDDP (2-ethylidene-1,5-dimethyl-3,3-diphenylpyrrolidine)	278.3	234.2/186.2	2.92	100	2.05	6.20
	Methadone	310.2	265.2/105	3.07	100	0.97	2.94
MDA	MDA	180.1	105/133	1.7	100	3.44	10.42
	MDEA	208.2	163.2/105.2	1.99	100	2.61	7.91
	3,4-Methylenedioxyamphetamine (MDMA)	194.1	163.2/105.2	1.84	100	0.98	2.97
Methylphenidate	Methylphenidate	234.1	84.1/91.1	2.24	25	0.32	0.96
Muscle relaxant	Carisoprodol	261.2	176.2/97.2	2.78	25	1.44	4.35
	Meprobamate	219.1	158.2/97.1	2.28	25	1.39	4.20
Nicotine	Cotinine	177.1	80/98.1	1.32	25	0.21	0.62
Opiates	Codeine	300.1	152.1/115.1	1.7	25	1.29	3.90
	Hydrocodone	300.1	199.1/128.1	1.84	25	1.12	3.39
	Hydromorphone	286.2	185/128	1.36	25	0.63	1.91
	Morphine	286.2	152/165	1.24	25	1.73	5.25
	Norcodeine	286.4	152.3/165.2	1.52	25	1.73	5.24
	Norhydrocodone	286.4	199.3/128.2	1.72	25	0.79	2.41
	Dihydrocodeine	302.4	199.2/128.3	1.66	25	0.42	1.26
Opioids & opiate analogues	Meperidine	248.2	220/174.1	2.27	25	0.46	1.40
Opioid, antagonist	Naloxone	328.1	212.2/253.1	1.62	25	2.03	6.15
	Naltrexone	342.16	212.2/267.2	1.8	25	0.86	2.60
Opioids, partial	Pentazocine	286.2	218.1/69.2	2.42	25	0.36	1.10
	Nalbuphine	358.3	340.3/272	2.06	25	0.85	2.58
	Butorphanol	328.3	310.3/131.2	2.49	25	0.22	0.66
Opioids, synthetic	Sufentanil	387.1	111.1/238	2.86	25	0.10	0.31
Other, antitussive, psychedelic	Dextromethorphan	272.1	171.1/215.1	2.78	25	1.34	4.06
	LSD	324.3	223.1/208	2.46	3	0.06	0.19

(continued on next page)

Table 5
(continued)

Group	Analyte	Q1 Mass (Da)	Q3 Mass (Da)	RT (min)	Cutoff (ng/mL)	LOD (ng/mL)	LOQ (ng/mL)
Oxycodone	Oxycodone	316.2	241/256	1.79	25	0.58	1.76
	Oxymorphone	302.1	227/198.1	1.28	25	0.74	2.24
	Noroxycodone	302.3	227.2/187.2	1.68	25	0.67	2.04
	Noroxymorphone	288.4	213.3/184.1	1.08	25	1.37	4.15
PCP	PCP	244.3	91/159.3	2.79	25	1.07	3.23
Pregabalin	Pregabalin	160.1	97/83	1.3	100	3.26	9.89
Propoxyphene	Propoxyphene	340.2	266.2/58.2	2.79	25	1.19	3.62
Sedative hypnotics	Zaleplon	306.2	236.3/264.2	3.3	25	0.91	2.75
	Zolpidem	308.2	235.1/236.1	2.61	10	0.41	1.24
	Zopiclone	389	245.1/217	2.37	25	2.10	6.36
Stimulant, synthetic	Phentermine	150.2	91.1/133.1	1.65	25	0.35	1.05
	Methcathinone	164.1	131.1/130	1.48	25	0.23	0.71
Synthetic cannibinoids	JWH-018N-Pentanoic acid	372.15	155/126.9	3.68	15	0.19	0.58
	JWH-073-4OH butyl	344.07	155/127	3.55	15	0.25	0.76
	JWH-073-N-butanoic acid	358.2	155/127	3.66	15	1.73	5.24
Tapentadol	Tapentadol	222.2	107.1/121.1	2.1	25	0.70	2.14
Tramadol	Tramadol	264.1	58.1/42.1	2.19	25	1.41	4.28
Tricyclic antidepressants	Nortriptyline	264.2	91/191.2	2.91	25	0.63	1.91
	Amitriptyline	278.2	91/191.2	2.94	25	0.67	2.04
	Imipramine	281.1	85.9/57.6	2.89	25	0.23	0.69
	Desipramine	267.2	72.1/193.2	2.86	25	0.54	1.62

time, thus avoided decreasing dwell times for each MRM transitions by reducing the numbers of concurrent MRMs being monitored. Target scan time was set as 0.2 seconds, and the MRM detection window was 30 seconds.

In summary, MRM methods of 2 large testing panels were presented as an example to demonstrate the benefit of using LC-MS/MS analysis to provide a fast and accurate tool for clinical testing. LC-MS/MS is one of the most suitable technologies for clinical toxicology applications toward rapid, highly selective, and robust testing of known drug analytes from human biofluids.

The advantages and disadvantages of liquid chromatography–tandem mass spectrometry

Advantages As shown in the above applications, LC-MS/MS offers superior specificity, sensitivity, and throughput, compared with other most commonly used techniques, such as IAs, UV-based chemical analysis, GC-MS, or conventional HPLC. LC-MS/MS offers much better specificity for a target molecule, because the quadrupole recognizes not only the original ionized molecule but also all the fragments derived from the original ionized molecule. Combined with the HPLC technique, the separation of the analytes is much easier and the retention time is another characteristic factor that enhances the selectivity of the mass spectrum.

The LC-MS/MS exhibits flexibility and versatility for the clinical laboratories to develop and validate new assays in house within a short time. LC-MS/MS assays, as laboratory developed tests, are highly attractive for target analytes where no commercial IAs are available. In contrast to GC/MS, which is limited to volatile molecules, LC-MS/MS has much wider range of applications because most biologically active molecules are polar, thermolabile, and nonvolatile. In addition, the LC-MS/MS sample preparation is simpler and does not require derivatization techniques.

A single LC-MS/MS run is able to provide a large number of quantitative or qualitative results. Thus, LC-MS/MS offers a far higher sample throughput. Another approach to increase the high throughput is to use the "multiplexed LC system." The Thermo Fisher TLX4 online sample preparation system and the Sciex MPX system are 2 examples of such an endeavor. Basically, the concept of a multiplex system is to maximize the use of MS by introducing specimens to MS from multiple chromatographic systems in a staggered fashion. Multiplexing allows the "spare time" of MS, which is the LC starting time before the first analyte elutes and the end time after the last analyte elutes, to be used by detecting analytes on the second LC stream. Depending on the optimized chromatography separation condition for a give group of analytes, multiplex systems can generally increase the throughput to 1.5- to 2-fold.

Another advantage of using LC-MS/MS in clinical toxicology applications is the possibility of identifying adulterated samples. Usually, IA only provides information on the drug category with semiquantitative data, but does not specify the exact drugs. For example, a screen test only provides the information that the sample contains opioids or benzodiazepines, but does not specify exactly which opioid drugs or benzodiazepine drugs are detected. As the diversion of opioid medications by the patients to other people for use and sale is not rare, a more robust approach to drug testing can help identify drug adulteration of urine samples as a portal for drug diversion. LC-MS/MS gives quantitative data for prescribed drugs and their metabolites, thereby providing objective ancillary assistance to the clinician to help assess if the patient takes their medication regularly versus adulteration of the specimen. For example, ingested hydrocodone would normally convert hydromorphone as well as dihydrocodiene and norhydrocodone, all of which would likely

Table 6
List of 52 psychiatric drugs and their categories, precursor and transition ions, retention time, cutoff concentration, as well as method validation results for limit of detection and limit of quantitation

Drug Group	Analyte	Q1 Mass (Da)	Q3 Mass (Da)	RT (min)	Cutoff (ng/mL)	LOD (ng/mL)	LOQ (ng/mL)
Alkaloid	Mitragynine	399.2	174.1/159.1	1.7	25	2.67	8.08
Antidepressants, serotonergic	Trazodone	372.2	176.1/148.1	1.59	25	0.65	1.97
	Vilazodone	442.5	197.3/425	1.52	25	5.17	15.65
	Citalopram	325.2	109.1/262.2	1.56	25	0.71	2.15
	Desmethylmirtazapine	252	195/209	1.46	25	0.53	1.62
	Duloxetine	298.1	44.1/154.2	1.73	25	17.15	52
	Fluoxetine	310.1	44/148	1.59	25	1.87	5.67
	Mirtazapine	266.2	195.2/194.2	1.48	25	0.46	1.4
	Paroxetine	330.1	69.9/135.1	1.8	25	0.44	1.32
	Sertraline	306.1	159/275.1	1.8	25	1.32	4
	Venlafaxine	278.2	58/121.1	1.56	25	1.08	3.26
	O-Desmethylvenlafaxine	264.1	58.1/107	1.11	25	1.64	4.98
Antidepressants, tricyclic	Desipramine	267.2	72.1/193.2	1.7	25	0.88	2.65
	Imipramine	281	85.9/57.6	1.73	50	1	3.02
	Amitriptyline	278.2	91.0/191.2	1.83	25	1.38	4.19
	Clomipramine	315.2	86.1/58	1.83	25	0.5	1.51
	Doxepin	280.2	107.1/235.1	1.72	25	0.42	1.28
	Nortriptyline	264.2	91.0/191.2	1.73	25	1.33	4.02
Antidepressants, other	Bupropion	239.8	184/166	1.52	25	1.84	5.57
	Selegiline	188.3	91.1/119.1	1.2	25	0.62	1.88
Antiepileptics	Carbamazepine epoxide	253.1	210.2/180.1	1.79	25	1.04	3.16
	Carbamazepine	237.1	194.1/165	1.81	25	0.75	2.29
	Hydroxycarbamazepine	255.1	237/194.1	1.52	25	3.85	11.67
	Lamotrigine	256.02	211.1/157	1.38	25	5	15.16
	Oxcarbazepine	253.1	180.2/208.2	1.66	25	1.1	3.33

Category	Compound						
Antipsychotics	Ziprasidone	413.2	194.1/130	1.67	25	2.14	6.49
	Norquetiapine	296.12	210.1/139.1	1.66	25	0.79	2.41
	Olanzapine	313.1	256.2/198.1	1.22	25	0.72	2.19
	7-Hydroxyquetiapine	400.3	269/208	1.26	25	1.78	5.39
	9-Hydroxyrisperidone	427.2	207.2/110	1.48	25	0.7	2.11
	Aripiprazole	448.1	285.2/176.2	1.94	25	1.68	5.08
	Asenapine	286.2	165.1/229.1	1.78	25	0.6	1.83
	Clozapine	327.1	270.1/192.2	1.64	25	0.26	0.8
	Desmethylolanzapine	299.1	256.1/198.1	1.22	25	1.25	3.79
	Fluphenazine	438.3	171.1/143.2	1.86	25	0.8	2.43
	Haloperidol	376.1	123/358.2	1.59	25	0.43	1.3
	Iloperidone	427	261/190.1	1.71	25	0.41	1.25
	Lurasidone	493.7	166.3/220.2	2.59	50	0.61	1.86
	Quetiapine	384.2	221.2/253.2	1.66	25	1.89	5.73
	Risperidone	411.2	191.1/148.2	1.63	25	2.07	6.27
Ketamine	Ketamine	238.1	125/220.2	1.5	25	0.12	0.36
Methylphenidate	Ritalinic acid	220.1	84.1/56.2	1.22	25	1.04	3.16
Skeletal muscle relaxant	Cyclobenzaprine	276.2	215.1/216.1	1.73	25	1.49	4.51
Stimulant, synthetic	MDPV (Methylenedioxypyrovalerone)	276.2	126.1/135	1.42	25	1.51	4.59
	Mephedrone	178.3	145.0/144.0	1.14	3	0.08	0.25
	Methylone	208.1	160.1/132.1	1.03	3	0.51	1.54
	Methcathinone	164.1	131.0/130.0	0.89	25	0.35	1.05
Other, adrenergic agonist, antihistamine, antitussive, anxiolytic	Ephedrine	166.1	91.1/115.0	0.91	25	1.93	5.85
	Diphenhydramine	256.1	167/152.1	1.68	25	3.9	11.82
	Dextromethorphan	272.1	171.1/215.1	1.77	25	0.33	1
	Buspirone	386.3	122.1/95	1.77	25	1	3.03
Other, nicotinic agonist	Varenicline	212.091	169.1/168.1	0.93	25	2.62	7.95

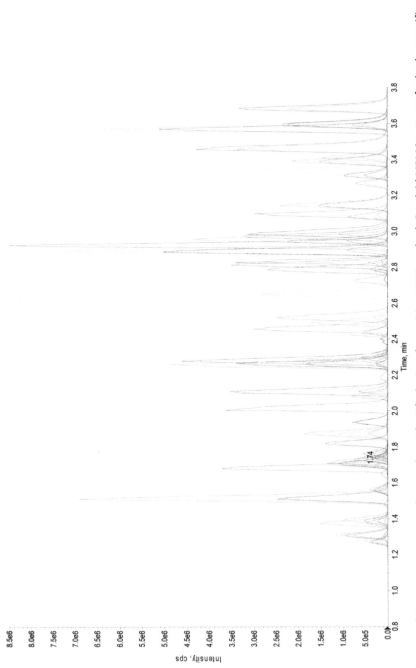

Fig. 8. Chromatogram of 72 pain management drug analytes identified using the positive MRM method. Overlaid MRM ion traces for both quantifier and qualifier transition ions are shown in different colors. MRM detection window was 3 minutes.

be detected in the urine with varying concentrations depending on time of ingestion, hydration status, liver and kidney function, among other factors. However, if hydrocodone is the only analyte detected in a urine specimen with a positive concentration that is over the high range cutoff value, whereas the expected metabolites (hydromorphone, dihydrocodiene and norhydrocodone) are negative or below the lower limits of detection cutoff, there would be a suspicion of specimen adulteration where the patient may have added hydrocodone directly into the urine sample, as a means of testing positive for the clinician while diverting the rest of the medication for economic incentives.

Disadvantages One major concern of the LC-MS/MS technique is ion suppression. Signal intensity obtained from a clean "standard" can differ significantly from human matrix samples, especially when the samples were not properly processed. Ion suppression presents a challenge in LC-MS/MS quantitation. However, using more selective extraction procedures for sample preparation and improving chromatographic retention to separate analytes from the highly polar matrix component can minimize the effect. Although LC-MS/MS offers the flexibility of developing assays to meet the clinical needs, the shortcoming of the flexibility is that method development, validation, and quality control may vary among different laboratories because most of the LC-MS/MS methods used in the clinical laboratories are often laboratory developed. Accuracy experiments are a prerequisite step in method validation to ensure the result variance is less than 20% from laboratory to laboratory. However, concern still exists regarding data discrepancies among different laboratories even with small variations like selecting different internal standards. The instrument itself is relatively more expensive compared with other technologies. Also, in addition to the expense of setting up and maintaining an LC-MS/MS laboratory, there is the understanding that highly qualified staff is required for method development, maintaining the instrument, as well as the day-to-day operation and data processing.

FUTURE PERSPECTIVES

MS technology has achieved an unprecedented maturation and development in the past few decades toward toxicology and other clinical applications. Many exciting new applications and developments are underway for clinical MS.[19] Advances in instrumentation, interfaces, software, and sample preparation techniques will all enable faster, better, and less-expensive testing. At the same time, integration of this technology into clinical automated systems shows promise toward moving the technology into a more automated setting. To reach that point, standardization of method development and validation processes, especially for laboratory developed tests, will need to take place.

Currently, most quantitative clinical analyses use tandem quadrupole mass spectrometers. The desire for increased sensitivity and robustness will drive instrument-related improvements, particularly in source design and ion transmission. Similarly, instrument development in LC continues, allowing faster chromatographic run times and greater resolution. Advances in both LC and MS will drive improvement in laboratory metrics, coupling decreased turnaround times with increased sensitivity.[56]

Although tandem quadrupoles will continue to be a dominant instrument in clinical chemistry analysis for some time, advances in instrumentation that enable the coupling of higher-resolution detection with the precise quantification available in triple quadrupoles will likely become available. Specifically, quadrupole TOF and orbitrap mass spectrometers show great promise in adding the additional capability of high-resolution/accurate mass detection to clinical analyses, which will allow greater specification in the analysis.[57] High-resolution instruments provide both quantitative and qualitative analyses while acquiring high-resolution full scan or MS/MS data. Furthermore, high-resolution full scan data acquisition provides a more complete description of the content of a sample. The quantitative performance of current high-resolution instruments is reported to be similar to that of current triple quadrupole mass spectrometers.[58–60]

An additional venue for instrumental development is increased automation; this is taking place on several fronts simultaneously. The need for reduced cost drives advances in automation and the simplification of sample preparation, particularly for sample sets with relatively low numbers of samples. Integration of automated sample preparation with LC-MS/MS systems will reduce the effort and time required for sample preparation and will reduce the possibility of error as more sample information is passed electronically from one stage of analysis to the next. Similarly, the reduction of human intervention in the review of data will drive efficiency, as will the integration of data reporting from the analyst to the clinical laboratory information system. Bidirectional information transfer will also be a productivity tool. Ultimately, the integration of LC-MS/MS into clinical chemistry analyzers may provide access to the already-established technologies currently implemented for sample preparation and information handling.

Another pathway for MS that is heavily based on automation and miniaturization would be the introduction of MS systems in point-of-care venues for rapid testing of bodily fluids for therapeutic and illicit drugs, peptides, and hormones.[61] Before that goal can be accomplished, much work needs to be done to standardize the method development and validation processes, with a potential end of having US Food and Drug Administration (FDA)-approved tests using LC-MS/MS. The current guidelines provide an excellent framework for laboratory developed tests, but greater homogenization of methods between laboratories will provide more consistent results. The FDA is moving to increasing oversight on laboratory developed tests; any forthcoming regulation will greatly impact the role of LC-MS/MS in the clinical laboratory.

The future of MS in clinical analysis is promising and bright. Opportunities for research and improvement are constantly maturing. At the same time, the impact of LC-MS/MS in the health care community continues to grow, making this technology interesting and impactful.

REFERENCES

1. Aston FW, LIX. The mass-spectra of chemical elements. The London, Edinburgh, and Dublin Philosophical Magazine and Journal of Science 1920;39(233): 611–25.
2. Thomson JJ. The discharge of electricity through gases. New York: Charles Scribner's Sons; 1898.
3. Thomson JJ. Rays of positive electricity and their application to chemical analysis. London: Longmans Green; 1913.
4. Thomson JJ. On the appearance of helium and neon in vacuum tubes. Science 1913;37:360–4.
5. Nier AO. Some reminiscences of mass spectrometry and the Manhattan Project. J Chem Educ 1989;66(5):385–8.
6. Rayward WBB, Ellen M. The history and heritage of scientific and technological information systems: Proceedings of the 2002 conference. Medford (NJ): Information Today, Inc; 2004.

7. Drew CM, Smith SR. ASTM E-14 Meeting on Mass Spectrometry. San Francisco, May 1955. p. 36.
8. Comisarow MB, Marshall AG. Fourier transform ion cyclotron resonance spectroscopy. Chem Phys Lett 1974;25(2):282–3.
9. Blakley CR, Carmody JJ, Vestal ML. Liquid chromatograph-mass spectrometer for analysis of nonvolatile samples. Anal Chem 1980;52(11):1636–41.
10. Carroll DI, Dzidic I, Stillwell RN, et al. Subpicogram detection system for gas phase analysis based upon atmospheric pressure ionization (API) mass spectrometry. Anal Chem 1974;46(6):706–10.
11. Yamashita M, Fenn JB. Electrospray ion source. Another variation on the free-jet theme. J Phys Chem 1984;88(20):4451–9.
12. Yost RA, Enke CG. Selected ion fragmentation with a tandem quadrupole mass spectrometer. J Am Chem Soc 1978;100(7):2274–5.
13. Millington DS, Kodo N, Norwood DL, et al. Tandem mass spectrometry: a new method for acylcarnitine profiling with potential for neonatal screening for inborn errors of metabolism. J Inherit Metab Dis 1990;13(3):321–4.
14. Budzikiewicz H, Schaefer M. Mass spectrometry: an introduction. 6th edition. Weinheim, Germany: Wiley-VCH; 2012.
15. Zeleny J. Instability of electrified liquid surfaces. Phys Rev 1917;10(1):1–7.
16. Carroll DI, Dzidic I, Stillwell RN, et al. Atmospheric pressure ionization mass spectrometry. Corona discharge ion source for use in a liquid chromatograph-mass spectrometer-computer analytical system. Anal Chem 1975;47(14):2369–72.
17. Short LC, SS, Syage JA. APPI: the second source for LC-MS. 2008. Available at: http://www.chromatographyonline.com/appi-second-source-lc-ms. Accessed March 24, 2016.
18. Hanold KA, Fischer SM, Cormia PH, et al. Atmospheric pressure photoionization. 1. General properties for LC/MS. Anal Chem 2004;76(10):2842–51.
19. Grebe SK, Singh RJ. LC-MS/MS in the clinical laboratory—where to from here? Clin Biochem Rev 2011;32(1):5–31.
20. Ahmadzai H, Huang S, Hettiarachchi R, et al. Exhaled breath condensate: a comprehensive update. Clin Chem Lab Med 2013;51(7):1343–61.
21. Josko D. Updates in immunoassays: introduction. Clin Lab Sci 2012;25(3):170–2.
22. Ouchterlony O. Handbook of immunodiffusion and immunoelectrophoresis. With appendices by three other authorities, and an equipment section. Ann Arbor (MI): Ann Arbor Science Publishers; 1968.
23. Yalow RS, Berson SA. Immunoassay of endogenous plasma insulin in man. J Clin Invest 1960;39:1157–75.
24. McPherson R. Henry's clinical diagnosis and management by laboratory methods. St. Louis (MO): Elsevier; 2011.
25. McClatchey KD. Clinical laboratory medicine. Philadelphia: Lippincott Wiliams & Wilkins; 2002.
26. George S. Position of immunological techniques in screening in clinical toxicology. Clin Chem Lab Med 2004;42(11):1288–309.
27. George S, Braithwaite RA. Use of on-site testing for drugs of abuse. Clin Chem 2002;48(10):1639–46.
28. Abuelzein E, Institute for New T. Trends in Immunolabelled and Related Techniques. 2012. Available at: http://www.intechopen.com/books/trends-in-immunolabelled-and-related-techniques. Accessed April 20, 2016.
29. Chung HS, Lee ST, Lee SY. Evaluation of Viva-E drug testing system [in Korean]. Korean J Lab Med 2007;27(5):330–7.

30. Wu AH, French D. Implementation of liquid chromatography/mass spectrometry into the clinical laboratory. Clin Chim Acta 2013;420:4–10.

31. Kricka LJ. Human anti-animal antibody interferences in immunological assays. Clin Chem 1999;45(7):942–56.

32. Leung KS, Fong BM. LC-MS/MS in the routine clinical laboratory: has its time come? Anal Bioanal Chem 2014;406(9–10):2289–301.

33. Horie H, Kidowaki T, Koyama Y, et al. Specificity assessment of immunoassay kits for determination of urinary free cortisol concentrations. Clin Chim Acta 2007; 378(1–2):66–70.

34. Taieb J, Benattar C, Birr AS, et al. Limitations of steroid determination by direct immunoassay. Clin Chem 2002;48(3):583–5.

35. Simonick TF, Watts VW. Preliminary evaluation of the Abbott TDx for screening of D-methamphetamine in whole blood specimens. J Anal Toxicol 1992;16(2):115–8.

36. Bertholf RL. Gas chromatography and mass spectrometry in clinical chemistry. Encyclopedia of analytical chemistry. Hoboken (NJ): John Wiley & Sons, Ltd; 2006.

37. James AT, Martin AJ. Gas-liquid chromatography: the separation and identification of the methyl esters of saturated and unsaturated acids from formic acid to n-octadecanoic acid. Biochem J 1956;63(1):144–52.

38. Maurer HH. Systematic toxicological analysis of drugs and their metabolites by gas chromatography-mass spectrometry. J Chromatogr 1992;580(1–2):3–41.

39. Maurer HH. Systematic toxicological analysis procedures for acidic drugs and/or metabolites relevant to clinical and forensic toxicology and/or doping control. J Chromatogr B Biomed Sci Appl 1999;733(1–2):3–25.

40. Kraemer T, Theis GA, Weber AA, et al. Studies on the metabolism and toxicological detection of the amphetamine-like anorectic fenproporex in human urine by gas chromatography-mass spectrometry and fluorescence polarization immunoassay. J Chromatogr B Biomed Sci Appl 2000;738(1):107–18.

41. Maurer HH. Role of gas chromatography-mass spectrometry with negative ion chemical ionization in clinical and forensic toxicology, doping control, and biomonitoring. Ther Drug Monit 2002;24(2):247–54.

42. Fitzgerald RL, Rexin DA, Herold DA. Benzodiazepine analysis by negative chemical ionization gas chromatography/mass spectrometry. J Anal Toxicol 1993; 17(6):342–7.

43. Maurer HH. Position of chromatographic techniques in screening for detection of drugs or poisons in clinical and forensic toxicology and/or doping control. Clin Chem Lab Med 2004;42(11):1310–24.

44. Schutz H, Gotta JC, Erdmann F, et al. Simultaneous screening and detection of drugs in small blood samples and bloodstains. Forensic Sci Int 2002;126(3): 191–6.

45. Weinmann W, Renz M, Vogt S, et al. Automated solid-phase extraction and two-step derivatisation for simultaneous analysis of basic illicit drugs in serum by GC/MS. Int J Legal Med 2000;113(4):229–35.

46. Polettini A, Groppi A, Vignali C, et al. Fully-automated systematic toxicological analysis of drugs, poisons, and metabolites in whole blood, urine, and plasma by gas chromatography-full scan mass spectrometry. J Chromatogr B Biomed Sci Appl 1998;713(1):265–79.

47. Lacassie E, Dreyfuss MF, Gaulier JM, et al. Multiresidue determination method for organophosphorus pesticides in serum and whole blood by gas chromatography-mass-selective detection. J Chromatogr B Biomed Sci Appl 2001;759(1):109–16.

48. Lacassie E, Marquet P, Gaulier JM, et al. Sensitive and specific multiresidue methods for the determination of pesticides of various classes in clinical and forensic toxicology. Forensic Sci Int 2001;121(1–2):116–25.
49. Maurer H, Pfleger K, Weber A. Mass spectral and GC data of drugs, poisons, and their metabolites. 3rd edition. Deerfield Beach (FL): Wiley-VCH; 1985.
50. Mills S, Torrance N, Smith BH. Identification and management of chronic pain in primary care: a review. Curr Psychiatry Rep 2016;18(2):22.
51. Nahin RL. Estimates of pain prevalence and severity in adults: United States, 2012. J Pain 2015;16(8):769–80.
52. Dubois MY, Follett KA. Pain medicine: the case for an independent medical specialty and training programs. Acad Med 2014;89(6):863–8.
53. Gaskin DJ, Richard P. The economic costs of pain in the United States. J Pain 2012;13(8):715–24.
54. Mitchell PB. Therapeutic drug monitoring of psychotropic medications. Br J Clin Pharmacol 2001;52(Suppl 1):45S–54S.
55. Mitchell PB. Therapeutic drug monitoring of psychotropic medications. Br J Clin Pharmacol 2000;49(4):303–12.
56. Annesley T, Diamandis E, Bachmann L, et al. A spectrum of views on clinical mass spectrometry. Clin Chem 2016;62(1):30–6.
57. Grund B, Marvin L, Rochat B. Quantitative performance of a quadrupole-orbitrap-MS in targeted LC–MS determinations of small molecules. J Pharm Biomed Anal 2016;124:48–56.
58. Fedorova G, Randak T, Lindberg RH, et al. Comparison of the quantitative performance of a Q-Exactive high-resolution mass spectrometer with that of a triple quadrupole tandem mass spectrometer for the analysis of illicit drugs in wastewater. Rapid Commun Mass Spectrom 2013;27(15):1751–62.
59. Kadar H, Veyrand B, Antignac JP, et al. Comparative study of low- versus high-resolution liquid chromatography-mass spectrometric strategies for measuring perfluorinated contaminants in fish. Food Addit Contam Part A 2011;28(9):1261–73.
60. Morin L-P, Mess J-N, Garofolo F. Large-molecule quantification: sensitivity and selectivity head-to-head comparison of triple quadrupole with Q-TOF. Bioanalysis 2013;5(10):1181–93.
61. Ferreira CR, Yannell KE, Jarmusch AK, et al. Ambient ionization mass spectrometry for point-of-care diagnostics and other clinical measurements. Clin Chem 2016;62(1):99–110.

Common Interferences in Drug Testing

Michael P. Smith, PhD[a,b,*], Martin H. Bluth, MD, PhD[c,d]

KEYWORDS

- False positive • False negative • Drugs • Toxicology • Forensic • Workplace
- Laboratory

KEY POINTS

- Interferences relating to laboratory toxicology testing refer to results which differ from their true value and are often encountered in the setting of a drug screen compared with confirmatory testing results.
- Interferences fall into two general categories; those that cause false positive results (when a drug screen is positive but confirmatory testing is negative) and those that cause false negative results (when a drug screen is negative when in reality the sample donor has ingested the tested substance).
- Interferences can result from differences in laboratory testing methodology, reagent and analyte cross reactivity, limits of analyte detection, instrument resolution, reporting cutoff, sample processing, tissue type and sample adulteration among others.
- Awareness of the possible causes of such interferences are integral to proper laboratory result interpretation and patient management.

Interferences with toxicology testing fall into two categories: those that cause false-positive results and those that cause false-negative results. The terms *false positive* and *false negative* in the context that follows refers to the screening test result as compared with the true result; that is, a false-positive result is a result that is screen positive for a particular class of drugs, when in reality, the donor has not ingested any of those substances. Conversely, a false-negative result is when a sample screens negative for a class of drugs, when in reality, the donor has ingested one of the tested substances.[1]

False-positive screen results are not a major concern for most toxicology laboratories, as confirmatory testing will resolve the screening discrepancy. Conformation

The authors have no commercial or financial conflict of interest.
[a] Oakland University William Beaumont School of Medicine, Rochester, MI, USA; [b] Toxicology and Therapeutic Drug Monitoring Laboratory, Beaumont Laboratories, Beaumont Hospital-Royal Oak, 3601 West 13 Mile Road, Royal Oak, MI 48073, USA; [c] Department of Pathology, Wayne State University School of Medicine, 540 East Canfield, Detroit, MI 48201, USA; [d] Consolidated Laboratory Management Systems, 24555 Southfield Road, Southfield, Michigan 48075, USA
* Corresponding author. Toxicology and Therapeutic Drug Monitoring Laboratory, Beaumont Laboratories, Beaumont Hospital-Royal Oak, 3601 West 13 Mile Road, Royal Oak, MI 48073.
E-mail address: michaelp.smith@beaumont.org

Clin Lab Med 36 (2016) 663–671
http://dx.doi.org/10.1016/j.cll.2016.07.006
0272-2712/16/© 2016 Elsevier Inc. All rights reserved.

testing is always more sensitive and specific than the initial screening test. False-negative results are a significant concern, however, as a sample that screens negative will not be sent for confirmatory testing. This issue becomes a concern because if the donor has intentionally masked the ingestion of a drug, the testing will not reveal it.

It should be noted that interferences only occur with the initial testing, which is usually immunoassay. Mass spectrometry confirmation tests are not affected by interfering substances or cross-reacting drugs.[2]

FALSE POSITIVE

False-positive interferences are usually drugs or other substances that are often structurally related to the class of drugs that is being screened for. Antibodies in the screening reagent are designed to detect common epitopes, particularly in drug classes with many substances (opioids, benzodiazepines, sympathomimetic amines). This design allows the test to be able to detect the many different drugs within a particular class. However, sometimes substances may be structurally similar to the intended class and, thus, are inadvertently detected by the assay. There is most often no intent on the part of the sample donor to cause a false-positive result.[3,4] **Table 1** describes commonly known drug interferences.[4,5]

FALSE NEGATIVE

False-negative interferences may or may not be intentionally ingested to attempt to mask the ingestion of a drug patients do not want to be detected. False-negative tests are more of a concern because, based on most toxicology laboratories' testing scenarios, negative screening samples are not investigated further.

Dilution

The simplest of these interferences involves diluting one's urine to the point that the concentration of the drug is less than the detection limits of the test. Patients either add additional liquid to the urine sample or drink something that causes their urine to be very dilute. Although this is a very effective technique, it is easily detected by the testing facility when they test the creatinine and specific gravity or observe the collection process. A normal urine has a creatinine greater than 20 mg/dL, along with a specific gravity that is greater than 1.030. If a urine specimen has both creatinine and specific gravity values less than these cutoffs, the urine is considered to be dilute.[6]

Substitution

Patients can attempt to substitute their urine with either someone else's urine or with a urinelike liquid. This type of interferences is detected with an observed collection, recording the temperature of the urine immediately after collecting, and/or the testing facility testing the creatinine and specific gravity of the sample. A sample that is not between 90°F and 100°F is not humanly possible and should be questioned as to the source of the specimen (Nuclear Regulatory Commission, Regulations Title 10, Code of Federal Regulations, part § 26.111). Additionally, a creatinine that is less than 2 mg/dL with a specific gravity that is less than or equal to 1.0010 or greater than or equal to 1.030 is not physiologically possible and is, thus, considered to be substituted.[6]

Adulterated

Another way a sample can be tampered with is by the addition of a substance that interferes with screening test that is causing the antibody to not bind to the drug. Specimen validity testing for oxidative substances and the pH of the sample usually detects

Table 1
Drugs that cause false-positive immunoassay screens

Drug Screen	Interfering Substance
Amphetamines	Amantadine
	Benzphetamine
	Bupropion
	Chlorpromazine
	Clobenzorex
	l-deprenyl
	Desipramine
	Dextroamphetamine
	Ephedrine
	Fenproporex
	Isometheptene
	Labetalol
	MDMA
	Methamphetamine
	L-Methamphetamine (Vick's inhaler)
	Methylphenidate
	Phentermine
	Phenylephrine
	Phenylpropanolamine
	Promethazine
	Pseudoephedrine
	Ranitidine
	Ritodrine
	Selegiline
	Thioridazine
	Trazodone
	Trimethobenzamide
	Trimipramine
Benzodiazepines	Oxaprozin
	Sertraline
Cannabinoids	Dronabinol
	Efavirenz
	Hemp-containing food
	NSAIDs
	Proton pump inhibitors
	Tolmetin
Cocaine	Coca leaf tea
	Topical anesthetics containing cocaine
Opioids	Dextromethorphan
	Heroin
	Poppy seeds
	Quinine
	Quinolones
	Rifampin
	Verapamil

(continued on next page)

Table 1 (continued)	
Drug Screen	**Interfering Substance**
PCP	Dextromethorphan
	Diphenhydramine
	Doxylamine
	Ibuprofen
	Ketamine
	Meperidine
	Mesoridazine
	Thioridazine
	Tramadol
	Venlafaxine

Abbreviations: MDMA, 3,4-methylenedioxymethamphetamine; NSAIDs, nonsteroidal antiinflammatory drugs; PCP, phencyclidine.

Data from Johnson-Davis KL, Sadler AJ, Gnzen JR. A retrospective analysis of urine drugs of abuse immunoassay true positive rates at a national reference laboratory. J Anal Toxicol 2016;40:97–107; and Brahm NC, Yeager LL, Fox MD, et al. Commonly prescribed medications and potential false-positive urine drug screens. Am J Health Syst Pharm 2010;67:1344–50.

these and other types of interferences.[7] A specimen will be reported as substituted when one of the following criteria is met:

- pH less than 3 or 11 or greater
- Nitrite ≥500 mcg/mL
- Chromium (VI) is present
- A halogen (eg, bleach, iodine, fluoride) is present
- Glutaraldehyde is present
- Pyridine is present
- A surfactant is present

Collection Process

The observed collection is the process of searching patients before the collection process as well as observing the patients providing the urine specimen. For obvious reasons, this process can cause both the patients and the collector to become uncomfortable. It is the collector's responsibility to strictly adhere to the observed collection protocols to ensure the sample is valid. This protocol includes asking potentially difficult or embarrassing questions as well as ensuring items, such as prosthetic limbs, do not contain substituted urine or other adulterating substances.[8] There is variability among clinical collection sites with regard to adherence to ascertaining whether strict collection protocols are part of a standard operating procedure and enforced. Thus, careful assessment of collection processes in light of an inconsistent laboratory toxicology result can often shed light as to whether adulteration or specimen mishandling, including accidental patient specimen mix-up, may have taken place.

Sample Processing

Once the sample reaches the laboratory, noting any odors or unusual appearance can be clues that the sample has been tampered with. Excessive foam, lack of color or a greenish-blue color, or the odors of bleach are all indications that the sample has been tampered with.[8]

Besides intentionally creating a false-negative response, many questions can arise from the unintentional false-positive result. This result most often occurs because of cross reactivity between substances within the same class or a structurally similar drug. This cross reactivity causes a difficult situation for health care providers or law enforcement/probation officers, particularly when the person being tested has a history of drug abuse. There are also issues that arise when samples are stored for extended amounts of time as well as when multiple different sample types are submitted for analysis on the same individual. Adherence to a strict standard operating procedure with respect to collection, affirmation of patient/sample pairing, packaging and processing as well as accounting for human fatigue can help obviate such types of preanalytical sample procurement errors.

There is nothing that can replace the information that is obtained by taking a thorough history and background. Additionally, the laboratory cannot be tasked with carrying the entire burden of the drug testing result. It must be clearly understood that the clinical toxicology laboratory provides objective ancillary support, which should be used in concert with other clinical parameters toward the effective management of patients and should not be a standalone measurement in this regard. It is the responsibility of the provider to investigate when the testing result is not what was expected. Literature review, requestioning patients, or even a call to the laboratory to ask for clarity in unusual situations may be warranted. In most such situations the error can be identified through careful inspection of the process. However, there are times when such assessment does not yield clarity. In such cases, retesting of the patients, either scheduled and/or unscheduled with careful attention to their drug ingestion scheduling, polypharmacy, collection of sample, and so forth can help in this regard.

Sample Type

The use of different sample types can lead to confusion when performing drug testing. The reason is simple human physiology. The different sample types represent different phases of the absorption, distribution, metabolism, and excretion (ADME) process. Depending on the time of ingestion, not all sample types can be expected to be positive. The sample types most often submitted for analysis are urine, blood, hair, and oral fluid. There are more if postmortem analysis is considered, but that is beyond the scope of this review.

If multiple different specimen types are submitted for testing on the same patient/subject, it is possible for some to misinterpret the results. For example, the most common dual specimen submission is urine and blood. The window of detection for blood can differ from that of urine for many analytes. One only has to consider the principles of ADME to understand why a urine test could be positive at the same time a blood test is negative. Blood passes through the liver at an approximate rate of 1.5 to 1.8 L/min.[9] Thus, in the typical 70-kg patient with an anticipated blood volume of about 5 L, the total blood volume would traverse the liver every 2.8 to 3.3 minutes. Further, each drugs half-life (in addition to variations in catabolic enzyme type and efficiency) would affect the rate of catabolism. The liver is one of the principal organs that removes the drug from the blood and can further metabolize the parent drug to something that the body can easily excrete in the urine. Certain unique parent-metabolite profiles are often detectable, thus, making urine an ideal specimen for testing for recent use of substances, up to 96 hours after ingestion, for most analytes. For example, ethanol detection in urine does not correlate with a similar presence and concentration in blood. Studies by Winek and colleagues[10] reported a disparity in the ethanol urine/blood ratios ranging from 0.7:1 to 21:1 demonstrating that presence and concentration in one fluid cannot necessarily predict such in another fluid. Similarly, buprenorphine analysis can be affected by disease states, such as end-stage renal failure, whereby blood/plasma concentrations of the two inactive metabolites, norbuprenorphine and buprenorphine-3-glucuronide, were found to be increased by 4 and 15 times, respectively, in subjects with renal failure, whereas urine concentrations were not reported to be affected. This finding is likely because renal elimination plays a relatively small role (less than 30% after intravenous administration) in the overall clearance of buprenorphine.[11] Such an understanding would be necessary for interpretation in patients with such disease states as discussed later in this review. **Table 2** lists the characteristics of the 4 most common specimen types used in toxicology testing.[12,13]

Instrumentation

Questioning a drug screen result is not uncommon and neither is repeating said test at a different facility. However, before comparing results from 2 different laboratories, it is imperative that the physician knows the technology each laboratory uses. A growing trend is for laboratories to forgo the immunoassay screen and perform only a Liquid

Table 2			
Characteristics of the 4 most common specimen types			
Specimen Type	**Window of Detection**	**Benefits**	**Limitations**
Oral fluid	0–50 h	No need for medical facility Can be done anywhere Difficult to adulterate sample	Detection limited to single-dose studies, limited/no controlled studies in prolonged users Not all possible adulterants tested, particularly those effecting the pH of the sample Oral ingestion/hygiene and drug exposure duration can affect results
Blood	0–48 h	Only specimen that is accepted by courts of law for ethanol	Medical professional needed for collection Invasive Usually have to rely on detection of parent compound, metabolites usually of minimal benefit
Urine	0–96 h Up to 30 d for THC	Most-established sample type No need for medical professional	Requires restroom for collection Can be adulterated/tampered with
Hair	1–12 mo	Ability to detect ingestion for up to 1 y	Extensive sample preparation needed by laboratory Testing not available immediately Can have higher amount of false positives if sample preparation done incorrectly Extensive training required for collector Possible hair damage from chemicals used for styling and/or grooming

Abbreviation: THC, tetrahydrocannabinol.

Chromatography with Tandem Mass Spectrometry (LCMS/MS) confirmatory analysis, using either multiple transitions or 2 different prepared samples. The LCMS/MS is significantly more sensitive than immunoassay and, thus, will potentially be able to detect substances that are less than immunoassay cutoffs.

Thus, it is not uncommon for a clinician to question the laboratory when a patient's urine results as negative using the screen (Immunoassay [IA]) technology and positive (ie, 156 ng/mL) on confirmatory (LCMS/MS) technology, often performed by 2 different laboratories, thereby casting doubt on the proficiency of one laboratory over another. This is erroneous, because in such a case it could be that the IA screen lower limits of detection (LOD) could be 300 ng/mL, whereas the LCMS/MS confirmatory LOD could be 50 ng/mL, thus explaining the negative screen and positive confirmation of a concentration of 156 ng/mL, in addition to other interfering factors that can affect the IA result.

Therefore, it is the responsibility of the provider to know what testing platforms are used at the laboratories and what the differences are between the laboratories before making decisions on the results.[2,14]

Interpretation

The toxicology result is often called on to render a decision of whether patients are taking their prescribed medications, taking other nonprescribed medications, and/or illicit substances. Although the detecting technologies and the inherent interferences have been discussed, there is also another layer of interrogation and thought that needs to be manifest to interpret a toxicology laboratory result. The laboratory's purpose is to detect or not detect and, where applicable, provide a concentration of the analyte. It is not the position of the routine (vs forensic) clinical toxicology laboratory to render a unilateral decision of whether patients diverted, surreptitiously administered, or overdosed on a medication or illicit substance. Such an assessment should be made in the context of integrating many other aspects of the patient-physician relationships (ie, track marks on the arm, "meth head" countenance, inconsistencies in patient history, and so forth). Indeed there have been reports of secondhand exposure to various narcotics, such as cocaine,[15,16] marijuana,[17–19] and other agents, through ventilation, passive exposure, skin, and other means,[15,16,20,21] as well as ingestion of herbal remedies that were unknowingly tainted with analgesic and illicit substances, such as benzodiazepines and opiates, among others.[22,23] A positive result may avail itself depending on which technology and which cutoff values are in place and can differ among laboratories. To this end, ElSohly[15] reported the presence of cocaine in the urine after the handling of cocaine-laced money, with a peak concentration of 72 ng/mL over a 24-hour period. As stated in vignettes earlier in this review, such a concentration would test negative using screening immunoassay technology with a cutoff of 300 ng/mL, yet test positive with confirmatory (Liquid chromatography (LC) or gas chromatography (GC) MS/MS) technology with a cutoff of 25 ng/mL.[15] Thus, the laboratory results can foster questions to explain inconsistencies rather than unilaterally vilify them.[24,25]

SUMMARY

In terms of providing the accurate final result, a false-positive screening testing is not a concern for a toxicology laboratory that routinely provides screen tests that reflex to confirmation tests. However, false-positive screening results become a significant problem when confirmation testing is not offered, performed, or requested. The laboratory can only perform testing that is ordered by a client, be that a physician or other non–health care entity (human resources department, hiring agency, and so forth). If the ordering entity chooses to save money by not requesting mandatory confirmation testing, those parties should be aware of the false-positive rate for all drug classes they are screening for.[1] Such false-positive results have resulted in confusion as well as employment termination and legal proceedings, which have been rectified with appropriate confirmations studies and better understanding of toxicology testing in general. Ordering entities should also be aware of the cross-reactivity rates of the screening tests they are ordering or using. Point-of-care testing units, such as all-in-one cup tests or other dipstick-type testing device, have been documented as having significantly higher cross-reactivity rates and, thus, higher false-positive rates than laboratory-run immunoassay tests. Additionally, the same precautions should be evaluated if an ordering entity does not request all positive screening tests be sent for confirmatory testing. In conclusion, it is the ordering entities' responsibility to understand the advantages and limitations of the drug testing they are ordering and use such objective ancillary results in the context of other information obtained during the clinical assessment to support and facilitate appropriate clinical management. The clinical toxicology laboratory can be an invaluable asset[26] in facilitating understanding and education in assisting the clinician with respect to laboratory testing and resulting to achieve this end point.

REFERENCES

1. Johnson-Davis KL, Sadler AJ, Gnzen JR. A retrospective analysis of urine drugs of abuse immunoassay true positive rates at a National Reference Laboratory. J Anal Toxicol 2016;40:97–107.
2. Manchikanti L, Malla Y, Wargo BW, et al. Comparative evaluation of the accuracy of immunoassay with liquid chromatography tandem mass spectrometry (LC/MS/MS) of urine drug testing (UDT) opioids and illicit drugs in chronic pain patients. Pain Physician 2011;14:174–87.
3. Saitman A, Park H, Fitzgerald RL. False-positive interferences of common urine drug screen immunoassays: a review. J Anal Toxicol 2014;38:387–96.
4. Brahm NC, Yeager LL, Fox MD, et al. Commonly prescribed medications and potential false-positive urine drug screens. Am J Health Syst Pharm 2010;67:1344–50.
5. Moeller KE, Lee KC, Kissack JC. Urine drug screening: practical guide for clinicians. Mayo Clin Proc 2008;83:66–76.
6. Federal Register/Vol. 80. No. 94/pg. 28101–28151.
7. Kirsh KL, Christo PJ, Heit H, et al. Specimen validity testing in urine drug monitoring of medications and illicit drugs: clinical implications. J Opioid Manag 2015;11:53–9.
8. SAMHSA. Medical review officer manual for federal agency workplace drug testing programs, 2010. Available at: http://www.samhsa.gov/sites/default/files/mro-manual.pdf. Accessed August 25, 2016.
9. Dobson EL, Warner GF, Finney CR, et al. The measurement of liver circulation by means of the colloid disappearance rate: I. Liver blood flow in normal young men. Circulation 1953;7:690–5.
10. Winek CL, Murphy KL, Winek TA. The unreliability of using a urine ethanol concentration to predict a blood ethanol concentration. Forensic Sci Int 1984;25:277–81.
11. European Medicines Agency. Suboxone- EPAR-Scientific Discussion; 2006. Available at: http://www.ema.europa.eu/docs/en_GB/document_library/EPAR_-_Scientific_Discussion/human/000697/WC500058497.pdf. Accessed August 25, 2016.

12. Cone EJ, Huestis M. Interpretation of oral fluid tests for drugs of abuse. Ann N Y Acad Sci 2007;1098:51–103.
13. Verstraete AG. Detection times of drugs of abuse in blood, urine, and oral fluid. Ther Drug Monit 2004;26:200–5.
14. Reisfield GM, Bertholf R, Barkin RL, et al. Urine drug test interpretation: what do physicians know? J Opioid Manag 2007;3:80–6.
15. ElSohly MA. Urinalysis and casual handling of marijuana and cocaine. J Anal Toxicol 1991;15:46.
16. Baselt RC, Chang JY, Yoshikawa DM. On the dermal absorption of cocaine. J Anal Toxicol 1990;14:383–4.
17. Niedbala RS, Kardos KW, Fritch DF, et al. Passive cannabis smoke exposure and oral fluid testing. II. Two studies of extreme cannabis smoke exposure in a motor vehicle. J Anal Toxicol 2005;29:607–15.
18. Mulé SJ, Lomax P, Gross SJ. Active and realistic passive marijuana exposure tested by three immunoassays and GC/MS in urine. J Anal Toxicol 1988;12:113–6.
19. Niedbala S, Kardos K, Salamone S, et al. Passive cannabis smoke exposure and oral fluid testing. J Anal Toxicol 2004;28:546–52.
20. Herrmann ES, Cone EJ, Mitchell JM, et al. Non-smoker exposure to secondhand cannabis smoke II: effect of room ventilation on the physiological, subjective, and behavioral/cognitive effects. Drug Alcohol Depend 2015;151:194–202.
21. Cone EJ, Bigelow GE, Herrmann ES, et al. Nonsmoker exposure to secondhand cannabis smoke. III. Oral fluid and blood drug concentrations and corresponding subjective effects. J Anal Toxicol 2015;39:497–509.
22. Bogusz MJ, Hassan H, Al-Enazi E, et al. Application of LC-ESI-MS-MS for detection of synthetic adulterants in herbal remedies. J Pharm Biomed Anal 2006;41:554–64.
23. Liu SY, Woo SO, Koh HL. HPLC and GC-MS screening of Chinese proprietary medicine for undeclared therapeutic substances. J Pharm Biomed Anal 2001;24:983–92.
24. Piekoszewski W, Florek E. The role of laboratory examinations in medical toxicology. Przegl Lek 2005;62:954–9.
25. Chen P, Braithwaite RA, George C, et al. The poppy seed defense: a novel solution. Drug Test Anal 2014;6:194–201.
26. Ward MB, Hackenmueller SA, Strathmann FG, Education Committee of the Academy of Clinical Laboratory Physicians and Scientists. Pathology consultation on urine compliance testing and drug abuse screening. Am J Clin Pathol 2014;142:586–93.

Toxicology in Pain Management

Daniel A. Schwarz, MD[a],*, M.P. George, MS[b], Martin H. Bluth, MD, PhD[c,d]

KEYWORDS

- Pain management • Pain medicine • Toxicology • Drug testing

KEY POINTS

- Urine toxicology testing can prove very useful for drug assessment, prescribing and monitoring approaches in pain management.
- Drug testing provides an objective measure of assessing risk stratification in conjunction with the patient's medical, psychiatric and compliance history.
- Understanding drug metabolism, biological fluid matrices as well as the differences and limitations of presumptive (screen) versus definitive (confirmatory) testing methods are critical to effective and appropriate patient management.

INTRODUCTION

Toxicology monitoring has become the standard of care in providing objective laboratory data toward managing chronic pain patients, whether cancer or chronic noncancer pain (CNCP). Recent guidelines issued by the Centers for Disease Control and Prevention (CDC) for prescribing opioids for chronic pain recommend urine drug testing before starting opioid therapy and periodically monitoring for prescribed medications as well as controlled prescription drugs and illicit drugs. The literature is extensive regarding the frequency and general methods of testing in the pain medicine journals,[1–3] by the American Pain Society (APS) and the American Academy of Pain Medicine[4] (AAPM), plus the more recently formed subspecialty board for interventional pain, established under the American Society of Interventional Pain Physicians[5] (ASIPP). The main difference among these societies is regarding the definition of chronic pain; APS and AAPM define chronic pain as persisting beyond the normal tissue healing time of 3 months,[4] whereas ASIPP originally defined it as 6 months[6,7] and then adjusted it to 3 months.[8] Regardless, the goal of this review is to present an

Disclosures: None.
[a] The Center for Pain Recovery, 18444 West, 10 Mile Road, STE 102, Southfield, MI 48075, USA;
[b] Laboratory Operations, Alere Toxicology, 9417 Brodie Lane, Austin, TX 78748, USA;
[c] Department of Pathology, Wayne State University School of Medicine, 540 East Canfield, Detroit, MI 48201, USA; [d] Consolidated Laboratory Management Systems, 24555 Southfield Road, Southfield, MI 48075, USA
* Corresponding author.
E-mail address: Dr@painrecoverymd.com

Clin Lab Med 36 (2016) 673–684
http://dx.doi.org/10.1016/j.cll.2016.07.007
0272-2712/16/© 2016 Elsevier Inc. All rights reserved.
labmed.theclinics.com

overview on the indications for toxicology testing primarily in CNCP, including frequency based on risk stratification, select medications, or drugs and their metabolism, regulatory and legal oversight that impact testing approaches, differences, and limitations in screening versus confirmatory testing methodologies, as well as sample matrices, and some algorithms the clinician may apply to insure medical necessity and evidence-based standard of care.

General Approaches to Toxicology Monitoring in Pain Medicine

Drug testing is vastly misunderstood and underutilized in health care. In addition, the term "urine drug testing" has generically been used for all types of drug testing. Urine drug testing is somewhat of a catch-all term because there are various types of urine drug testing the physician can use to monitor pain management patients.[9,10] Urine drug testing is used to monitor compliance with prescription medication and to identify substances prescribed as well as those that are not expected to be present. There are hundreds of chemicals, both licit and illicit, used today, especially with the emergence of synthetic psychoactive drugs; thus, it is impossible to test each drug in every patient. The most prevalent abused classes of drugs are marijuana, opiates, opioids, cocaine, benzodiazepines, and other sedatives.

Drug testing is performed in diverse settings, such as employment, criminal justice, clinical diagnosis, and monitoring of addiction patients in treatment. Each of these settings is intended for distinct purposes. For example, the Department of Transportation and the Federal Employee Drug Testing systems use the Mandatory Guideline (CFR 49, Part 40), the gold standard in the employment setting.[11] It is a deterrent program and safeguards against potential false positives. The Federal Workplace Program mandates administrative cutoffs and any drug at or above that set cutoff is reported positive, and any drug below the established cutoff is reported negative. However, a negative result does not mean the patient has no drug in their system; it simply says the drug level is below the cutoff. It is important to note that a laboratory cutoff is established by standard controls that determine the range of concentration that is allowed to be reported to the clinician; these operational aspects are tightly regulated by governmental and accrediting bodies, and nonadherence to such can result in fines, penalties, and laboratory suspension or closure. Therefore, the Federal workplace protocol can been misleading in the clinical setting, where a negative result could be positive in the realm of a lower limit of detection cutoff. Furthermore, the pain management drug test must eliminate false positive and false negative results for patient care.

The Federal Program only tests for 6 classes of drugs: amphetamines, marijuana metabolite, cocaine metabolite, opiates (codeine, morphine (M), and heroin metabolites only), ecstasy, and phencyclidine. However, pain management testing is a clinical test which includes illicit drugs, opiates, opioids, benzodiazepines, sedatives, and muscle skeletal relaxants. Thus, clinical drug testing is mainly used in pain management, addiction treatment, and psychiatry. Physicians may prescribe opiates and/or opioids in a wide range of doses to treat a patient's pain. These prescribed drugs can also interact with illicit drugs, other psychoactive drugs, sedatives, and alcohol, which could be lethal in patients on chronic pain medications, where higher doses of opiates or opioids are often prescribed as tolerance builds. As a result, the physician needs to monitor these patients periodically for the presence of the prescribed medication as well as other nonprescribed opioid and/or sedatives in the patient's system. The detection time is longer when the drug cutoffs are lower in accordance with absorption, distribution, metabolism, and excretion and steady-state kinetics. For example, cocaine can be detected up to 5 days at a 25-ng/mL cutoff versus 2 days at a 300-ng/mL cutoff. Further, illicit drugs, benzodiazepines, and/or alcohol, along with psychoactive drugs, can put health and safety at risk due to drug interaction. To this end, although toxicology testing can provide objective assessment of drug profiles to aid the physician in narcotic/analgesic prescribing options, understanding the testing cutoffs and the differences in reporting that they may avail will provide greater utility to patient management.

There is an "opioid epidemic" described as overprescribing, with a decade-long national trend of increased prescription opiate deaths, often in concert with other narcotics/analgesics/anxiolytics (ie, benzodiazepines). Currently, some states, Florida being the first, because of the Oxycontin pill mills, have already passed aggressive legislation, and others are rapidly in the midst of similar bills, limiting amounts of prescription opioids (morphine equivalent dosage [MED]) to board-certified pain specialists, percentage of pain patients per total practice allowed, mandatory Prescription Drug Monitoring Programs (PDMPs) (49 states, Missouri being the exception), and even initial limits on first-time opioid prescriptions to 7 days (with exceptions). Washington was the second state to have similar legislation, specifically "Do not exceed 120 mg of oral morphine equivalents/day without either demonstrated improvements in function and pain or first obtaining a consultation with a pain management expert," and has had their third revision since June 2015, including functional assessments like the Oswestry Disability Scale.[12]

This field is ever changing. However, the focus should remain on the core evidence-based practice of clinical toxicology as it relates to Pain Medicine rather than the epidemiologic study of opioid abuse.

INDICATIONS FOR MEDICATION MONITORING/DRUG TESTING

The key reasons behind toxicology testing in pain management patients are based on the principles that lead to drug interaction, overdose, and basic patient safety issues. The following list shows the reasons the overall mortality has increased significantly over the past decade from prescription medications:

1. Increase in total opioid prescriptions
     Americans, who account for 4.6% of earth's population, consume 80% of the
        world's produced prescription opioids and 99% of total hydrocodone, according to the ASIPP fact sheet (www.asipp.org)
2. Methadone
     5% of opioid prescriptions = one-third of opioid-related deaths
     Physician errors in methadone prescribing (eg, initial dosing, dose titration, opioid rotation to methadone).
     Payers promote methadone as first-line therapy (significantly lower cost vs other opioids)
     Torsades de pointes
3. Coadministration of other central nervous system depressants (may be with or without prescriber knowledge)
     Benzodiazepines
     Alcohol
     Antidepressants
4. Unanticipated medical or psychiatric comorbidities
     Depression
     Substance-use disorders
     Sleep apnea
5. Patient nonadherence to regimens
     Escalating doses without prescriber knowledge

Risk Stratification

Before prescribing opioids to any patient, the standard of care requires that the physician undergo risk stratification using basic history with simple screening tools to assess personal and family history of substance use disorder, mental illness, tobacco use disorder, or alcoholism. Failure to do this is below the standard of care in the community and is leading to increased scrutiny by the State Medical Boards, the Drug Enforcement Agency, which can now request patient records in addition to dispensing logs,[13] as well as civil litigation.[14] The most common and well-validated screening tools for opioid-naïve patients include the Opioid Risk Tool developed by Dr Lynn Webster[15] with the Screener and Opioid Assessment for Patients with Pain, which has been revised to include aberrant behaviors[16] and can then be subsequently cross-validated to included chronic pain patients.[17] Patients with alcohol history initially should be screened with any of the alcohol risk screening tools: CAGE (Cut down, Annoyed by criticism, Guilty, and need Eye-opener next morning), MAST (Michigan Alcoholism Screening Test), and AUDIT (Alcohol Use Disorders Identification Test).[18] However, pain management practices may not routinely perform the alcohol screening tests.

Compliance history

Any patient should have a review of risk factors to help guide the frequency of toxicology testing, and which substances to test for based on prior compliance history. Risk assessment by compliance history should occur whether for an existing patient, or a referred patient, based on the referring physicians records. Obviously, accepting a discharged patient for compliance issues will most likely continue to be a high-risk patient. Having the toxicology records will help direct the type of testing and initial frequency. It will also support the "Medical Necessity," which is an important component. The physician and the laboratory must justify which tests to order and frequency of such tests. Toxicology testing must be based on risk stratification, regardless of presumptive or definitive testing.

Psychiatric history

Comorbid disorders are a commonly missed cause of opioid misuse and are associated with, or lead to, overdose deaths. A common scenario is that the patient is concurrently seeing a psychiatrist that, despite the standard of medical care, is also being prescribed alprazolam for chronic anxiety rather than acute anxiety. Toxicology testing is done for patient safety, because many patients are not aware of the high risk that opioids and benzodiazepines have in combination. Several co-occurring mental illness disorders are frequently associated with substance misuse or abuse and need to be screened before proceeding with opioids in CNCP patients.[19,20] Utilization of the brief General Anxiety Disorder 7-item scale and Patient Health Questionnaire 9-item for depression screening, two common aspects in pain management, goes far in helping diagnose and treat common comorbid mental health aspects of chronic pain. They are a critical component of risk stratification to help determine frequency of toxicology testing and risk of compliance.

Medical necessity

An initial baseline drug test should be performed before prescribing opioid medication, and certain medications should be verified using definitive ("confirmed" or "quantitative") rather than presumptive ("screened" or "qualitative") testing. Overall, most of the literature quotes around 11% of all pain patients of any sex, demographic, race, or age are using an illicit drug. Nonprescription, or sometimes called, nonmedical opioid use, occurs between 20% and 40% in an average pain management population, regardless of the same demographics noted. Thus, the initial toxicology test needs to include any and all opioids, opiates, illicit, benzodiazepines, sedatives, cannabis, common synthetics for the demographic and geographic range and should be definitively tested, where appropriate, at the laboratory level.

The Center for Medicare and Medicaid Services indications The following indications are directly from the Center for Medicare and Medicaid Services (CMS) Web site as indications for a presumptive drug test (immunoassay):

> *In whom illicit drug use, non-compliance or a significant pre-test probability of non-adherence to the prescribed drug regimen is suspected and documented in the medical record; and/or In those who are at high risk for medication abuse due to psychiatric issues, who have engaged in aberrant drug-related behaviors, or who have a history of substance abuse.*

In the case of chronic pain, specifically as discussed here, CMS further describes its indications as such:

- Determine the presence of other substances before initiating pharmacologic treatment
- Detect the presence of illicit drugs
- Monitor adherence to the plan of care

These same guidelines are suggestions that follow commercial payers as well, in terms of medical necessity for medical reimbursement. Basically, toxicology testing affords safety of the patient to insure they are not taking medication or psychoactive drugs, which, combined with prescription pain medication, can lead to toxic levels and/or overdose. In addition, such testing insures the patient is being compliant by taking the prescriptions as directed under the guidance of the physician, rather than taking other nonprescribed pain medication, illicit substances, or diverting. Unfortunately, despite the best science, today's toxicology, regardless of the matrix, will not provide an actual steady-state pharmacokinetic value. However, the combination of pill count, random testing and specimen validity will provide the closest metric to curb diversion and help prevent such activity. It is important, in this instance, to highlight that toxicology testing provides objective ancillary data to the clinician to help manage the patient in concert with other components of the medical gestalt, which differs with each patient.

Metabolism of common medications

Understanding the metabolism of the pain medication is integral to knowing what parent drug and metabolites to test for in plasma, oral fluid, and urine. These pathways are briefly reviewed for the most common medications used, and the parent-metabolite relationships that will show in the urine, which currently represent the ideal evidenced-based clinical matrix, although a plethora of literature has been published in the last few years validating oral fluid testing.

Morphine

Morphine (M) is the mainstay drug with which most others are compared, for purposes of many state regulations. It is produced from codeine and heroin metabolism. Primary metabolism is via phase II hepatic pathway by glucuronide (G) conjugation via uridine 5'-diphosphoglucuronosyltransferase (UGT) using several variations of the enzyme to morphine-6-glucoronide, M-6-G (active), morphine-3-glucoronide, M-3-G (inactive), and an array of several metabolites, including morphine 3,6-diglucoronide,

M-3,6-G, normorphine (via N-demethylation), and others. Finally, of interest is that M, through a yet unknown pathway, can metabolize into hydromorphone (HM) as a minor metabolite.

A case example is a Caucasian female patient using opioid rotation to wean down from overprescribed oxycodone 720 mg/24 hours (1080 morphine equivalent dosage [MED]) by 25% reduction for cross-tolerance to M dosed 800 mg/24 hours using opioid rotation. The objective urine definitive report using liquid chromatography coupled with tandem mass spectrometry (LC-MS/MS) shows HM. This pathway is more common in women on higher doses of M, but usually does not exceed 6% of the M concentration. In the urine, one should find 75% as M-3-G, 10% free M, 4% conjugated normorphine, 1% free normorphine, and trace M-6-G, M-3,6-G, M-3-sulfate plus HM.[21] However, others quote 55% M-3-G, 10% free M, 15% M-6-G plus 6% HM[22]; such variations can also be observed within and between patients and can be due to differences in liver/kidney function, polypharmacy, hydration status, dosing among others.

Codeine

Codeine is a prodrug (the only opioid/opiate formal prodrug), which has no analgesic effect until activated by the liver. The primary activation is phase I: (1) O-demethylation via cytochrome P450 enzyme (CYP2D6) to M and (2) N-demethylation via CYP3A4 with minimal HM from M.[23] Other metabolites, as described later in this review, include hydrocodone, which further metabolizes to dihydrocodiene and norhydrocodone as well as HM. An example wherein a patient on codeine only demonstrates hydrocodone and HM may be due to their being a fast metabolizer as well as the time of ingestion, hydration status, and the like, although diversion and surreptitious ingestion of hydrocodone cannot be excluded. Such a result can be elucidated with focused patient dialogue, scheduled or unscheduled retesting, as well as switching to another medication that should not result in any metabolites being present in the urine.

Hydrocodone

Hydrocodone, an active analgesic, undergoes (1) O-demethylation via CYP2D6 into HM and (2) N-demethylation into minimally active norhydrocodone. A minor pathway for both hydrocodone and HM is 6-keto-reduction as (1) hydrocodone into 6α and 6β hydrocol and (2) HM into 6α and 6β hydromorphol.[21] Finally, HM is further metabolized by phase II via UGT into hydromorphone-3-glucoronide (HM-3-G).[24]

In blood and oral analysis, the primary metabolite is parent hydrocodone followed by norhydrocodone, and significantly less HM.[25] The benefit of oral analysis is the consistent presence of norhydrocodone with a hydrocodone:norhydrocodone (HC:norHC) ratio of 1:16, and minimal HM, which helps delineate the patient is taking hydrocodone rather than HM.[26] Urine analysis reveals 26% hydrocodone eliminated in 72 hours, with results as follows: (1) hydrocodone, 9% to 12%; (2) norhydrocodone, 5% to 19%; (3) HM-3-G, 2% to 4%; (4) 6α and β hydrocol, 1% to 3%.[21] HM is always present in its conjugated form.[27]

Hydromorphone

Hydromorphone (HM) is primarily metabolized by UGT at the 3 position to HM-3-G, and some 6-keto-reductase into 6α and 6β hydromorphol as noted in the prior section. One opioid review mentions HM-6-G,[28] which is a minimal amount, verified by the original article,[29] in conjugation with any 6-moeity that is not supported due to the presence of a ketone at the 6 position,[30] which is the key differentiation between M (hydroxyl at 6) and HM. Blood concentration finds HM-3-G ~ 25 times parent HM, whereas oral fluid is highly variable and inconsistent with significantly lower thresholds required.[26] Most data unfortunately are from hydrocodone studies, because there is a paucity of HM metabolism data in oral fluid. Urine finds at least 35% conjugated at HM-3-G, 6% free HM, and the remainder at H-3-sulfate, H-3-glucoside, the 6-keto forms, while chronic pain patients may find primarily HM-3-G without free HM.[21] A final note, in renal failure, both M and HM, being conjugated into 3-glucuronide, have been found to build up to potentially neurotoxic levels. One must take caution with M and HM in renally compromised patients of the M-3-G and HM-3-G levels, which lead to neuroexcitatory toxic responses in those individuals.

Matrices

Urine is the preferred biological fluid for drug testing for many years, and it is a matured technology. It is widely used in toxicology testing for years using various analytical techniques. Typically, the concentrations of drugs in urine are multiples higher than other matrices, and the drugs can be detected for 2 to 3 days. It is important to note that urine drug concentration, however, does not correlate to the dose. Unfortunately, urine is easier to adulterate than most other matrices. Hair, oral fluid, and blood are good biological matrices; however, the drug concentrations are low.[31] As a result, the matrices other than urine testing require highly sensitive LC-MS/MS instrumentation and scientists with more training in the technology.

Oral fluid is becoming a viable matrix for illicit and prescription drugs. Drug concentrations in oral fluid are 50-fold lower than in urine, and a highly sensitive analytical technique with high level of expertise is required to perform drug testing in oral fluid samples. Oral fluid collection is easy and noninvasive, and it is difficult to adulterate. Recent studies show that oral fluid has some correlation to the blood concentration, although not a direct correlation, and it varies with the drug. The notable difference is that cannabis detection time is significantly longer in urine when compared with oral fluid. The reason is because cannabis metabolites are detected in urine, whereas oral fluid detects the active parent compound, Δ-9-tetrahydrocannabinoid. Overall, oral fluid is the least invasive collection and is a viable biological matrix in clinical drug testing. However, oral fluid testing can be affected by ingestion of other items, hygiene, pH, and transport among others.[32]

Drug concentrations in blood have therapeutic, toxic, and impairment values; however, blood collection is highly invasive and requires a licensed phlebotomist to collect the blood. Furthermore, urine drug concentration does not correlate directly to the blood-drug concentration.

All these biological matrices have been used in clinical drug testing. Typically, drug detection in urine is 2 to 3 days, and certain drugs can be detected in hair for 30 to 90 days. Oral fluid and blood may have shorter detection windows, and the lower drug cutoff concentrations could match oral fluid detection window close to the urine detection window for opiates, benzodiazepines, sedatives, and stimulants. However, the oral fluid and blood marijuana detection window is only 1 to 2 days compared with 3 to 30 days in urine. Appreciating that there are differences in parent/metabolite relationships when testing different fluid matrices helps in matrix test selection and subsequent result interpretation. For example, urine marijuana test is for the carboxylic acid metabolite of the active compound delta-9-tetrahydrocannabinoid (Δ9THC-COOH), and oral fluid and blood test is for the active compound delta-9-tetrahydrocannabinoid (Δ9THC).

Presumptive Versus Definitive

Clinical drug testing typically uses two testing technologies: (1) point-of-care testing (POCT) using strips or cups, or instrument-based immunoassay test (analyzer), and

(2) the laboratory-based chromatography coupled with mass spectrometry tests (GC-MS and LC-MS/MS). The POCT and analyzer give immediate results to the physician for immediate treatment decisions. Both analyzer and POCT are formulated with specific drug antibodies for competitive binding with labeled drugs to the drugs in the urine specimen. The POCT and analyzer are immunoassays and are formulated for a specific drug in a class of drugs such as opiates and benzodiazepines. As a result, some of the drugs in that class have poor cross-reactivity with the assay and give false negative results (**Fig. 1**). There are various immunoassays that are US Food and Drug Administration (FDA) 510K cleared today, such as Enzyme Multiple Immunoassay, Kinetic Interaction of Microparticle in Solution, and Cloned Enzyme Donor Immunoassay. All immunoassays are identical as a general principle, and there may be some cross-reactivity, with one drug better than another. The immunoassays are formulated with one drug in a class of drugs for 100% cross-reactivity, and the other drugs in that class vary with the antibody the manufacturer has produced. For example, opiate immunoassay is formulated with M, and benzodiazepine immunoassay is formulated with oxazepam. As a result, for the opiate immunoassay where M is the principal drug used in the formulation, in testing for HM, hydrocodone, and oxymorphone, all have very poor cross-reactivity and may give false negative results. Furthermore, one type of immunoassay may have lower cross-reactivity for hydrocodone than the other immunoassays, and none of the immunoassays are formulated or FDA 510K cleared for hydrocodone, oxycodone, HM, or oxymorphone. For this

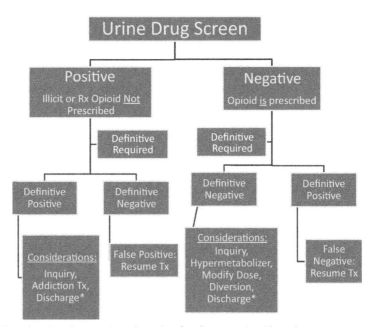

Fig. 1. Sample urine drug testing algorithm for discrepancies. Flow chart represents possible approach when urine drug screen expectations do not correlate with medical prescription documentation. Scenario depicts opioid drugs but can be extrapolated for other drug classes. "Screen" refers to POCT or EIA and "definitive" refers to LC/MS confirmation testing methods as described in the text. Inquiry refers to discussion with patient on drug administration, compliance, dosing, consistency, etc., as described in the text. *Patient discharge depends upon the relationship with the patient, risk assessment and other factors described in the text.

reason, a false negative result for many drugs can occur with immunoassay in certain drug class. Because POCT cups and strips are also immunoassays, similar limitations exist.

Benzodiazepines are another class where immunoassay has similar variation in cross-reactivity with one benzodiazepine drug to another benzodiazepine drug. Similarly, for the benzodiazepine immunoassay where oxazepam is the principal drug used in the formulation, testing for lorazepam and clonazepam has very poor cross-reactivity and may give false negative results for these drugs. For the end result, all laboratory-based immunoassays and POCT strips or cups have the same limitations and can provide similar misleading results. However, single-drug assays, like marijuana, cocaine, amphetamine, methamphetamine, and phencyclidine, are mostly reliable for immunoassay detection, and it may be best and economical to screen patients for illicit drug use.

In addition, POCT and analyzer have poor selectivity and also give false positive results (see **Fig. 1**). All these immunoassays are FDA 510K cleared for screening specific drugs in the urine at the specified cutoff in the package insert. Another caveat with laboratory-based immunoassay is in lowering the cutoff from the FDA 510K–cleared cutoffs. The FDA 510K–cleared cutoffs are based on the performance of the assay at the cutoff, and it has to meet 98% or better confidence in calling a drug negative or positive. However, the same assay may provide enough information to suspect some activity for the drug below the FDA 510K cleared cutoff, and one can then use definitive testing technology (GC-MS and LC-MS/MS) to further confirm the presence or absence of drugs. Although there are a few non-FDA 510K–cleared assays in many clinical laboratories, full caution must be taken in developing and validating these assays based on the laboratory-based test regulations. Whether FDA 510K cleared or laboratory developed, it should be understood that POCT and analyzer results are presumptive and that GC-MS and LC-MS/MS are "definitive" testing technologies.

The GC-MS and the LC-MS/MS are highly sophisticated analytical technologies for the analysis of organic compounds in trace amounts. The LC-MS/MS revolutionized diagnostic testing. The GC-MS testing requires extensive sample cleanup and derivatization before analysis, and the GC-MS technology is not amicable to analyzing many drugs in one injection. The modern LC-MS/MS technology allows changing the mobile phase during a run, and this gives the capability of analyzing multiple similar compounds in one injection. The LC-MS/MS uses 3 technologies in one instrument. First, the high-pressure LC separates the compound by changing the mobile phase; second, the MS filters the masses based on the molecular weight and charge; third, the molecules are fragmented, and the fragments are measured for each drug and their metabolites. Each sample could take 2 to 15 minutes on the LC-MS/MS, and the analysis time depends on the number of compounds. Typically, fewer compounds take less time, and many compounds need a longer time of analysis to achieve chromatographic separation and an adequate mass spectral scan. An isotopic deuterium–labeled internal standard is used to validate the presence of each of the compounds tested. Whether quantitative or qualitative, the LC-MS/MS test is a definitive test for drugs and their metabolites by measuring the molecular weight and their fragmentations along with the chromatographic retention time, thus providing a unique molecular fingerprint for the analyte being assessed. The biological specimens have to be hydrolyzed and cleaned up before injecting into the LC-MS/MS to minimize the matrix effect. The LC-MS/MS method of development and analysis involves a high level of technology expertise and skill. The resource requirements such as GC-MS or LC-MS/MS instrumentation, technical expertise, cost, and the time that it takes to perform qualitative or quantitative testing by LC-MS/MS (definitive testing) are considerably greater than conventional POCT and IA testing, thus justifying them as high-complexity testing methodologies.

It must be stressed that toxicology testing is to be used as an objective ancillary test for the clinical provider. For example, a patient on oxycodone may be ingesting as prescribed and/or "pill scraping" directly into the urine. In such a case, the patient with oxycodone as well as the presence of its metabolites oxymorphone (in addition to noroxycodone and noroxymorphone) in the urine is consistent with oxycodone ingestion, whereas an elevated oxycodone urine concentration and no oxycodone metabolites (oxymorphone or noroxycodone) may alert the physician that the patient may not have taken the pill as prescribed; rather, the patient scraped the pill into his/her urine. However, it could also be that the patient recently ingested the oxycodone and did not yet convert the parent drug into the metabolites. In such a case, noting the time of ingestion with serial toxicology testing (both scheduled and unscheduled) would help the clinician determine the likelihood of compliance versus diversion. It can be more difficult where prescription drugs like M and its metabolite HM are both individually prescribed pharmaceutical opiate drugs because both drugs would appear in urine. Furthermore, for some illicit drugs, concentration may not have much clinical value.

Clinical drug testing laboratories are under CLIA (Clinical Laboratory Improvement Amendments) guidance, which has no set standards for methodologies and laboratory protocols, and there is no FDA oversight on the Laboratory Developed Tests (LDT). The FDA has a proposal for the oversight of LDT assays, which is not in effect today. The certifying agencies such as the College of American Pathologists or COLA do not have guidelines for best practices in clinical drug testing and their inspection checklist is to verify the CLIA requirement. Therefore, some clinical laboratories may screen by immunoassay and confirm the positive results on GC-MS or LC-MS/MS, whereas other laboratories may perform the definitive test on LC-MS/MS at detection levels without using the immunoassay screening. The clinical laboratories performing the immunoassay screen first and reflexing to LC-MS/MS or GC-MS confirmation are using the SAMHSA (The Substance Abuse and Mental Health Services Administration) model. This laboratory protocol is more economical; however, this misses many psychoactive drugs (SAMSHA Household Survey List) in the patient specimen. There are 3 reasons for this: (1) the POCT and analyzer do not cross-react with all the drugs in a class of druglike opiates and benzodiazepines; (2) the analyzer and the POCT have high cutoffs and miss low concentrations; (3) not all the psychoactive drugs have commercial POCT and analyzer reagent kits and these laboratories are not including these drugs in their test menu. Therefore, definitive testing by LC-MS/MS whether qualitative or quantitative may be the best practice protocol in pain and addiction testing to screen for all the opiates, opioids, benzodiazepines, stimulants, and sedatives. Nonetheless, analyzer or POCT can provide a very economical way to screen for illicit drugs like marijuana, cocaine and methamphetamine.

Specimen Validity Test

Specimen validity is very important in the detection process for the evaluation of drug use for proper diagnosis and treatment.[33] Oral fluid, hair, and blood are direct-observed collection. Urine specimens are subject to adulteration or substitution. There are many adulterants available on the Internet to beat the drug test. Most of them are oxidants to interfere with immunoassay test. Some of these oxidants change the structure of the marijuana metabolite and make it undetectable by immunoassay and LC-MS/MS. The characteristics of the urine specimen are based on its appearance, temperature, pH, creatinine concentration, and specific gravity. Normal urine has a temperature of 90°F to 100°F and a pH between 4.5 and 8.1. Urine specimens at room temperature may increase the pH due to micro-organism growth. Normal urine has a creatinine concentration of 20 mg/dL or higher and specific gravity greater than 1.003. It is also known that patients may bring someone else's urine to avoid drug detection. Therefore, observed urine collection is the best practice.

SUMMARY

Pain management continues to pose a challenge to the clinician who walks the tightrope of providing appropriate pain relief while also monitoring the signs and potential for abuse and diversion. Although the relationship of the clinician and patient remains paramount for appropriate trust and management in this regard, appropriate utilization of toxicology testing provides an objective measure of ancillary support to facilitate such management. Understanding when to test, how often, and which fluids to sample, in addition to the variability and differences in methodology, as well as human physiologic variability can help the clinician with respect to testing approaches and interpretation for effective pain management.

REFERENCES

1. Manchikanti L, Manchukonda R, Pampati V, et al. Does random urine drug testing reduce illicit drug use in chronic pain patients receiving opioids? Pain Physician 2006;9(2):123–9.
2. Pesce A, West C, Rosenthal M, et al. Illicit drug use in the pain patient population decreases with continued drug testing. Pain Physician 2011;14(2):189–93.
3. Gilbert JW, Wheeler GR, Mick GE, et al. Urine drug testing in the treatment of chronic noncancer pain in a Kentucky private neuroscience practice: the potential effect of Medicare benefit changes in Kentucky. Pain Physician 2010;13(2):187–94.
4. Chou R, Fanciullo GJ, Fine PG, et al. Clinical guidelines for the use of chronic opioid therapy in chronic noncancer pain. J Pain 2009;10(2):113–30.
5. Manchikanti L, Abdi S, Atluri S, et al. American Society of Interventional Pain Physicians (ASIPP) guidelines for responsible opioid prescribing in chronic noncancer pain: part 2–guidance. Pain Physician 2012;15(3 Suppl):S67–116.
6. Manchikanti L, Boswell MV, Singh V, et al. Comprehensive evidence-based guidelines for interventional techniques in the management of chronic spinal pain. Pain Physician 2009;12(4):699–802.
7. Manchikanti L, Singh V, Datta S, et al. Comprehensive review of epidemiology, scope, and impact of spinal pain. Pain Physician 2009;12(4):E35–70.
8. Manchikanti L, Abdi S, Atluri S, et al. American Society of Interventional Pain Physicians (ASIPP) guidelines for responsible opioid prescribing in chronic noncancer pain: part I–evidence assessment. Pain Physician 2012;15(3 Suppl):S1–65.
9. Heltsley R, Depriest A, Black D, et al. Oral fluid drug testing of chronic pain patients. II. Comparison of paired oral fluid and urine specimens. J Anal Toxicol 2012;36(2):75–80.
10. Melanson SE, Ptolemy AS, Wasan AD. Optimizing urine drug testing for monitoring medication compliance in pain management. Pain Med 2013;14(12):1813–20.
11. Phan HM, Yoshizuka K, Murry DJ, et al. Drug testing in the workplace. Pharmacotherapy 2012;32(7):649–56.
12. Washington State Association of State Medical Directors. Interagency guideline on prescribing opioids for pain. 2015. p. 105.

13. United States v. Zadeh. 2014, U.S. Dist. LEXIS 181500, ×1.
14. Debbrecht-Switalski J. Evidence-based best practice for opioid prescribing and monitoring: medicolegal pain management expert symposium. International Conference on Opioids. Boston, June 6, 2016.
15. Webster LR, Webster RM. Predicting aberrant behaviors in opioid-treated patients: preliminary validation of the opioid risk tool. Pain Med 2005;6(6):432–42.
16. Butler SF, Fernandez K, Benoit C, et al. Validation of the revised screener and opioid assessment for patients with pain (SOAPP-R). J Pain 2008;9(4):360–72.
17. Butler SF, Budman SH, Fernandez KC, et al. Cross-validation of a screener to predict opioid misuse in chronic pain patients (SOAPP-R). J Addict Med 2009;3(2): 66–73.
18. Reid MC, Fiellin DA, O'Connor PG. Hazardous and harmful alcohol consumption in primary care. Arch Intern Med 1999;159(15):1681–9.
19. Pade PA, Cardon KE, Hoffman RM, et al. Prescription opioid abuse, chronic pain, and primary care: a Co-occurring Disorders Clinic in the chronic disease model. J Subst Abuse Treat 2012;43(4):446–50.
20. Goldner EM, Lusted A, Roerecke M, et al. Prevalence of axis-1 psychiatric (with focus on depression and anxiety) disorder and symptomatology among non-medical prescription opioid users in substance use treatment: systematic review and meta-analyses. Addict Behav 2014;39(3):520–31.
21. DePriest AZ, Puet BL, Holt AC, et al. Metabolism and disposition of prescription opioids: a review. Forensic Sci Rev 2015;27(2):115–45.
22. Hughes MM, Atayee RS, Best BM, et al. Observations on the metabolism of morphine to hydromorphone in pain patients. J Anal Toxicol 2012;36(4):250–6.
23. Yee DA, Atayee RS, Best BM, et al. Observations on the urine metabolic profile of codeine in pain patients. J Anal Toxicol 2014;38(2):86–91.
24. Barakat NH, Atayee RS, Best BM, et al. Urinary hydrocodone and metabolite distributions in pain patients. J Anal Toxicol 2014;38(7):404–9.
25. Cao JM, Ma JD, Morello CM, et al. Observations on hydrocodone and its metabolites in oral fluid specimens of the pain population: comparison with urine. J Opioid Manag 2014;10(3):177–86.
26. Cone EJ, DePriest AZ, Heltsley R, et al. Prescription opioids. IV: disposition of hydrocodone in oral fluid and blood following single-dose administration. J Anal Toxicol 2015;39(7):510–8.
27. Cone EJ, Heltsley R, Black DL, et al. Prescription opioids. II. Metabolism and excretion patterns of hydrocodone in urine following controlled single-dose administration. J Anal Toxicol 2013;37(8):486–94.
28. Mercadante S. Opioid metabolism and clinical aspects. Eur J Pharmacol 2015; 769:71–8.
29. Smith HS. The metabolism of opioid agents and the clinical impact of their active metabolites. Clin J Pain 2011;27(9):824–38.
30. Wright AW, Mather LE, Smith MT. Hydromorphone-3-glucuronide: a more potent neuro-excitant than its structural analogue, morphine-3-glucuronide. Life Sci 2001;69(4):409–20.
31. Verstraete AG. Detection times of drugs of abuse in blood, urine, and oral fluid. Ther Drug Monit 2004;26:200–5.
32. Crouch DJ. Oral fluid collection: the neglected variable in oral fluid testing. Forensic Sci Int 2005;150:165–73.
33. Kirsh KL, Christo PJ, Heit H, et al. Specimen validity testing in urine drug monitoring of medications and illicit drugs: clinical implications. J Opioid Manag 2015;11:53–9.

Toxicology in Addiction Medicine

Daniel A. Schwarz, MD[a],*, M.P. George, MS[b], Martin H. Bluth, MD, PhD[c,d]

KEYWORDS

• Pain • Addiction • Management • Drug • Testing • Toxicology

KEY POINTS

- Toxicology testing in addiction medicine varies across the spectrum yet remains a powerful tool in monitoring addictive patients.
- There are many reference laboratories offering toxicology testing, and physicians should have some understanding of laboratory, methodology, testing portfolio, and customer support structure to aid them in selecting the best toxicology laboratory for their patients.
- The definitive drug testing by gas chromatography coupled with mass spectrometry and high-performance liquid chromatography coupled with tandem mass spectrometry are highly accurate if the tests are performed in a good laboratory with technical and toxicology expertise.
- Patients with substance disorders may need to be tested for a wider spectrum of drugs, with greater frequency, over a longer period of time to discourage and identify relapse. In certain instances utilizing oral fluid testing can minimize specimen adulteration-substitution concerns.
- Consultation with a clinical pathologist/toxicologist in conjunction with the consideration of monitoring large numbers of illicit and psychoactive drugs in the addictive patient may provide important clinical information for their treatment.

INTRODUCTION

Toxicology testing is an important standard of care in monitoring the addictive patient. Toxicology tests offer reproducible, unbiased, and objective evidence of chronically relapsing disorder for clinical observation. Drug tests do not provide diagnostic information to identify substance use disorders or physical dependence.[1–3] It is a common observation that drug users minimize or deny drug use. In some instances, drug users provide a partial list of the drugs that they are abusing and hide the other drug use to

[a] The Center for Pain Recovery, 18444 West 10 Mile Road, Suite 102, Southfield, MI 48075, USA; [b] Laboratory Operations, Alere Toxicology, 9417 Brodie Lane, Austin, TX 78748, USA; [c] Department of Pathology, Wayne State University School of Medicine, 540 East Canfield, Detroit, MI 48201, USA; [d] Consolidated Laboratory Management Systems, 24555 Southfield Road, Southfield, MI 48075, USA
* Corresponding author.
E-mail address: dr@painrecoverymd.com

Clin Lab Med 36 (2016) 685–692
http://dx.doi.org/10.1016/j.cll.2016.07.009
0272-2712/16/© 2016 Elsevier Inc. All rights reserved.

labmed.theclinics.com

cause a "smoke-screen effect."[1] Drug tests also can improve the communication between the health care provider and the patient. Although a positive drug test result often means that patient had taken a drug, a negative test result does not always mean that the patient did not abuse any drugs. Drug testing is also an important tool in monitoring patients for adherence to their prescribed medications. Urine and oral fluid drug concentration has some limited value but it does not often correlate to the blood concentration.[4] Blood is the only biological matrix that provides therapeutic and toxic concentrations of drugs. The overdose mortality and prescription drug addiction rates in the United States have been increasing due to diverted prescribed opiates, opioids, and benzodiazepines, and we are in the midst of a National Prescription Drug overdose and prescription drug addiction epidemic.[5–8] Often health care providers do not completely trust the drug test results due to the assumption that a drug test gives false-positive and false-negative results. Although there are certain cases in which interfering variables can affect laboratory toxicology results,[9] the clinical toxicology laboratory is capable of providing accurate results for the presence of drugs that are tested, using specific and/or conformational methodologies at the specified cutoff. It is important to note that all clinical laboratories are not the same and there are no set standards on the testing protocols used in clinical drug testing. Furthermore, more than 200 clinical toxicology laboratories appeared in the past 5 years as a result of the lucrative reimbursement system.[10] Thus, as in any profession, it is important to develop an understanding and trust with the laboratory with which a physician chooses to partner toward providing these ancillary services for patient care. In general, clinically relevant reasons for a negative result include the following:

1. The patient has not used that drug.
2. The test did not include that drug.
3. Drug concentration in the biological fluid (urine, oral fluid, or blood) is below the laboratory-established cutoffs.

There are also opportunities for adulteration of a sample, which can also yield a negative result (eg, dilution, oxidants); however, various modalities can be incorporated into a clinical setting to mitigate such possibilities (eg, specimen validity testing,[11] monitored collections). There are multiple technologies available for drug testing. Some of them are simple spot tests that can be performed in the physician's office and they are called Clinical Laboratory Improvement Amendments (CLIA) Waved Point of Care Testing (POCT), an allocation afforded to low-complexity tests. Some of the drug tests are performed on highly sophisticated analytical technique, such as gas chromatography coupled with mass spectrometry (GC-MS) or high-performance liquid chromatography coupled with tandem mass spectrometry (LC-MS/MS), which are considered high complexity and are therefore not usually available in a physician's office. Each one of these technologies is useful in clinical testing and the physician needs to understand the limitations of these tests. The POCT and the instrumental drug tests are immunoassays; the tests are limited to fewer drugs and these tests also produce false-positive and false-negative results.[12–14] On the other hand, the GC-MS and LC-MS/MS are confirmatory tests and provide definitive presence of the drug and their metabolites at low concentration cutoffs. In addition, there are various kinds of toxicology testing, such as workplace, forensic, performance enhancement, and criminal justice testing.[1,14]

Due to the complexities of various drug tests and technologies, many experts have concluded that most physicians do not have the proficiency in ordering and interpretation of these tests.[1,2,15] The technology in toxicology testing has changed over the past few years and some of the highly difficult analysis of drugs and chemicals that were previously allocated for pharmaceutical industry use have been applied for use in clinical laboratories with the additional benefit of cost containment to assess multiple drugs and metabolites in one analysis. As a result, the Centers for Medicare and Medicaid Services (CMS) has revised the toxicology testing fee schedule in 2016 and simplified the toxicology testing codes.[16] Although maturation of the technology has afforded a less costly alternative to order large number of drug panels, private health insurance companies are still trying to understand toxicology testing and their applications to the clinical setting in certain respects.

SUBSTANCES OF ABUSE
Legal Versus Illicit

Potentially, more than 130 psychoactive compounds are readily available in the United States, and this includes conventional illicit drugs like cannabinoids, cocaine, meth-amphetamines, ecstasy, phencyclidine, and heroin, as well as psychoactive prescription drugs like opiates, opioids, benzodiazepines, sedatives, stimulants, and muscular relaxants.[1,2,5] Over the past few years, designer drugs, including stimulants such as bath salts, and synthetic cannabinoid compounds such as K2 spice, have emerged. There are more than 15 synthetic stimulants and more than 35 synthetic cannabinoids on the illegal drug market. These compounds came into the market to mask detection of conventional prescription drug abuse through toxicology testing. It has been observed that as the drug test becomes available for the detection of these com-pounds, the compounds disappear and new drugs appear,[1] which has provided a new concern for addictionologists as well.

Inpatient Versus Outpatient

It may not be cost justifiable to perform testing on all drugs every time one engages a patient, and the physician may evaluate the necessity for testing rather than provide a blanket test order. Inpatients in a treatment facility may require frequent tests and may include a larger panel, and in the outpatient setting there may not be a need to test the extensive list. However, testing for commonly abused illicit drugs and prescription opi-ates, opioids, and benzodiazepines are cost-effective based on the 2016 CMS fee schedule, where pricing is based on a tier pricing system (group of drug classes) and not a stacking pricing system that was used until January 2016 for each drug. The true effective drug test is a random drug test, because patients can often abstain from drugs if a predictable time is set for specimen collection.

   The addictive patient may change from one drug to another drug if the patient wants to conceal the drug use during a scheduled collection. Therefore, a random test for illicit drugs, opiates, opioids, stimulants, and benzodiazepine may be a reasonable approach. Outpatient testing has more risk, because the patient has a significantly greater chance to relapse as well as access substances of abuse.[1]

Medical Necessity

Any health care test or procedure is required by law to be medically necessary to treat the patient. CMS has published extensive instructions on medical necessity and it is beyond the scope of this article to include detailed regulations on medical necessity. However, a few reminders of medical necessity are as follows: (1) document the test or-der in the patient medical records; (2) avoid blanket test orders; (3) match the test order with appropriate International Classification of Diseases, 10th Revision coding; (4) re-view test results and make a clinical decision regarding patient management and docu-ment the finding and the decision in the patient medical records. Finally, the physician needs to use risk stratification.[5,13] For example, if the patient is older and a known alcoholic, then breathalyzer testing with intermittent alcohol and/or ethel glucuronide/ethel sulfate (EtG/EtS) may be appropriate and more cost-effective.[1] Alternatively, if the patient is younger and tests positive for heroin, cannabis, and alprazolam, and is prescribed buprenorphine medication with a concurrent mood disorder prescribed quetiapine after phenobarbital detoxification, then the risk of ingesting synthetic cannabis, and relapse to misusing other benzodiazepines remains a real concern. That patient will require definitive confirmatory (GC/MS or LC/MS) testing for benzodiazepines, because screening (immunoassay) testing may not detect clonazepam, lorazepam, and alprazolam, depending on the antibody construct used in the screening testing method. In addition, the patient will require periodic definitive confirmatory testing for synthetic cannabinoids, although the frequency of such testing is not clear.[1,16]

Forensic Drug Testing Versus Clinical Drug Testing

Different toxicology tests are used in various settings. Workplace drug testing started in the 1980s, and the federal government mandated the testing for federal employees, instituted safety (drug) testing for transportation workers in 1990, and specific drug-testing standards from specimen collection to reporting have been implemented. The program is designed to withstand legal challenges and the system is set to eliminate false positives. A strict chain of custody documentation is followed from collection of the specimen to disposal of the specimen. Extensive guidelines on specimen collection, transport, chain of custody, testing, and reporting have been published in the Federal Register (49 CFR Part 40). Federally mandated workplace drug testing is only for 6 drug classes: cannabinoids, cocaine, amphetamines (amphetamine, methamphetamine), phencyclidine, ecstasy (MDMA, MDA, MDEA), and opiates (heroin, codeine, and morphine only). The testing protocol is a screen by laboratory-based immunoassay (EIA) at the specified cutoff and confirmation of any presumptive positives (via EIA) using definitive tests like GC-MS or LC-MS/MS. All results are reported to a medical review officer (MRO) to make the final decision on a positive result. The MRO may turn a positive result to negative if there is a legitimate prescription for the positive drug. All these protocols are to legally defend the positive drug test in an administrative or court hearing.[1]

Clinical drug testing is part of a patient's examination performed by a clinician with whom the patient is in a therapeutic relationship. The clinical toxicology test is used to identify the presence of drugs and chemicals in the patient, which provides ancillary objective information to aid the clinician in partnership with the patient in appropriate patient management. The clinical drug test must eliminate false-positive and false-negative results. The drug detection window is inversely proportional to the cutoff concentration: the lower the cutoff the longer the detection window. The cutoff concentration should be as low as the technology can provide, in concert with the clinical application value; extremely low cutoff values run the risk of false positives, which occur as a result of methodological interferences[17,18] rather than presence of the actual drug, and must be accounted for when cutoff values differ from laboratory to laboratory. Addiction patients should be tested at zero-tolerance level, which is the limit of detection for the test. The clinical drug test often includes many more drugs than workplace drug testing. Therefore, the workplace drug testing model is not always appropriate for the clinical setting.[1,10]

Medically Assisted Treatment

Medication-assisted treatment (MAT) often refers to addiction intervention with pharmacopeia, such as methadone or buprenorphine. In both cases, the toxicology test is used to ensure that the patient is (1) taking the prescribed drugs, (2) not taking another nonprescribed opiate or schedule II-V medication, and (3) not taking an illicit substance or alcohol. Unlike pain management, or other disciplines, a positive test in addiction medicine is handled much differently.

A positive test for a nonprescribed schedule II-V medication or illicit substance is addressed with intervention rather than discharge, just as would absence of the MAT opiate (buprenorphine or methadone). However, without getting into details, due to federal regulations, it may take at least one week before a methadone patient can be titrated up to their maintenance dose. Therefore, it is not uncommon for them to be "chipping" away at heroin until they can receive the full amount of MAT needed to cut the heroin craving. Thus, their urine will still test positive for opioid under "OPI" or "MOP" (depending on the presumptive cup or dipstick POCT that is used) and 6-acetylmorphine, the metabolite specific for heroin which should be sent to the laboratory for LC-MS/MS or GC-MS for definitive confirmation.

Toxicology testing serves to determine if MAT is effective, or requires a higher dose or application of the American Society of Addiction Medicine Criteria,[5] to increase the level of care to the next appropriately elevated treatment level. Rarely is a toxicology test result used to discharge a patient in addiction medicine, but rather warnings, and adjustments to the treatment plan are implemented. In the outpatient setting, toxicology testing is more dependent on the type of environment. For example, an Opioid Treatment Program (OTP) usually has the staffing to administer and monitor drug testing, whereas an office-based buprenorphine provider managed by a solo practitioner may have limited to no staff. In addition, methadone OTP uses the toxicology results as a reward, as compliance allows the patient "take home" privileges, whereas the office-based buprenorphine provider often starts off at 30 days, based on the level of training, which varies. Of interest is that there still remains a significant number of other illicit drugs, similar to pain management patients, at any time in the MAT outpatient setting, that may be detected by toxicology testing. A review found at least 30% of patients in methadone recovery tested positive for cocaine on average,[19] thus further highlighting the importance of toxicology testing in such risk-oriented settings. Finally, the known history of co-occurring disorders in substance abuse, including anxiety, depression, attention-deficit/hyperactivity disorder, bipolar disorder, and others, leads to higher incidence of patients being treated by physicians who do not know about the patients' methadone ingestion and/or may not yet participate in their state specific Prescription Drug Monitoring Program (PDMP). Thus, toxicology testing can help assess other medications that (1) the patient fails to disclose (PDMP can have a 2–3-week delay) and (2) is newly published as abuse potential, like gabapentin.[20]

SUBSTANCES

Although there are multiple substances that are available as a source for potential addiction, either as subsequent abuse in the course of pain management or via recreational means, the following represents common agents that are normally associated with addiction as well as those related to MAT to manage their use.

Alcohol

Blood is the ideal specimen for monitoring recent use of alcohol, and the detection window of alcohol in blood is only few hours.[21] Urine alcohol also has a short window, and diabetic patients may produce alcohol by fermenting the sugar in the urine. EtG and EtS are metabolites of alcohol and the detection window can be longer commensurate with alcohol ingestion: ≤24 hours after intake of ≤0.25 g/kg ethanol, and for

≤48 hours after intake of ≤0.50 g/kg ethanol. Patients who are alcohol dependent can increase the detection times for urinary EtG and EtS from 75 to more than 90 hours during recovery from heavy drinking, thereby dubbing EtG/EtS the "80-hour" alcohol markers.[22] Care must be taken to interpret the EtG and EtS results because exposure to alcohol from various sources (wipes, mouthwash, alcohol-containing cold remedies, and some fermented drinks) could cause positive ethanol, EtG, and EtS.[23,24]

Heroin

Heroin metabolizes immediately to 6-monoacetyl morphine (6-MAM) and morphine. In a very small percentage of patients, only 6-MAM was detected, and the morphine concentration was very low or undetectable. Therefore, the 6-MAM test is important in the addiction treatment setting. A small amount of codeine may present in most of the heroin preparations, and the typical ratio of morphine to codeine is 2:1 or less. In addition, there is a concomitant increase in heroin deaths, with evidence of a mixed-in component of nonprescription (illicit manufactured) fentanyl.[14,25] Ascertaining whether mortality occurred due to prescription fentanyl versus illicitly produced fentanyl cannot be deduced through forensic toxicology, although prescription records can clarify whether the deceased had a valid prescription, along with cause-of-death police reports.

Although prescription opioid mortality still exceeds heroin mortality nationally by almost 4:1, Ohio, having been 1 of the first 2 states after Florida, to implement such legislation in 2012 (House Bill 93), has seen an interesting statistical outcome. The Centers for Disease Control and Prevention's Morbidity and Mortality Report for 2013 actually had heroin deaths significantly exceeding prescription opioid deaths, but then in 2014 they approximated each other, only because fentanyl was classified under the rubric of prescription opiate (synthetics) even if "illicit."[26] Such changes in classification can affect trend bias and reporting since another detailed study showed that a crime scene sample could delineate illicit versus pharmaceutical fentanyl in certain cases.[25]

Methadone

Methadone metabolizes to normethadol and 2-ethylidene-1,5-dimethyl-3,3-diphenyl-pyrrolidine (EDDP), and both methadone and EDDP metabolize to glucuronide conjugate. Methadone without EDDP is most likely due to pill scraping. Most of the POCT is formulated for methadone, and there is an immunoassay reagent available for the metabolite EDDP. Therefore, EDDP may be a better test in monitoring methadone patients. At any time across the United States, there is an approximately 30% incidence of cocaine use in patients at methadone clinics. Also, currently, methadone clinics do NOT report on the state PDMPs, so more often than not, patients with comorbid addiction/pain who cease with their methadone treatment will end up back in a pain practice transition to oxycodone with the explanation that the oxycodone was obtained from a friend or relative (~55% of nonprescribed opioids/opiates). This also supports the need for a very broad-based definitive toxicology testing approach on the initial intake for recovery patients.

Buprenorphine

Buprenorphine metabolizes to norbuprenorphine, and both buprenorphine and norbuprenorphine form a glucuronide conjugate. Immunoassays, both POCT and laboratory-based tests, do not cross-react with glucuronide metabolites and could give false-negative results. Definitive testing by LC-MS/MS may be ordered on these false-negative specimens. Pill scraping (or putting a fraction of the "Suboxone" strip into the urine) is commonly used by these patients to falsely demonstrate that they are taking their medication as prescribed. However, in such cases, the presence of buprenorphine without the metabolite norbuprenorphine can indicate that the patient added a small portion of the pill into their urine.

Overall, toxicology testing in addiction medicine varies across the spectrum, yet remains a powerful tool in monitoring addictive patients. There are various types of drug-testing devices available for a physician's in-house office testing requirements and most of these are useful testing devices. However, these devices have limitations, and the physicians should understand their limitations. Also, there are many reference laboratories offering toxicology testing and physicians should have some understanding of laboratory, methodology, testing portfolio, and customer support structure to aid them in selecting the best toxicology laboratory for their patients. The definitive drug testing by GC-MS and LC-MS/MS is highly accurate if the tests are performed in a good laboratory with technical and toxicology expertise. Moving from urine to oral fluid testing reduces the privacy concerns and minimizes the specimen adulteration-substitution issue. Patients with substance disorders need to be tested for a wider spectrum of drugs over a longer period of time to discourage and identify relapse. Drug testing should be similar to general clinical diagnostic testing in which patients are monitored for diseases like diabetes and hypertension.[27,28] Furthermore, the new CMS fee schedule made it possible to monitor a large number of drugs at a reasonable cost. To this end, consultation with a clinical pathologist/toxicologist[29] in conjunction with the consideration of monitoring large numbers of illicit and psychoactive drugs in the addictive patient may provide important clinical information for their treatment.

REFERENCES

1. Dupont RL. Drug Testing: a white paper of the American Society of Addiction Medicine. Chevy Chase (MD): ASAM; 2013. p. 5–108.
2. Kirsh KL, Baxter LE, Rzetelny A, et al. A survey of ASAM members' knowledge, attitudes, and practices in urine drug testing. J Addict Med 2015;9:399–404.
3. Tenore PL. Advanced urine toxicology testing. J Addict Dis 2010;29:436–48.
4. Cone EJ, DePriest AZ, Heltsley R, et al. Prescription opioids. IV: disposition of hydrocodone in oral fluid and blood following single-dose administration. J Anal Toxicol 2015;39:510–8.
5. Mee-Lee D, American Society of Addiction Medicine. The ASAM criteria: treatment for addictive, substance-related, and co-occurring conditions. 3rd edition. Chevy Chase (MD): American Society of Addiction Medicine; 2013. p. xv, 460.
6. Washington State Agency Medical Directors' Group. Interagency guideline on prescribing opioids for pain. 3rd edition. 2015.
7. Ohio Department of Health. 2014 Ohio Drug Overdose Data: General Findings; 2016. p. 1–10.
8. U.S. Department of Health and Human Services, Centers for Disease Control and Prevention, Drug-Poisoning Death Involving Opioid Analgesics. NCHS Data Brief, No.166, September 2014.
9. Saitman A, Park HD, Fitzgerald RL. False-positive interferences of common urine drug screen immunoassays: a review. J Anal Toxicol 2014;38:387–96.
10. Manchikani L, Malla Y, Wargo BW, et al. Protocol for accuracy of point of care (POC) or in-iffice unrine drug testing (immunoassay) in chronic pain patients: a prospective analysis of immunoassay and liquid chromatography tandem mass spectrometry (LC/MS/MS). Pain Physician 2010;13:E1–22.

11. Kirsh KL, Christo PJ, Heit H, et al. Specimen validity testing in urine drug monitoring of medications and illicit drugs: clinical implications. J Opioid Manag 2015;11:53–9.
12. Reisfield GM, Goldberger BA, Bertholf RL. 'False-positive' and 'false-negative' test results in clinical urine drug testing. Bioanalysis 2009;1:937–52.
13. Starrels JL, Fox AD, Kunins HV, et al. They don't know what they don't know: internal medicine residents' knowledge and confidence in urine drug test interpretation for patients with chronic pain. J Gen Intern Med 2012;27:1521–7.
14. Markway CE, Baker SN. A review of the methods, interpretation, and limitations of the urine drug screen. Orthopedics 2011;34(11):877–81.
15. Reisfield GM, Bertholf R, Barkin RL, et al. Urine drug test interpretation: what do physicians know? J Opioid Manag 2007;3:80–6.
16. Centers for Medicare and Medicaid, Calendar Year (CY) 2016 Clinical Laboratory Fee Schedule (CLFS), Final Determination, November 2015.
17. Yuan C, Heideloff C, Kozak M, et al. Simultaneous quantification of 19 drugs/metabolites in urine important for pain management by liquid chromatography-tandem mass spectrometry. Clin Chem Lab Med 2012;50:95–103.
18. Yuan C, Lembright K, Heideloff C, et al. Quantification of buprenorphine, norbuprenorphine and 6-monoacetylmorphine in urine by liquid chromatography-tandem mass spectrometry. J Chrom Separ Tech 2013;4:174.
19. Kosten TR, Wu G, Huang W, et al. Pharmacogenetic randomized trial for cocaine abuse: disulfiram and dopamine beta-hydroxylase. Biol Psychiatry 2013;73: 219–24.
20. Schifano F. Misuse and abuse of pregabalin and gabapentin: cause for concern? CNS Drugs 2014;28:491–6.
21. Furr-Holden CD, Milam AJ, Nesoff ED, et al. Not in my back yard: a comparative analysis of crime around publicly funded drug treatment centers, liquor stores, convenience stores, and corner stores in one mid-Atlantic city. J Stud Alcohol Drugs 2016;77(1):17–24.
22. Helander A, Böttcher M, Fehr C, et al. Detection times for urinary ethyl glucuronide and ethyl sulfate in heavy drinkers during alcohol detoxification. Alcohol Alcohol 2009;44:55–61.
23. Reisfield GM, Goldberger BA, Pesce AJ, et al. Ethyl glucuronide, ethyl sulfate, and ethanol in urine after intensive exposure to high ethanol content mouthwash. J Anal Toxicol 2011;35:264–8.
24. Costantino A, Digregorio EJ, Korn W, et al. The effect of the use of mouthwash on ethylglucuronide concentrations in urine. J Anal Toxicol 2006;30:659–62.
25. Marinetti LJ, Ehlers BJ. A series of forensic toxicology and drug seizure cases involving illicit fentanyl alone and in combination with heroin, cocaine or heroin and cocaine. J Anal Toxicol 2014;38:592–8.
26. Cone EJ, Heltsley R, Black DL, et al. Prescription opioids. II. Metabolism and excretion patterns of hydrocodone in urine following controlled single-dose administration. J Anal Toxicol 2013;37:486–94.
27. Moeller KE, Lee KC, Kissack JC. Urine drug screening: practical guide for clinicians. Mayo Clin Proc 2008;83:66–76.
28. Dowell D, Haegerich TM, Chou R. CDC guideline for prescribing opioids for chronic pain—United States, 2016. MMWR Recomm Rep 2016;65:1–49.
29. Ward MB, Hackenmueller SA, Strathmann FG, Education Committee of the Academy of Clinical Laboratory Physicians and Scientists. Pathology consultation on urine compliance testing and drug abuse screening. Am J Clin Pathol 2014; 142:586–93.

Precision Medicine in Toxicology

Daniel A. Schwarz, MD[a],*, M.P. George, MS[b], Martin H. Bluth, MD, PhD[c,d]

KEYWORDS

- Precision medicine • Pharmacogenetics • Pharmacogenomics • Toxicology
- Metabolism • Cytochrome

KEY POINTS

- Precision medicine applies primarily to pharmacokinetics in toxicology and relates to basic hepatic metabolism, the common substrates, inducers and inhibitors of cytochrome P450 along with genetic variants which affect enzyme function.
- Mastering hepatic metabolism through an understanding of the genetics behind Phase I, or oxidation/reduction and some Phase II, or conjugation, enhances the scientific and clinical application of common drug toxicology.
- Evidence based research and clinical correlations conclude that knowledge of inducers and inhibitors, in conjunction with genetic variations, are integral components for applied precision medicine in toxicology.

INTRODUCTION

Precision medicine, also referred to as *personalized medicine,* is a recently assigned banner to depict the amalgam of the disciplines of pharmacogenetics and pharmacogenomics (PGx) as they apply to clinical medicine. The US Food and Drug Administration (FDA) has amassed a large almost decade old Web site of data under its Drugs tab (http://www.fda.gov/Drugs/DevelopmentApprovalProcess/DevelopmentResources/DrugInteractionsLabeling/default.htm) devoted to this topic, primarily as it relates to adverse drug reactions. This review is principally devoted to the metabolism of substances commonly measured by toxicology testing that may be used to avoid misuse or abuse and result in deleterious clinical effects. These include the opioids, opiates, sedatives/hypnotics (benzodiazepines and others), cannabinoids, cocaine, and psychostimulants. This article reviews (1) the phase I, or P450 direct enzyme-mediated oxidative/reduction pathway and (2) the phase II, or conjugation pathway. Next, this

[a] The Center for Pain Recovery, 18444 West 10 Mile Road, Suite 102, Southfield, MI 48075, USA; [b] Laboratory Operations, Alere Toxicology, 9417 Brodie Lane, Austin, TX 78748, USA; [c] Department of Pathology, Wayne State University School of Medicine, 540 East Canfield, Detroit, MI 48201, USA; [d] Consolidated Laboratory Management Systems, 24555 Southfield Road, Southfield, MI 48075, USA
* Corresponding author.
E-mail address: dr@painrecoverymd.com

Clin Lab Med 36 (2016) 693–707
http://dx.doi.org/10.1016/j.cll.2016.07.010   labmed.theclinics.com

article reviews single nucleotide polymorphisms (SNPs), or isolated regions of the DNA, in various regions including the promoter, and their activity, including terminology and known metabolic pathways' effects on substrates. Subsequently, this report addresses the inducers and inhibitors of the enzymes affecting the phase I metabolism, which can, in certain respects, play a more significant role than the SNPs.

A clinical summary supports the minimal role PGx variant SNP testing has on opioid pharmacodynamics and the significant role it carries in psychiatric toxicology and the knowledge of inhibitor/inducer PGx required for appropriate pain management and addiction toxicology today.

Phase I metabolism covers the cytochrome P450 (CYP) enzymes that include oxidative, reduction and hydrolysis of drugs into a more polar metabolite, usually active, by adding $-OH$, $-SH$ or $-NH_2$ moieties. A common example would be O or N-demethylation of oxycodone by CYP2D6 and CYP3A4, respectively. These are catalyzed by the common CYP hepatic enzymes that can be affected by SNPs. However, not every enzyme may be affected by a SNP, and not every medication or drug may be affected, especially if it is metabolized by several enzyme pathways. The more common CYP enzymes affecting metabolism for purposes of substances tested by toxicology for this series are as follows: CYP2C19, CYP2D6, CYP2C9, CYP3A4 and 3A5, CYP1A2, and CYP2B6. Although there are others, these are the primary ones of study for our purpose. **Fig. 1** shows the most common CYP enzymes, and **Fig. 2** shows the number of drugs metabolized per CYP enzyme.

Phase II metabolism represents a subsequent conjugation of either parent drug or metabolite that has already undergone phase I metabolism into an even more polar, hydrophilic moiety. The new structure usually undergoes renal excretion. This conjugation is done by glucuronidation, sulfation, or hydroxylation. One of the common enzymes is UDP-glucuronosyltransferase (UGT), which exists in multiple subclasses, including a major one affecting opioid toxicology, UGT2B7*2, and its metabolism of morphine,[1] which is reviewed toward the end of this article.

Pharmacokinetics is the primary concern of this review and deals with the absorption, metabolism, distribution, and excretion of a drug. Toxicology testing depends on all these factors, as we measure analytes in the plasma, oral fluid, urine, sweat, hair, or other matrices. PGx affects the metabolism of the compound either through an SNP variation or because another drug either induced or inhibited the same enzyme,

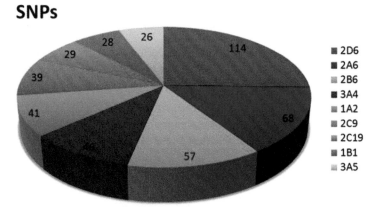

Fig. 1. SNPs in CYP. (*From* Preissner SC, Hoffmann MF, Preissner R, et al. Polymorphic cytochrome P450 enzymes (CYPs) and their role in personalized therapy. PLoS One 2013;8(12):e82562; with permission.)

Drugs

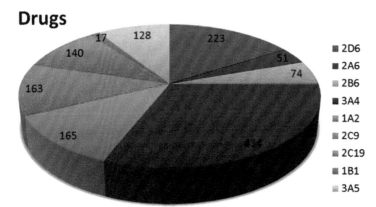

Fig. 2. Number of drugs metabolized per SNP. (*From* Preissner SC, Hoffmann MF, Preissner R, et al. Polymorphic cytochrome P450 enzymes (CYPs) and their role in personalized therapy. PLoS One 2013;8(12):e82562; with permission.)

thus, affecting its metabolism. This is the core aspect of how PGx is integral to our study of toxicology.

Pharmacodynamics, on the other hand, is the affect the drug will have on the body, often with a focus at the organ or tissue site, and can be subject to drug concentration levels. Although pharmacokinetics also has a role at the tissue site, pharmacodynamics primarily focuses on the effect in relation to receptor binding, effect on the cell, secondary messenger, or positive/negative feedback inhibition/induction of receptors after drug/receptor binding. Thus, another separate topic is PGx and how SNPs affect coding for central nervous system receptors such as the μ-opioid and catechol-*O*-methyltransferase receptors, which is beyond the scope of general toxicology testing.

Table 1 is a chart containing the most common substrates categorized by the CYP enzymes. The most important aspect the reader must understand is this subject matter is continuously changing and is not an exact science. **Table 2** depicts the common inducers, whereas **Table 3** depicts inhibitors of select enzymes.

It is important to understand the interaction between the inducers, inhibitors, and the substrate before any SNP variations. This on its own is analogous to understanding the basics of microbiology before learning which antibiotic one would use to treat an infection and whether it should attack the cell membrane, cell wall, or DNA or if its action is bacteriostatic or bacteriocidal. PGx is similar, and the knowledge of the enzyme or substrate should be mastered before assessing genetic variations. In fact, most drugs are metabolized through CYP3A4 and 3A5, yet only 4 substrates are clinically affected by genetic variation (highlighted in **Table 1**) that we know of at this time.[2]

With respect to SNP variants, the phenotypic enzymatic activities that result from such are classified into 4 categories of metabolism based upon kinetics: rapid, normal, intermediate, or poor. The authors prefer to use this direct, more clinically applicable nomenclature because the current system tends to be redundant, less cohesive, and, at times, confusing. What the authors refer to as *rapid* is currently known as *ultra-rapid*, whereas our reference to *normal* is currently labeled *extensive-normal*. Intermediate metabolizers vary, which makes it difficult for physicians to apply the clinical science. However, the authors refer the reader at this time to focus on the substrates, inducers, and inhibitors and the free link: Medscape's Drug Interaction checker (http://reference.medscape.com/drug-interactionchecker). Any health care professional may use the drug-interaction portion, which is the only site that currently provides PGx

Table 1
Phase I common substrates

CYP2C19		CYP2D6		CYP2C9	
Psychotropics	Proton pump	ADHD	Opioids	Hypoglycemics	NSAIDS
Amitriptyline (1°)	Omeprazole	Modafinil	*Hydrocodone*	Glipizide	Celecoxib
Clomipramine (2°)	Lansoprazole	*Amphetamine*	*Codeine (P)*	Glimepiride	Diclofenac
Imipramine	Pantoprazole	Atomoxetine	*Tramadol*	Tolbutamide	Meloxicam
Citalopram	Cardiovascular	*Methylphenidate*	Oxycodone (2°)	Glyburide	Naproxen
Escitalopram	Clopidogrel (P)	Psychotropics	β blockers	Anti-coagulants	Ibuprofen
Sertraline	Prasugrel	Aripiprazole	Carvedilol	S-warfarin	Indomethacin
Anticonvulsant	Other	Risperidone	Metoprolol	Diuretic	Anticonvulsant
Phenobarbital (<25%)	*Carisoprodol*	Haloperidol	Propranolol	Torsemide	Valproic acid
Diazepam	Proguanil/(P)	Thioridazine	Antiarrythmics	ARBs	Phenytoin (1°)
Clobazam (2°)	Atovaquone	Clozapine	Flecainide	Losartan (P)	Other
Phenytoin (2°)	Nelfinavir	Olanzapine (2°)	Propafenone	Irbesartan	Sildenafil
Oncology	Tolbutamide	Donepezil	Quinidine	Statins	Hypnotics
Cyclophosphamide (P)		Tricyclics	Oncology	Fluvastatin	*Zolpidem (2°)*
		Nortriptyline	Tamoxifen (P)	Rosuvastatin	
		Clomipramine (1°)	Doxorubicin		
		Desipramine	SNRIs		
		SSRIs	Duloxetine		
		Fluoxetine (1°)	Venlafaxine		
		Paroxetine (1°)			
		Sertraline			

CYP3A4/5	CYP1A2	CYP2B6
Psychotropics	**Psychotropics**	Opioids
Carbamazepine	Clomipramine	*Methadone*
Aripiprazole	Imipramine	
Quetiapine	Fluvoxamine	
Mirtazapine	**Antipsychotics**	
Trazodone	Haloperidol	
Sertraline	Clozipine	
Oncology	Olanzapine	
Vincristine	**Muscle relaxant**	
Vinblastine	Cyclobenzaprine	
Imatinib	Tizanidine	
Erlotinib (1°)	**Hypnotics**	
Doxorubicin	*Zolpidem (2°)*	
Cardiovascular	**Ardiovascular**	
Amlodipine	Mexiletine	
Diltiazem	Propranolol (2°)	
Nifedipine	**Oncology**	
Verapamil	Erlotinib (2°)	
Amiodarone	**Other**	
Other	Theophylline	
Tacrolimus	Caffeine	
Cyclosporin	Zolmitriptan	
Hydrocortisone	Ondansetron (2°)	
Dexamethasone	Acetaminophen	
Ondansetron (2°)		
Donepezil		
Erythromycin		
Statins		
Atorvastatin		
Lovastatin		
Simvastatin		
Sex hormones		
Finasteride		
Estradiol		
Progesterone		
Ethinylestradiol		
Testosterone		
HIV		
Amprenavir		
Efavirenz		
Atripla		
Atazanavir		
Ritonavir		
Opioids		
Buprenorphine		
Fentanyl		
Methadone		
Oxycodone (1°)		
Tranquilizers		
Alprazolam		
Midazolam		
Hypnotics		
Zolpidem (1°)		
Eszopiclone		

Bold, affected by SNP in 3A4; italic, toxicology tested.
Abbreviations: (1°), primary metabolic pathway; (2°), secondary metabolic pathway; ADHD, attention deficit hyperactivity disorder; ARBs, angiotensin receptor blockers; HIV, human immunodeficiency virus; NSAID, nonsteroidal anti-inflammatory drug; SNRI, serotonin and norepinephrine reuptake inhibitors; SSRI, selective serotonin reuptake inhibitors.

| Table 2 | | | | | |
| Inducers | | | | | |
2C19	2D6	2C9	3A4	1A2	2B6
Carbamazepine	None	Carbamazepine	Carbamazepine	Carbamazepine	Carbamazepine
Norethindrone	known	Phenytoin	Dexamethasone	Omeprazole	Phenytoin
Prednisone		Phenobarbitol	Glucocorticoids	Phenytoin	Phenobarbitol
Rifampicin		Rifampicin	Nafcillin	Phenobarbitol	Rifampicin
St John's Wort		St John's Wort	Nelfinavir	Polycyclic	St John's Wort
			Oxycarbazepine	–aromatic/	
			Phenytoin	hydrocarbons	
			Phenobarbitol	Rifampicin	
			Progesterone		
			St John's Wort		
			Topiramate		

inducer/inhibitor clinical PGx information. This information should be interrogated before prescribing medications.

There are several databases that include SNPs, variants, the substrates, and quoted literature with the best aims at their functional variants (**Box 1**). However, there are discrepancies within the literature, in demographics, and over time as new publications arise. Thus, the viewer should not take any set publication as the gold standard by any means. The authors encourage the reader to search the listed databases and carefully review any publications including the type of study (isolated SNPs or genomewide association study using thousands of patients with a set marker and known trait) and inclusion of demographics.

CYP2C19 primarily only affects the metabolism of diazepam and the muscle relaxer carisoprodol as highlighted in **Table 1**. However, the current literature provides some laboratory evidence of the interaction of substrates and inhibitors/inducers, but there are not many significant studies showing clinical relevance in toxicology at this time.[3–5] It is suggested to check for interactions prior to prescribing these medications.

CYP2D6

Codeine (C) is the only formal opioid prodrug that has no analgesic effect until activated by the liver. The primary activation is phase I; (1) O-demethylation via

| Table 3 | | | | | |
| Inhibitors | | | | | |
2C19	2D6	2C9	3A4/5	1A2	2B6
Fluoxetine	Bupropion	Fluconazole	Indinavir	Fluoroquinolones	Thiotepa
Fluvoxamine	Fluoxetine	Amiodarone	Nelfinavir	Fluvoxamine	Ticlopidine
Ketoconazole	Paroxetine	Isoniazid	Ritonavir	Ticlopidine	
Lansoprazole	Quinidine		Clarithromycin		
Omeprazole	Duloxetine		Erythromycin		
Ticlopidine	Chlorpheniramine		Itraconazole		
	Clomipramine		Ketoconazole		
	Doxepin		Nefazodone		
	Haloperidol		Grapefruit Juice		
	Methadone		Verapamil		
	Mibefradil		Diltiazem		
	Ritonavir		Amiodarone		
			Fluvoxamine		

> **Box 1**
> **Databases of single nucleotide polymorphisms**
>
> Human CYP allele: http://www.cypalleles.ki.se/
>
> PharmGKB: http://www.pharmgkb.org/
>
> dbSNP: http://www.ncbi.nlm.nih.gov/projects/SNP/
>
> 1000 Genomes Project: http://browser.1000genomes.org/index.html
>
> SNPedia: http://www.snpedia.com/index.php/SNPedia
>
> Gene Cards: http://www.genecards.org/index.shtml

CYP2D6 to morphine (M) and (2) *N*-demethylation via CYP3A4 to norC. A blood sample will contain M and its metabolites along with norC, whereas oral fluid will reveal C and norC.

Urine drug testing is based on CYP2D6 activity and includes genetic variants or P450 inducers and inhibitors as follows:

A rapid 2D6 variant (*1/*2) will activate C into M exceeding the standard dosing. This dosing resulted in overdose of children, leading several children's hospitals to remove codeine from their formularies and a general review published by the Clinical Pharmacogenetics Implementation Consortium in 2012, updated in 2014.[6,7] Overall, the rapid variant SNP resulted in excess formation of M in mothers breast milk leading to overdose of neonates, in post-tonsillectomy patients with or without sleep apnea,[8] and even in some cases in which only 1 allele carried the *2 variant (heterozygous),[7] leading the FDA to come out with extensive black box warnings about codeine in the pediatric, neonatal/breast feeding population, along with the Consortium as noted. Similarly, any potential 2D6 inducer could have the same effect, although at this time there are no known in vivo or in vitro inducers of CYP2D6.

Hydrocodone (HC) undergoes (1) *O*-demethylation via 2D6 into hydromorphone (HM) and (2) *N*-demethylation by 3A4/5 into minimally active norHC. HM also undergoes phase II metabolism by UGT into HM-3-G.[9]

In blood and oral analysis, the primary metabolite is parent HC followed by norHC and significantly less HM.[10] The benefit of oral analysis is the consistent presence of norHC with an HC/norHC ratio of 1:16, and minimal HM, which helps delineate the patient is taking HC rather than HM.[11] Urine analysis finds 26% HC eliminated within 72 hours, with results as follows: (1) HC 9% to 12%, (2) norHC 5% to 19%, (3) HM-3-G 2% to 4%, and (4) 6 α and β Hydrocol 1% to 3%.[12] The importance of norHC in urine, as in oral fluid, is to delineate the use of HC versus ingestion of HM, which is always present in its conjugated form.[13]

Despite the phase I CYP2D6 metabolism of HC, a review of the literature and the Consortium have not found inhibitors[14] or PGx variants in either poor or rapid metabolizers to affect toxicology results from a laboratory metric of clinical relevance.[7]

Oxycodone (OC) primary metabolism ($\sim$85%) is *N*-demethylation by CYP3A4/3A5 to noroxycodone (NOC), which has minimal analgesic activity and secondarily ($\sim$15%) is *O*-demethylation by CYP2D6 to oxymorphone (OM), which has more analgesic activity than its parent compound. NOC then converts into noroxymorphone (NOM) via CYP2D6. OM and NOM undergo phase II conjugation to OM-3-G.[15] Finally, OC, NOC, and OM undergo some keto-reduction to the 6 α and β metabolites.[12,15] In both blood and oral fluid, the primary analytes found in descending order are OC, NOC, and OM, with blood/oral ratios fairly uniform.[16] Of importance is that oral testing finds NOC in 80%–90% of specimens, helping discern patients taking OC and not

OM.[16] One experimental urine study reported 8% free OC with 23% free NOC then 10.4% conjugated OM, 8.6% conjugated NOM, and approximately 6% of various keto metabolites.[17] The authors, having experience with millions of human pain management specimens and review of evidence-based clinical research, support urine metabolites as primarily free OC, NOC with conjugated OM to a lesser extent based on genetic variability, and inducers/inhibitors of CYP2D6 and 3A4.[18] Clinically, the message is (1) free OC and NOC; (2) conjugated OM, which varies with metabolism; (3) less NOM only 39% conjugated; and (4) creatinine correction, where applicable, should be done for final levels.[19]

OC would require both a grapefruit diet (3A4 inhibition) and a CYP2D6 poor metabolizer (*3-*9 homozygous variant) or inhibitorlike paroxetine (see **Table 2**) to create complete metabolic inhibition to create toxic levels of OC. This would appear in the urine as minimal OC, no NOC or OM, and with elevated OC in the plasma. An actual small clinical study proved the above case by combining itraconazole, a potent 3A4 azole antifungal with paroxetine, a strong 2D6 inhibitor. The study found a minimal pharmacokinetic effect with 2D6 inhibition alone, although not statistically significant. However, the combined 3A4/2D6 inhibition was significant in both pharmacokinetic and pharmacodynamic effects from OC-reduced metabolism.[20]

The opposite, however, in which a rapid 2D6 variant could potentially increase OM production by urine drug testing, or clinically, any evidence-based increased risk has not been found in the literature to date. Thus, the Consortium has not included OC in its warning or risk, stating the data are conflicting and attributes any current analgesia side effects to the parent compound.[7]

OM is primarily metabolized through conjugation, which is phase II, or UGT into OM-3-glucuronide (OM-3-G) and some keto-reduction into the 6α/β-hydroxy-OM (6-HOM) with urine as follows: greater than 40% OM-3-G, less than 5% free and conjugated 6-HOM, and less than 5% parent OM.[12] In plasma, one finds a similar result with primarily OM-3-G at 90% greater levels than free OM.[15] Any precision medicine in toxicology would be based on urine drug toxicology (UDT) as described in that section in this review.

3A4

As briefly noted during the introduction, precision medicine in toxicology primarily affects most metabolism through inhibitors and inducers through the 3A4 enzyme; similarly, currently only the 3 common statins and tacrolimus are known to be affected by SNPs. Fentanyl, methadone, tramadol, buprenorphine and OC are some of the key opiates metabolized by this enzyme.[15]

2B6

Methadone is a complex opiate consisting of dual activity based on the racemic stereo-isomers: the (R) or "l"-isomer provides μ-opioid agonist activity for nociceptive pain, whereas the (S) or "d"-isomer provides N-methyl, D-aspartate receptor antagonist activity for neuropathic pain. Primary metabolism is N-demethylation by 3A4, 2B6 (and to a minor extent by 2D6 and 2C19) into 2- ethylidene-1,5-dimethyl-3,3-diphenylpyrrolidene (EDDP). In the urine, we commonly measure 2:1 EDDP to methadone, with the ratio increasing directly with urine pH. In a large series by Pesce and colleagues,[21] in part because of its lipophilic nature, they found a lack of consistency with the ratio in chronic pain patients as the dose varied,[22] although they were unable to conclude with certainty the causal relationship. However, an earlier PGx study showed a definite pharmacokinetic variation with the 2B6*6 allele as a poor metabolizer affecting methadone.[23]

Overall, the study found the (S) enantiomer was affected, which is associated more often with prolonged QT interval and respiratory depression, although because medications were a covariable, it could not rule out potential inhibitors. More recently, Levran and colleagues[24] excluded any medication confounders and accounted for ABCB1, an SNP variant, for the efflux p-glycoprotein blood–brain barrier transport protein associated with higher methadone dose requirements by the same author in 2008. In this study, Levran and colleagues[24] not only agreed with the findings of earlier study but actually found evidence-based clinical support for lower methadone dosing by the 2B6*6 homozygous allele.[24] Although a more recent study briefly attempted to state its inability to corroborate Levran's findings, it had multiple covariables, lacked the same power, and was not focused on the same specific aims but rather was more broadly focused.[25] The 2B6 data support the prior data with a scientifically sound stepwise research protocol within a set demographic profile and is a step toward isolating clinically relevant variant effects of phase I metabolism on methadone dosing.

Buprenorphine (Bup) is primarily N-dealkylated to norBup by 3A4 and 2C8. Bup and norBup undergo glucuronidation by UGT into Bup-G and norBup-G, however, not by UGT2B7 but primarily by UGT1A3.[26] In terms of 3A4, the important PGx for toxicology remains inducers and inhibitors. The most important aspects for this publication include use of the drug interaction tool. At the time of print, the authors are not aware of any EMR/EHR having PGx logic built into their system. Briefly, in pain management, it is gradually becoming more prevalent for multidisciplinary groups to have one or more physicians with a Bup "Data 2000" waiver, to prescribe Bup for opioid dependency. Otherwise, a transdermal patch using lower doses of Bup exists, which requires knowledge of precision medicine in toxicology.

The most common toxicology concern is false-negative findings in presumptive testing for Bup. Because even American Society of Addiction Medicine–certified physicians surveyed answered many questions incorrectly regarding immunoassay testing,[27] it can be inferred that most physicians would likely miss the approximately 20% to 25% false-negative rate from the average point-of-care on-site testing device used in the physician's office today. The reason for this is that Bup is quickly metabolized into the nor-form[28] then conjugated into the glucuronide format. In addition, many pain and even primary care patients will be on inducers (see **Table 2**) including carbamazepine, topiramate, glucocorticoids, and herbal supplements.

Patients in addiction medicine who may be simultaneously undergoing detoxification for benzodiazepine dependency along with opioid/opiates may utilize phenobarbital and Bup, respectively. If the phenobarbital is extended for a prolonged taper, it may induce CYP enzymes, 3A4, and 2C8, potentially reducing the Bup level, although no formal clinical studies have been done to support this. More common, however, is the opposite situation, in which inhibitors of 3A4 can lead to elevated doses of norBup. This situation occurs in comorbid diseases such as human immunodeficiency virus treatment or fungal infections. Thus, it is important to use the drug interaction tool on Medscape's site as noted.

At the time of this writing, there are both FDA approval of a new subcutaneous long-acting 8-mg Bup implant and approval of phase III clinical trials of a 28-day Bup subcutaneous injection. The injection has been published in a few pharmacokinetic studies, with data supporting steady levels achieving at least 70% receptor saturation, although PGx inducer/inhibitor data are pending.[29]

URINE DRUG TOXICOLOGY

Primary metabolism of morphine (M) is phase II glucuronide (G) conjugation via UGT using several variations of the enzyme to M-6-G (active), M-3-G (inactive), and other metabolites: M-3,6-G, norM (via CYP3A4 and CYP2C8), which are conjugated to norM-3-G and norM-6-G. Similarly, HM is primarily metabolized by UGT at the 3 position to HM-3-G, and some 6-keto-reductase into 6α and 6β hydromorphone as noted in prior discussion. Although one opioid review mentions HM-6-G,[30] which is a minimal amount verified by the original article,[15] conjugation into any 6-moeity is not supported because of the presence of a ketone at the 6 position,[31] which is the key differentiation between M (hydroxyl at 6) and HM. Blood concentration finds HM-3-G approximately 25 times the concentration of the parent HM, whereas oral fluid is highly variable and inconsistent with significantly lower required thresholds.[11]

Most data unfortunately are from HC studies, and a paucity of HM metabolism data in oral fluid exist at the date of this writing. Urine is at least 35% conjugated to HM-3-G and 6% free HM and the remainder as H-3-sulfate, H-3-glucoside, and the 6 keto forms, while chronic pain patients may find primarily HM-3-G without free HM.[12]

In renal failure, both M and HM, both conjugated into 3-glucuronide, can build up to potentially neurotoxic levels. One must take caution with M and HM in renally compromised patients, as M-3-G and HM-3-G levels, which lead to neuro-excitatory toxic responses, can be more common in those individuals.[32,33]

Despite all the metabolic findings, and one commercial laboratory offering PGx testing for UGT2B7 genetic SNP, aside from pharmacokinetic urine testing,[1] we were only able to find one evidence-based clinical study in which pharmacodynamics have been affected by UGT from PGx in advanced cancer patients with renal dysfunction,[34] in which, as noted above, M-3-G and HM-3-G may exhibit neurotoxic effects.

In addition to the common functional polymorphisms of the *p450* genes listed above (CYP1A2, CYP2B6, CYP2C9, CYP2C19, CYP2D6, CYP3A4 and 3A5), there are additional variations that differ among populations (**Table 4**). For example, the CYP 2D6 variant 6*10 corresponds to decreased enzymatic activity and is found most common among Asians (50%) when compared with African and white populations, thus, warranting consideration of modifying the dosing of opiates such as C. Furthermore, the UDT results of such a patient prescribed C may only detect the presence of C and not show the characteristic metabolites of HC and M. This finding is in contrast to the 2D6 variant (*1/*2), representing a gene duplication, translating into increased enzymatic activity (ultrametabolizer) with respect to C to HC and M conversion. Such a UDT result may have no presence of C rather only HC, M, and HM, posing the inappropriate suspicion of diversion of C and surreptitious administration of M.

In summary, despite hundreds of publications over the past two decades rapidly expanding on precision medicine, there remains a pressing need for greater pronounced support towards the utility and application of genetic testing in the discipline of clinical toxicology. One can observe a similar pattern in its educational limitations.[35] Specifically, the core knowledge of precision medicine is tantamount to clinical decision making for toxicology and prescribing, especially at the time of this article based on the continued increase in combination opioid/opiate with benzodiazepine death rates.[36–38] It is imperative that precision medicine be part of the basic educational curriculum, specifically, key enzymes and their substrates, inducers, and inhibitors before being eligible to prescribe, and mandatory for any certification for a medical review officer.

Table 4
Common naturally occurring functional polymorphisms in the major cytochrome *P450* genes: Allele frequency and functional effects for CYP1A2, CYP2B6, CYP2C9, CYP2C19, CYP2D6, CYP3A4 and 3A5

Common Allelic Variants	Polymorphism/Substitution	Allele Frequency (%)[a]			Functional Effect[b]
		Ca	As	Af	
CYP1A2					
CYP1A2*1C	−3860G>A	—	—	—	↓Inducibility
CYP1A2*1F	−163C>A	33	68	—	↑Inducibility
CYP1A2*1K	Haplotype (−63C>A, −739T>G, −729C>T)	0.5	—	—	↓Inducibility ↓Activity
CYP2B6					
CYP2B6*4	K262R	5	—	—	↑Activity
CYP2B6*5	R487C	11–14	1	—	↓Expression
CYP2B6*6	Q172H; K262R	16–26	16	—	↑Activity
CYP2B6*7	Q172H; K262R; R487C	13	0	—	↑Activity
CYP2C9					
CYP2C9*2	R144C	13–22	0	3	↓Activity
CYP2C9*3	I359L	3–16	3	1.3	↓Activity
CYP2C9*5	D360E	0	2	0	↓Activity
CYP2C19					
CYP2C19*2	Splicing defect; I331V	15	30	17	Abolished activity
CYP2C19*3	W212X; I331V	0.04	5	0.4	Abolished activity
CYP2C19*17	I331V	18	4	—	↑Transcription
CYP2D6					
CYP2D6*3	Frameshift	1–2	<1	—	Abolished activity (PM)

(continued on next page)

Table 4
(continued)

Common Allelic Variants	Polymorphism/Substitution	Allele Frequency (%)[a]			Functional Effect[b]
		Ca	As	Af	
CYP2D6*4	Splicing defect	20–25	1	6–7	Abolished activity (PM)
CYP2D6*5	Gene deletion	4–6	4–6	4–6	Abolished activity (PM)
CYP2D6*10	P34S; S486T	<2	50	3–9	↓Activity (IM)
CYP2D6*17	T107I; R296C; S486T	<1	—	20–34	↓Activity (IM)
CYP2D6*41	R296C; splicing defect; S486T	1.3	2	5.8	↓Activity (IM)
CYP2D6*1 × N, N ≥2	Gene duplication	—	—	—	↑Activity (UM)
CYP2D6*2 × N, N ≥2	Gene duplication	—	—	—	↑Activity (UM)
CYP3A4					
CYP3A4*1B	5' flanking region	2–9	0	35–67	Altered expression
CYP3A4*2	S222P	2.7–4.5	0	0	Substrate-dependent altered activity
CYP3A4*3	M445T	1.1	—	—	↓Activity
CYP3A4*17	F189S	2.1	—	—	↓Activity
CYP3A4*18	L293P	0	—	1	↑Activity
CYP3A5					
CYP3A5*3	Splicing defect	90	75	50	Abolished activity
CYP3A5*6	Splicing defect	0	0	7.5	Severely ↓ activity
CYP3A5*7	346 frameshift	0	0	8	Severely ↓activity

↑, indicates increased; ↓, indicates decreased.

Abbreviations: Af, African; As, Asian; Ca, Caucasian (white); IM, intermediate metabolizer; PM, poor metabolizer; UM, ultra-rapid metabolizer.

[a] Allele frequency data *from* Refs.[39–45]

[b] Functional effect data are obtained from the Human Cytochrome P450 (CYP) Allele Nomenclature Committee website (http://www.cypalleles.ki.se/).

From Li J, Bluth MH. Pharmacogenomics and personalized medicine. In: McPherson RA, Pincus MR, editors. Henry's clinical diagnosis and management by laboratory methods. 23rd edition. Elsevier: 2017; p. 1409–10; with permission.

REFERENCES

1. Chau N, Elliot DJ, Lewis BC, et al. Morphine glucuronidation and glucosidation represent complementary metabolic pathways that are both catalyzed by UDP-glucuronosyltransferase 2B7: kinetic, inhibition, and molecular modeling studies. J Pharmacol Exp Ther 2014;349(1):126–37.
2. Klein K, Zanger UM. Pharmacogenomics of cytochrome P450 3A4: recent progress toward the "Missing Heritability" problem. Front Genet 2013;4:12.
3. Bramness JG, Skurtveit S, Fauske L, et al. Association between blood carisoprodol:meprobamate concentration ratios and CYP2C19 genotype in carisoprodol-drugged drivers: decreased metabolic capacity in heterozygous CYP2C19*1/CYP2C19*2 subjects? Pharmacogenetics 2003;13(7):383–8.
4. Sim SC, Nordin L, Andersson TM, et al. Association between CYP2C19 polymorphism and depressive symptoms. Am J Med Genet B Neuropsychiatr Genet 2010;153B(6):1160–6.
5. Andresen H, Augustin C, Streichert T. Toxicogenetics–cytochrome P450 microarray analysis in forensic cases focusing on morphine/codeine and diazepam. Int J Legal Med 2013;127(2):395–404.
6. Crews KR, Gaedigk A, Dunnenberger HM, et al. Clinical pharmacogenetics implementation consortium (CPIC) guidelines for codeine therapy in the context of cytochrome P450 2D6 (CYP2D6) genotype. Clin Pharmacol Ther 2012;91(2):321–6.
7. Crews KR, Gaedigk A, Dunnenberger HM, et al. Clinical pharmacogenetics implementation consortium guidelines for cytochrome P450 2D6 genotype and codeine therapy: 2014 update. Clin Pharmacol Ther 2014;95(4):376–82.
8. Khetani JD, Madadi P, Sommer DD, et al. Apnea and oxygen desaturations in children treated with opioids after adenotonsillectomy for obstructive sleep apnea syndrome: a prospective pilot study. Paediatr Drugs 2012;14(6):411–5.
9. Barakat NH, Atayee RS, Best BM, et al. Urinary hydrocodone and metabolite distributions in pain patients. J Anal Toxicol 2014;38(7):404–9.
10. Cao JM, Ma JD, Morello CM, et al. Observations on hydrocodone and its metabolites in oral fluid specimens of the pain population: comparison with urine. J Opioid Manag 2014;10(3):177–86.
11. Cone EJ, DePriest AZ, Heltsley R, et al. Prescription opioids. IV: disposition of hydrocodone in oral fluid and blood following single-dose administration. J Anal Toxicol 2015;39(7):510–8.
12. DePriest AZ, Puet BL, Holt AC, et al. Metabolism and disposition of prescription opioids: a Review. Forensic Sci Rev 2015;27(2):115–45.
13. Cone EJ, Heltsley R, Black DL, et al. Prescription opioids. II. Metabolism and excretion patterns of hydrocodone in urine following controlled single-dose administration. J Anal Toxicol 2013;37(8):486–94.
14. Kapil RP, Friedman K, Cipriano A, et al. Effects of paroxetine, a CYP2D6 inhibitor, on the pharmacokinetic properties of hydrocodone after coadministration with a single-entity, once-daily, extended-release hydrocodone tablet. Clin Ther 2015;37(10):2286–96.
15. Smith HS. The metabolism of opioid agents and the clinical impact of their active metabolites. Clin J Pain 2011;27(9):824–38.
16. Cone EJ, DePriest AZ, Heltsley R, et al. Prescription opioids. III. Disposition of oxycodone in oral fluid and blood following controlled single-dose administration. J Anal Toxicol 2015;39(3):192–202.

17. Lalovic B, Kharasch E, Hoffer C, et al. Pharmacokinetics and pharmacodynamics of oral oxycodone in healthy human subjects: role of circulating active metabolites. Clin Pharmacol Ther 2006;79(5):461–79.

18. Fang WB, Lofwall MR, Walsh SL, et al. Determination of oxycodone, noroxycodone and oxymorphone by high-performance liquid chromatography-electrospray ionization-tandem mass spectrometry in human matrices: in vivo and in vitro applications. J Anal Toxicol 2013;37(6):337–44.

19. Cone EJ, Heltsley R, Black DL, et al. Prescription opioids. I. Metabolism and excretion patterns of oxycodone in urine following controlled single dose administration. J Anal Toxicol 2013;37(5):255–64.

20. Gronlund J, Saari TI, Hagelberg NM, et al. Exposure to oral oxycodone is increased by concomitant inhibition of CYP2D6 and 3A4 pathways, but not by inhibition of CYP2D6 alone. Br J Clin Pharmacol 2010;70(1):78–87.

21. Leimanis E, Best BM, Atayee RS, et al. Evaluating the relationship of methadone concentrations and EDDP formation in chronic pain patients. J Anal Toxicol 2012; 36(4):239–49.

22. Leimanis E, Best BM, Atayee RS, et al. Evaluating the relationship of methadone concentrations and EDDP formation in chronic pain patients. J Anal Toxicol 2012; 36(4):239–49.

23. Crettol S, Déglon JJ, Besson J, et al. Methadone enantiomer plasma levels, CYP2B6, CYP2C19, and CYP2C9 genotypes, and response to treatment. Clin Pharmacol Ther 2005;78(6):593–604.

24. Levran O, Peles E, Hamon S, et al. CYP2B6 SNPs are associated with methadone dose required for effective treatment of opioid addiction. Addict Biol 2013;18(4): 709–16.

25. Mouly S, Bloch V, Peoc'h K, et al. Methadone dose in heroin-dependent patients: role of clinical factors, comedications, genetic polymorphisms and enzyme activity. Br J Clin Pharmacol 2015;79(6):967–77.

26. Chang Y, Moody DE. Glucuronidation of buprenorphine and norbuprenorphine by human liver microsomes and UDP-glucuronosyltransferases. Drug Metab Lett 2009;3(2):101–7.

27. Kirsh KL, Baxter LE, Rzetelny A, et al. A Survey of ASAM Members' knowledge, attitudes, and practices in urine drug testing. J Addict Med 2015;9(5):399–404.

28. Depriest A, Heltsley R, Black DL, et al. Urine drug testing of chronic pain patients. III. Normetabolites as biomarkers of synthetic opioid use. J Anal Toxicol 2010; 34(8):444–9.

29. Nasser AF, Greenwald MK, Vince B, et al. Sustained-release buprenorphine (RBP-6000) blocks the effects of opioid challenge with hydromorphone in subjects with opioid use disorder. J Clin Psychopharmacol 2016;36(1):18–26.

30. Mercadante S. Opioid metabolism and clinical aspects. Eur J Pharmacol 2015; 769:71–8.

31. Wright AW, Mather LE, Smith MT. Hydromorphone-3-glucuronide: a more potent neuro-excitant than its structural analogue, morphine-3-glucuronide. Life Sci 2001;69(4):409–20.

32. Milne RW, McLean CF, Mather LE, et al. Influence of renal failure on the disposition of morphine, morphine-3-glucuronide and morphine-6-glucuronide in sheep during intravenous infusion with morphine. J Pharmacol Exp Ther 1997;282(2): 779–86.

33. Ravenscroft P, Schneider J. Bedside perspectives on the use of opioids: transferring results of clinical research into practice. Clin Exp Pharmacol Physiol 2000; 27(7):529–32.

34. Fladvad T, Klepstad P, Langaas M, et al. Variability in UDP-glucuronosyltransferase genes and morphine metabolism: observations from a cross-sectional multicenter study in advanced cancer patients with pain. Pharmacogenet Genomics 2013; 23(3):117–26.
35. American Society of Addiction Medicine Board of Directors. Drug testing: a white paper of the American society of addiction medicine. Chevy Chase (MD): ASAM; 2013. p. 108.
36. Group, W.S.A.M.D.s., Interagency Guideline on Prescribing Opioids for Pain. Washington State Agency Medical Director's Group; 2015. p. 105.
37. Health, O.D.o., 2014 Ohio Drug Overdose Data: General Findings. Ohio Department of Health; 2016. p. 1–10.
38. Dowell D, Haegerich TM, Chou R. CDC guideline for prescribing opioids for chronic pain - United States, 2016. MMWR Recomm Rep 2016;65(1):1–49.
39. Xie HG, Kim RB, Wood AJ, et al. Molecular basis of ethnic differences in drug disposition and response. Annu Rev Pharmacol Toxicol 2001;41:815–50.
40. Bradford LD. CYP2D6 allele frequency in european caucasians, asians, africans and their descendants. Pharmacogenomics 2002;3:229–43.
41. Mizutani T. PM frequencies of major CYPs in asians and caucasians. Drug Metab Rev 2003;35:99–106.
42. Solus JF, Arietta BJ, Harris JR, et al. Genetic variation in eleven phase I drug metabolism genes in an ethnically diverse population. Pharmacogenomics 2004;5:895–931.
43. Roy JN, Lajoie J, Zijenah LS, et al. CYP3A5 genetic polymorphisms in different ethnic populations. Drug Metab Dispos 2005;33:884–7.
44. Suarez-Kurtz G. Pharmacogenomics in admixed populations. Trends Pharmacol Sci 2005;26:196–201.
45. Sistonen J, Sajantila A, Lao O, et al. CYP2D6 worldwide genetic variation shows high frequency of altered activity variants and no continental structure. Pharmacogenet Genomics 2007;17:93–101.

Toxicology in Reproductive Endocrinology

Roohi Jeelani, MD[a],*, Martin H. Bluth, MD, PhD[b,c], Husam M. Abu-Soud, PhD[a]

KEYWORDS

- Infertility • Reproductive outcomes • Subfertility • Toxicology • Alcohol • Drugs
- Environmental exposure • Health consequences

KEY POINTS

- Fertility relies on a series of time-dependent events, which are regulated by hormones. These hormones can be altered through exposure of consumed and environmental toxins.
- Reproductive dysfunction and infertility require laboratory evaluation, which involves serum hormone measurements.
- Infertility can be treatable through various assisted reproductive technologies. These can involve retrieval of the oocytes and insemination with sperm; however, if oocyte quality itself is disrupted through exposure through toxins, there is little that can be done to improve the quality.
- There are many toxins, including environmental, prescribed and illicit that can alter reproduction in the parent as well as future generations in a dose dependant manner.
- Currently there are no guidelines on laboratory testing for illicit drugs, alcohol, or environmental toxins in the scope of fertility testing. The best method remains to counsel and explain to patients at the first visit what impact it may have on their fertility.

INTRODUCTION

Reproduction is a dynamic process involving multiple pathways and signals throughout the body. If any of these steps are dysregulated, it can potentially lead to infertility. Many toxins and illicit drugs can impact and alter any part of these pathways, leading to difficulty in conceiving. Drugs such as opiates or cocaine have been known to disrupt oocyte quality, impacting fertilization and eventual fetal development and even childhood. Indeed, during in vitro fertilization, one may use genetic screening to biopsy and test the embryo for any chromosomal abnormalities, but other than that there is no laboratory test to detect the damage certain toxins may have caused. The

Disclosure: Nothing to disclose.
[a] Department of Obstetrics and Gynecology, The C.S. Mott Center for Human Growth and Development, Wayne State University School of Medicine, 275 East Hancock, Detroit, MI 48201, USA; [b] Department of Pathology, Wayne State University School of Medicine, 540 East Canfield, Detroit, MI 48201, USA; [c] Consolidated Laboratory Management Systems, 24555 Southfield Road, Southfield, MI 48075, USA
* Corresponding author.
E-mail address: rjeelani@med.wayne.edu

Clin Lab Med 36 (2016) 709–720
http://dx.doi.org/10.1016/j.cll.2016.07.011
0272-2712/16/© 2016 Elsevier Inc. All rights reserved.

labmed.theclinics.com

best and only intervention remains to consult patients at their first prenatal or even a preconception visit to discourage and eliminate potential exposure to any harmful toxins, drugs, or alcohol exposure because it may lead to detrimental effects on the fetus and even into adulthood for the child.

TOXICOLOGY AND REPRODUCTION

Behaviors such as illicit drug use, alcohol consumption, cigarette smoking, and excessive caffeine intake can alter reproductive health and fetal outcomes. Although the association remains loose and unclear, it is thought to be through the derangement of hormonal homeostasis and deterioration of oocyte milieu. In addition, toxin exposure to a variety of naturally occurring or man-made chemicals can alter hormone levels, resulting in an alteration in reproductive potential and possible fertility. Indeed, exposure to these toxins and its consequences are still not well understood, and many gaps still persist. As of yet, there are no guidelines regarding testing for these substances and at what level if any they can have an impact on reproduction. The optimal method to prevent any adverse effects on reproduction still remains to advise patients early on in their care to completely eliminate any substances of abuse and prevent any exposure to potential harmful toxins.

Illicit Drugs

Approximately 60% to 80% of adults use alcohol, and in addition to that, approximately 10% of adults may suffer from some type of substance use to the point of addiction.[1] In many instances there appears to be even higher rates of substance abuse as seen with analysis of meconium samples from newborns. Previously published studies, in certain cohorts, showed that neonates were 31% positive for cocaine, 18% positive for opiates, and 17% positive for cannabinoids, and out of these, many of them were positive for more than one of these drugs.[2,3] It becomes difficult to point to one drug to precipitate a certain outcome because many patients are multidrug abusers as noted by the study of meconium. Opiate and cocaine use while pregnant can lead to neonatal abstinence syndrome, which can persevere for months and lead to increased risk of neurobehavioral disorders and altered central nervous system (CNS) function later on.[4]

   In women, the strongest evidence of the adverse impact of cocaine on reproduction is demonstrated by adverse obstetric outcomes, which include early and late pregnancy loss and placental abruption. Reproductive disturbances in substance-abusing adult women are evidenced by menstrual abnormalities, which predominantly consist of amenorrhea in heroin abusers.[5] On the contrary, the fact that many of these women who are regular narcotic abusers achieve pregnancy and deliver implies that the degree of reproductive insult is not enough to prevent the birth of an exposed and affected baby. However, use of narcotics in women who were on the edge of being infertile may push them into the infertility zone. Previous work has established that in adult mammals opiates bind in the hypothalamus and cause inhibition of the secretion of luteinizing hormone (LH), which can lead to mild to moderate gonadal suppression.[6,7] Not only that, but these drugs can impact fertility; however, it remains difficult to attribute a particular outcome to the use of a certain drug. Drug dependence can lead to varying effects, including malnutrition, increased risk of infectious diseases, poor health care, and poor pregnancy outcomes. These patients also have increased risk of physical and verbal abuse, which also affects the probability of successful fertility and fetal health. People addicted to drugs may be so compromised that the steps essential for normal reproductive hemostasis will be adversely affected leading to reproductive failure. Currently, no specific guidelines have been developed in the field of reproductive endocrinology and toxicology because it remains very difficult to attribute a certain level or type of drug to a particular outcome. In addition, there has been sufficient evidence that addictive substances can pose a significant threat to the developing fetus and even continue throughout the neonatal period. Many disorders have been described, including but not limited to FAS, intrauterine growth restriction, and neonatal withdrawal syndrome. These insults not only alter the fetus in utero but also have been known to have a long-term impact on them as children.

Narcotics have a harmful impact on male reproduction as well. They have been shown to alter hormonal homeostasis through exerting their primary effect on the hypothalamic-pituitary axis, thus leading to effecting the gonads and sex accessory organs.[8] Narcotics can lead to a decrease in gonadotropin secretion and cause a stimulatory effect on prolactin secretion; both of these can cause an inhibitory effect on male sexual function. Previous studies have shown that in some patients, although hormone levels may remain normal or return to baseline after cessation of opiate use, semen parameters might still be altered. Men who abuse heroin have been shown to have asthenospermia and oligospermia.[9,10] An in vitro study done using human sperm and high concentrations of cocaine demonstrated a decrease in kinematics, straight line velocity, and linearity but no impact on overall sperm motility and fertilizing capability.[11] Many men have also claimed that abuse of cocaine leads to increased libido and sexual responsiveness.[12]

In animal models, adverse effects of drug use and fertility have been shown through a significant disturbance of spermatogenesis.[6] In addition to the impact of cocaine on reproductive function and sexual behavior of male rats, there has been some evidence for detrimental effects of long-term cocaine exposure on spermatogenesis and fertility in peripubertal male rats.[13] Chronic cocaine exposure in female rhesus monkeys also led to disruption of their menstrual cycles.[7] To summarize, the impact of narcotics and illicit agents such as cocaine on fertility still remain unclear and not well studied on human subjects. However, it is clear illicit drug use by individuals attempting to conceive is harmful and has consequences to their fertility, although the exact level of impact remains unknown. Furthermore, whereas the adverse effects of exposure to narcotics and illicit agents on the fetus are known, the specific future fertility effects of developmental exposure to these offspring remain unexplored. The relationship of selective agents and their effect on female and male reproductive health as well as general obstetrics, neonatology, and pediatrics, where applicable, follow.

Alcohol

Extensive evidence has shown that excessive ethanol consumption is harmful to both nongravid and gravid women in that even small amounts of exposure can adversely affect the fetus. Alcohol remains the substance most frequently abused by pregnant women, and fetal alcohol syndrome (FAS) has been well studied as well as described.[14] FAS is characterized by intrauterine growth retardation, facial abnormalities, congenital defects, musculoskeletal abnormalities, and dysfunction of the CNS.[14] Generally speaking, the amount of alcohol consumed will proportionally impact the fetus. An average daily maternal intake of 3 oz of alcohol is sufficient to significantly increase the incidence of FAS; however, consumption of less than 1 oz per day has little or no associated increased risk of FAS.[15] When taking into account birth defects, intake of 6 drinks of ethanol per day leads to a 50% chance of birth defects, or approximately 10 times the normal.[16] On the other hand, the impact of alcohol abuse and fertility remains uncertain. A study did show that if a woman consumed one or more drinks of ethanol per week, the probability of conception was reduced by about 50% in each menstrual cycle. The primary site of action is still not clear; however, acute effects of ethanol appear to be due to hypothalamic impacts.[17] Ethanol can act at the level of the CNS to inhibit LH secretion by the pituitary and therefore inhibit ovulation.[17] There is clear evidence of the reproductive toxicity of ethanol consumption; however, no clear testing guidelines and limitations have been developed. It is strongly advised to eliminate or cut down as much as possible on alcohol intake when attempting to achieve pregnancy.

Alcohol has been studied far more than any other substance of abuse. It has been known to have a feminizing effect on men who abuse alcohol because it is related to liver dysfunction and leads to reduced hepatic clearance of estrogens.[18] In men who consume lower amounts of ethanol, some effects on sex steroids can still occur.[19] It has been well established not only in male animals but also in humans that chronic ethanol exposure even at low levels can be associated with lower serum testosterone levels, increased levels of plasma sex hormone–binding globulin, and higher prolactin, leading to increased estrogen levels.[19] The reduction in plasma testosterone levels correlate with decreased responsiveness to human chorionic gonadotropin (hCG), alluding to the possibility that ethanol damages the Leydig cell compartment of the testis. In a more recent study, significantly reduced plasma concentrations of testosterone, LH, and follicle-stimulating hormone (FSH) were reported in male alcohol abusers.[20] Alcohol can cause significant deterioration in sperm concentration, semen volume, and sperm quality.[20,21] Adverse effects of chronic ethanol consumption on male fertility have been demonstrated in experimental animals and human studies; however, no clear correlation has yet been established.

In addition, in animal studies ethanol has been reported to inhibit ovulation and suppress plasma estradiol; progesterone levels are also suppressed. In a nonhuman primate study, female monkeys were given a 7- to 10-oz glass of alcohol a day for up to 6 months and were noted to have disruptions in reproductive function, as demonstrated by amenorrhea, uterine atrophy, decreased ovarian weights, and suppression of LH levels.[22] These clinical findings seemed to mimic the findings in clinical studies of alcoholic women. Thus, there is clear evidence of the reproductive toxic effects of chronic alcohol exposure; however, the consequences of moderate alcohol use on fertility remain unclear. Therefore, the American Society of Reproductive Medicine states, "The effects of alcohol, marijuana and other recreational drugs have not been clearly established. Nevertheless, such drug use generally should be discouraged for both men and women, particularly because they have well-documented harmful effects on the developing fetus." In addition, because there are no clear guidelines for when and who to test, it is always recommended to discourage such behavior at the initial fertility consult.

Cannabinoids

Cannabinoids have been extensively studied both in humans and in animal models. It has been proven that it or its major psychoactive constituent, tetrahydrocannabinol (THC), causes symptoms of neurobehavioral alterations, interrupts all phases of gonadal or reproductive function, and is toxic to the fetus. In women who abuse marijuana, they were noted to have shorter menstrual cycles (26.8 days) than those who did not (28.8 days).[23–25] In addition, marijuana users had more cycles that were anovulatory or had a shorter luteal phase when compared with nonusers. THC causes suppression of plasma LH levels and appears to be the primary mechanism by which THC exposure inhibits ovulation. Because gonadotropin-releasing hormone–induced LH secretion is not impacted by exposure to THC, the action of this drug appears at the hypothalamic axis rather than the actual hypophysial site. The antiovulatory effect of THC results from an inhibition of LH secretion that does not involve the direct blockade of LHRH (LH-releasing hormone). In addition, when evaluating the levels, they did not reveal any statistically significant differences in serum LH, FSH, estrogen, or progesterone levels between marijuana users and non-marijuana users even though there were decreased luteal phase progesterone levels. Of note, serum prolactin levels were reduced, and serum testosterone levels were noted to be increased in the marijuana users. It has been suggested that the impact of THC may vary on the hormonal status of women. In menopausal women, THC did not alter the LH levels; however, in premenopausal women, there was a suppression of LH levels during the lute phase.[26] Although no clear long-term impact on fertility has been established, it is still recommended to avoid all marijuana use when trying to achieve pregnancy.

Marijuana use can impact fertility in men by decreasing plasma testosterone levels with chronic use. In chronic marijuana users, it has been shown that they have abnormal sperm morphology, including reduced nuclear size, increased condensation of chromatin, disorganization of acrosomal structure, and absence of acrosomes.[27] A study reported decreased testosterone plasma levels in men who had been smoking marijuana for 6 months before testing. However, giving hCG to marijuana users can increase testosterone levels, which indicates a functional Leydig cell response. In addition to this, if the man has a 2-week period of abstinence following marijuana use, their testosterone levels have been shown to increase or improve from the suppression caused by this abuse.[28] However, there has been little shown on the impacts of cannabinoids on the male reproductive tract. Changes in testis function have been noted after treatment with cannabinoids.

In an animal model, more specifically in rats, seminiferous tubule degeneration and degenerative changes in spermatocytes and spermatids were seen after exposure to marijuana. In mice that were given THC for only 5 days, there was a dose-dependent increase in abnormal sperm. In female rabbits, THC administration resulted in inhibition of ovulation.[29] In female rats, THC was shown to cause a delay of onset of puberty and reduce the number of ova.[30] Also, it has been shown that marijuana agonists can interfere with implantation of the mouse embryo in vitro. There is sufficient evidence to show that THC can act directly and impact the ovary. It has been shown that THC exposure reduces ovarian responsivity to LH in experimental animal models. THC-inhibited progesterone synthesis was seen in rat luteal cell cultures in in vitro experiments; however, when this was done in vivo, daily administration of THC had no effect on plasma progesterone levels or luteal phase length.[31] Other animal studies showed that tolerance develops to the disruptive effects of THC on the primate menstrual cycle and that despite chronic use of THC, reversible suppressive effects of the drug on the menstrual cycle can occur.[32] Long-term exposure of sexually mature female rhesus monkeys to 3 weekly injections of THC resulted in a disruption of the menstrual cycle that persisted for several months. The disruption in the menstural cycle was noted by the absence of ovulation and decreased basal concentrations of gonadotropin and sex steroids levels in plasma. After several months, despite continued twice weekly administration with THC, normal cycles and hormone concentrations were restored. The restoration of a normal menstural cycle in the setting of regular THC exposure helps to explain the lack of cycle disruption in many women who are chronic users of cannabis. In addition to the impact on women, it can be safely stated that testicular and ovarian toxicity result with use of marijuana; however, the impact it has on future fertility remains unknown because their function does resume after discontinuation.

Caffeine

Caffeine, although a natural compound, has been noted to have a significantly negative impact on fertility and pregnancy. Once consumed, it can be readily absorbed and distributed throughout the body. It has been noted in saliva, breast milk, embryos, and even in the blood of neonates.[33] It is known to cause numerous amounts of biologic effects in the human, including CNS stimulation, increase in heart rate, relaxation of smooth muscles, and increased secretion of catecholamines. There are data, based both on animal and human studies, associating caffeine intake with spontaneous abortion, intrauterine growth retardation, birth defects, and possibly other toxic effects to the fetus. However, the impact of caffeine on other reproductive processes, including fertility itself, has been a focus of concern, yet there is no clear association. Biologic credibility for this theory is suggested by information that there are significant alterations in the reproductive hormone profile of users, that caffeine may hinder ovulation, and that its intake is positively correlated with sex hormone–binding globulin concentrations.[34] The impact of caffeine on human reproduction is proven by reports that show that daily consumption of the typical amount of caffeine found in a cup of coffee was associated with a 50% decrease in per menstrual cycle conception when compared with nonusers.[35] Women consuming greater quantities of caffeine had consistently lower pregnancy rates, thus demonstrating a dose-related effect. The association between ovulatory disorder infertility and consumption of caffeinated beverages failed to demonstrate any causality relationship between caffeine consumption, impaired ovulation, and decreased fertility.[35] Studies on the association between caffeine and miscarriages showed that an increase in daily caffeine intake may be associated with an increased risk of recurrent pregnancy loss. It has been shown by one study that an increased dose of daily caffeine intake of 200 mg or more during pregnancy increased the risk of miscarriage in the general population independent of pregnancy-related symptoms.[36] However, there are conflicting findings because other sources have failed to demonstrate the correlation between caffeine and miscarriage. The relationship between caffeine consumption by pregnant women and risk of miscarriage, low birth weight, preterm delivery, and congenital malformations found no evidence that caffeine consumption at moderate levels has any discernible adverse effect on pregnancy outcome.[37] It is considered that the previous warning on caffeine consumption and the risk of reproductive hazards were based on findings that gavage feeding of large doses of caffeine to rats resulted in a particularly high incidence of facial cleft palate. However, the latest review on the effects of restricted caffeine intake by mother on fetal, neonatal, and pregnancy outcome in Cochrane Database System Review found insufficient evidence to confirm or refute the effectiveness of caffeine avoidance on birth weight or other pregnancy outcomes.[36] Lack of scientific evidence showing any association between caffeine consumption and adverse effect on pregnancy outcome led the US Food and Drug Administration agency to conclude that caffeine, as currently used in foods, does not carry a health risk. However, the agency continues to recommend that pregnant women consume caffeine in moderation.

Caffeine could impact male fertility by changing sperm mobility and viability. There is a decrease in these parameters when consuming more than 699 mg/d of caffeine. In addition, a recent study showed that caffeinated soda and energy drink intake was associated with reduced fecundability in men.[38] In an animal model, male rats were shown to have decreased reproductive organ weight, sperm characteristics, LH/FSH levels, and also testicular cytoarchitecture; however, these effects were reversible after caffeine withdrawal.[39]

In summary, the data regarding the effects of caffeine on reproduction in humans are still conflicting. Although it is not possible to give a clear recommendation on specific amounts that are deemed safe for couples trying to conceive, it would be best to consume no more than 3 cups of coffee per day. This recommendation should be discussed at the first infertility visit and reassured with the patient because there is no way to monitor caffeine levels. The American College of Obstetricians and Gynecologists recommends that pregnant women limit consumption to the caffeine equivalent of 1 to 2 cups of coffee (200 mg of caffeine). Given the high prevalence of caffeine intake by women of childbearing age, it is clear that further research is required and guidelines on testing are needed.

Tobacco

Smokers expose themselves and people around them to numerous amounts of toxins and carcinogens. Cigarette smoke has many carcinogens, including, cadmium, arsenic, butane, ammonia, lead, acetone, carbon monoxide, pesticide residue, polycyclic aromatic hydrocarbons, and formaldehyde.[40] The most addictive component, nicotine, can lead to problems such as vasoconstriction, can cause decreased tissue oxygenation, remain in blood, urine, saliva, and follicular fluid, and impact other reproductive functions.[41] Previous measurements in the serum and follicular fluid of cigarette smokers show correlation with decreased pregnancy rates in women exposed to smoke as compared with nonsmokers. In addition, the presence of cadmium has also been shown in human ovaries and follicular fluid of smokers, proving that essential organs responsible for reproduction are exposed and affected by the products of tobacco smoke in smokers.[42] It has been shown that cigarette smoke can alter reproduction as evidenced by numerous animal and human studies.

Animal studies have shown that cadmium can impact cellular processes leading to chromosomal anomalies in both oocytes and embryos which can lead to a decrease in the number of oocytes, potentially alter embryo development and thus decreasing fertility. Also, many animal studies have proven that cigarette smoke leads to an increased rates of follicular destruction and accelerates ovarian aging leading to premature reproductive failure.[43] This reproductive failure has been proven by human studies showing that women who smoke have an increased loss of ovarian follicles and decreased ovarian reserve, leading to an earlier menopause[44] as well as high basal or stimulated FSH levels signifying decreased ovarian function. Cigarette smoke has also been shown to decrease human granulosa cell aromatase production, leading to decreased estrogen levels, which cause the elevated FSH.[45,46] Cigarettes can also alter meiotic maturation of oocytes, which may cause chromosomal abnormalities and alter fetal health or even cause spontaneous abortions.[47] Surveys have shown that it takes smokers longer to conceive than nonsmokers, as noted with the decrease in fertility with increasing numbers of cigarettes smoked per day. In utero exposure to cigarette smoke also can result in a decreased fecundability in the man.[48] Smoking cessation products that contain the same concentrations of nicotine can cause the same sequelae as smoking cigarettes, including risk of low birth weight, overweight offspring, insulin resistance, and hypertension.[49]

Women who smoke while being treated with assisted reproduction have decreased gonadotropin-stimulated estradiol production, resulting in fewer numbers of oocytes retrieved and resultant embryos, a 50% decrease in implantation and ongoing pregnancy rate.[50,51] Spontaneous abortion rates are also increased in these patients.[52] In addition, these patients have an increased risk of ectopic pregnancy.[53] However, this effect is temporary, because past smokers have pregnancy rates similar to non-smokers after 3 months of quitting.[54]

Smoking also impacts male fertility, causing decreased volume, sperm density, total count, and normal forms, although the impact of smoking might not be sufficient to impact male fertility in a functional capacity.[55] Nonetheless, evidence strongly suggests that cigarette smoking leads to a decrease in fertility and impacts assisted reproductive technology success and outcomes due to ovarian toxicity and decreased implantation rates. Because of the aforementioned, women pursuing conception should be advised to avoid exposure to cigarette smoke. Because quitting completely may be impossible for some smokers, decreasing the amount should be encouraged. Cessation of smoking is an integral part of preconception counseling and even at the first prenatal visit. Despite all these facts, no test has been established or required to test the level of nicotine in a patient's blood or other body fluids at either preconception or during pregnancy.

Endocrine Disorders and Toxicology

Polycystic ovarian syndrome (PCOS) is a common disorder characterized by features of hyperandrogenism, obesity, acanthosis nigrans, possible insulin resistance, and polycystic or enlarged ovaries on ultrasound. There is no theory behind why one may be prone to developing PCOS. One possible cause is that environmental contaminants may play a role in the development of PCOS. Environmental toxins have been noted in follicular fluid, and bisphenol A (BPA) was seen in both the serum and the follicular fluid with a concentration between 1 and 2 ng/mL fluid.[56] Serum BPA concentrations of patients with PCOS were also higher in women with PCOS when compared to aged matched controls. Interestingly, there is also a positive correlation between higher BPA and serum testosterone, androstenedione, and dehydroepiandrosterone sulfate, which are androgens and tend to be higher in PCOS patients as well.[57] This may possibly be due to the effect of androgens on the metabolism of BPA. Although there is strong evidence of higher BPA levels in patients with PCOS, the exact pathophysiology remains unknown. Further research needs to be conducted to reveal the underlying relationship between the development of PCOS and role of environmental toxins. Although patients are advised to limit exposure to environmental toxins, there are currently no laboratory screening tests nor guidelines to determine what analytes in particular, and levels of such may be detrimental to reproduction.

Endometriosis, another disease that may cause infertility or potentially subfertility, is characterized by endometrial glands and stroma outside the uterine cavity. It causes infertility and affects about 14% of women of all reproductive ages.[58] There are several theories leading to the development of endometriosis, including coelomic metaplasia, proliferation of a progenitor stem cell, or retrograde menstruation of endometrial cells.[59] Despite which theory one looks at, they all are thought to lead to the implantation and proliferation of ectopic endometrial cells outside the uterine cavity. Because this disease is estrogen dependent, the role of environmental toxins has gained much attention over the recent years. Several studies have reported a strong relationship between dioxin in the pathophysiology of endometriosis.[60,61]

Several occupations may have an increased risk of infertility due to exposure of toxins, such as those involved in the agriculture and chemical industries.[62] At the initial visit, it is crucial to ask about occupation and to counsel patients to limit interaction with any potential harmful toxins. Because there are no currently developed guidelines or laboratory tests available, counseling remains the best mode of action to improve reproductive outcomes.

SUMMARY

Human reproduction depends on a complex series of time-sensitive events. Despite the crucial and time-dependent integration of these events achieved by hormonal signaling, exogenous factors do play a role and may dysregulate this process. Because it remains almost impossible to attribute a single outcome to a single substance, as one may abuse multiple ones such as alcohol and caffeine, the crucial part lies in the dose and timing of exposures and the mechanism of action of the agent to determine the insult. It is not uncommon for many reproductive age humans to be exposed over multiple years to high doses of ethanol, opiates, cannabinoids, nicotine, and caffeine. However, exposure to environmental toxins still remains low, and the association of such toxins to reproductive health is still difficult to establish. There is strong support from data that alcohol, opiates, cannabinoids, cigarette smoke, and caffeine can negatively impact reproductive homeostasis. To this end, toxicology testing for established substances (alcohol, opioids, cannabinoids, and other illicit agents) can provide an objective understanding of a patient's ingestion and exposure habits as it relates to general health and fertility counseling, in particular. However, further research needs to be conducted to establish the levels at which select current and emerging new agents might start impacting reproductive capabilities and how toxicology laboratory tests should be incorporated into the workup and management of an infertile patient.

REFERENCES

1. Anderson K, Nisenblat V, Norman R. Lifestyle factors in people seeking infertility treatment—a review. Aust N Z J Obstet Gynaecol 2010;50(1):8–20.
2. Sadeu JC, Hughes CL, Agarwal S, et al. Alcohol, drugs, caffeine, tobacco, and environmental contaminant exposure: reproductive health consequences and clinical implications. Crit Rev Toxicol 2010;40(7):633–52.
3. Nair P, Rothblum S, Hebel R. Neonatal outcome in infants with evidence of fetal exposure to opiates, cocaine, and cannabinoids. Clin Pediatr (Phila) 1994; 33(5):280–5.
4. Finnegan LP, Wapner RJ. Your CE topic this month (no. 3). Drug abuse in pregnancy. J Pract Nurs 1984;34(2):14–23.
5. Oei J, Lui K. Management of the newborn infant affected by maternal opiates and other drugs of dependency. J Paediatr Child Health 2007;43(1–2):9–18.
6. Abel EL, Moore C, Waselewsky D, et al. Effects of cocaine hydrochloride on reproductive function and sexual behavior of male rats and on the behavior of their offspring. J Androl 1989;10(1):17–27.
7. Mello NK, Mendelson JH, Kelly M, et al. The effects of chronic cocaine self-administration on the menstrual cycle in rhesus monkeys. J Pharmacol Exp Ther 1997;281(1):70–83.
8. Smith CG. Drug effects on male sexual function. Clin Obstet Gynecol 1982;25(3): 525–31.
9. Ragni G, De Lauretis L, Bestetti O, et al. Gonadal function in male heroin and methadone addicts. Int J Androl 1988;11(2):93–100.
10. Ragni G, De Lauretis L, Gambaro V, et al. Semen evaluation in heroin and methadone addicts. Acta Eur Fertil 1985;16(4):245–9.
11. Yelian FD, Sacco AG, Ginsburg K, et al. The effects of in vitro cocaine exposure on human sperm motility, intracellular calcium, and oocyte penetration. Fertil Steril 1994;61(5):915–21.

12. Cone EJ, Kato K, Hillsgrove M. Cocaine excretion in the semen of drug users. J Anal Toxicol 1996;20(2):139–40.

13. George VK, Li H, Teloken C, et al. Effects of long-term cocaine exposure on spermatogenesis and fertility in peripubertal male rats. J Urol 1996;155(1):327–31.

14. Spohr HL, Willms J, Steinhausen HC. Fetal alcohol spectrum disorders in young adulthood. J Pediatr 2007;150(2):175–9.e1.

15. Rementeria JL, Bhatt K. Withdrawal symptoms in neonates from intrauterine exposure to diazepam. J Pediatr 1977;90(1):123–6.

16. Hakim RB, Gray RH, Zacur H. Alcohol and caffeine consumption and decreased fertility. Fertil Steril 1998;70(4):632–7.

17. Rettori V, Skelley CW, McCann SM, et al. Detrimental effects of short-term ethanol exposure on reproductive function in the female rat. Biol Reprod 1987;37(5): 1089–96.

18. Lloyd CW, Williams RH. Endocrine changes associated with Laennec's cirrhosis of the liver. Am J Med 1948;4(3):315–30.

19. Lester R, Van Thiel DH. Gonadal function in chronic alcoholic men. Adv Exp Med Biol 1977;85A:399–413.

20. Van Thiel DH, Gavaler JS, Lester R, et al. Plasma estrone, prolactin, neurophysin, and sex steroid-binding globulin in chronic alcoholic men. Metabolism 1975; 24(9):1015–9.

21. Kucheria K, Saxena R, Mohan D. Semen analysis in alcohol dependence syndrome. Andrologia 1985;17(6):558–63.

22. Mello NK, Bree MP, Mendelson JH, et al. Alcohol self-administration disrupts reproductive function in female macaque monkeys. Science 1983;221(4611): 677–9.

23. Brents LK. Marijuana, the endocannabinoid system and the female reproductive system. Yale J Biol Med 2016;89(2):175–91.

24. Mendelson JH, Mello NK, Ellingboe J, et al. Marijuana smoking suppresses luteinizing hormone in women. J Pharmacol Exp Ther 1986;237(3):862–6.

25. Alvarez S. Do some addictions interfere with fertility? Fertil Steril 2015;103(1): 22–6.

26. Mendelson JH, Cristofaro P, Ellingboe J, et al. Acute effects of marihuana on luteinizing hormone in menopausal women. Pharmacol Biochem Behav 1985;23(5): 765–8.

27. Hembree WC 3rd, Nahas GG, Zeidenberg P, et al. Changes in human spermatozoa associated with high dose marihuana smoking. Adv Biosci 1978;22–23: 429–39.

28. Kolodny RC, Masters WH, Kolodner RM, et al. Depression of plasma testosterone levels after chronic intensive marihuana use. N Engl J Med 1974; 290(16):872–4.

29. Asch RH, Fernandez EO, Smith CG, et al. Precoital single doses of delta9-tetrahydrocannabinol block ovulation in the rabbit. Fertil Steril 1979;31(3):331–4.

30. Wenger T, Croix D, Tramu G, et al. Marijuana and reproduction. Effects on puberty and gestation in female rats. Experimental results. Ann Endocrinol (Paris) 1992;53(1):37–43 [in French].

31. Symons AM, Teale JD, Marks V. Proceedings: effect of delta9-tetrahydrocannabinol on the hypothalamic-pituitary-gonadal system in the maturing male rat. J Endocrinol 1976;68(3):43P–4P.

32. Marks BH. Delta1-tetrahydrocannabinol and luteinizing hormone secretion. Prog Brain Res 1973;39:331–8.

33. Sieber SM, Fabro S. Identification of drugs in the preimplantation blastocyst and in the plasma, uterine secretion and urine of the pregnant rabbit. J Pharmacol Exp Ther 1971;176(1):65–75.
34. Petridou E, Katsouyanni K, Spanos E, et al. Pregnancy estrogens in relation to coffee and alcohol intake. Ann Epidemiol 1992;2(3):241–7.
35. Chavarro JE, Rich-Edwards JW, Rosner BA, et al. Caffeinated and alcoholic beverage intake in relation to ovulatory disorder infertility. Epidemiology 2009; 20(3):374–81.
36. Jahanfar S, Sharifah H. Effects of restricted caffeine intake by mother on fetal, neonatal and pregnancy outcome. Cochrane Database Syst Rev 2009;(2):CD006965.
37. Leviton A, Kuban KC, Pagano M, et al. Maternal toxemia and neonatal germinal matrix hemorrhage in intubated infants less than 1751 g. Obstet Gynecol 1988; 72(4):571–6.
38. Wesselink AK, Wise LA, Rothman KJ, et al. Caffeine and caffeinated beverage consumption and fecundability in a preconception cohort. Reprod Toxicol 2016;62:39–45.
39. Oluwole OF, Salami SA, Ogunwole E, et al. Implication of caffeine consumption and recovery on the reproductive functions of adult male Wistar rats. J Basic Clin Physiol Pharmacol 2016. [Epub ahead of print].
40. Jensen JA, Goodson WH, Hopf HW, et al. Cigarette smoking decreases tissue oxygen. Arch Surg 1991;126(9):1131–4.
41. Younglai EV, Foster WG, Hughes EG, et al. Levels of environmental contaminants in human follicular fluid, serum, and seminal plasma of couples undergoing in vitro fertilization. Arch Environ Contam Toxicol 2002;43(1):121–6.
42. Zenzes MT, Krishnan S, Krishnan B, et al. Cadmium accumulation in follicular fluid of women in in vitro fertilization-embryo transfer is higher in smokers. Fertil Steril 1995;64(3):599–603.
43. Watanabe T, Shimada T, Endo A. Mutagenic effects of cadmium on mammalian oocyte chromosomes. Mutat Res 1979;67(4):349–56.
44. Mattison DR, Singh H, Takizawa K, et al. Ovarian toxicity of benzo(a)pyrene and metabolites in mice. Reprod Toxicol 1989;3(2):115–25.
45. Sharara FI, Beatse SN, Leonardi MR, et al. Cigarette smoking accelerates the development of diminished ovarian reserve as evidenced by the clomiphene citrate challenge test. Fertil Steril 1994;62(2):257–62.
46. Barbieri RL, McShane PM, Ryan KJ. Constituents of cigarette smoke inhibit human granulosa cell aromatase. Fertil Steril 1986;46(2):232–6.
47. Windham GC, Von Behren J, Waller K, et al. Exposure to environmental and mainstream tobacco smoke and risk of spontaneous abortion. Am J Epidemiol 1999; 149(3):243–7.
48. Weinberg CR, Wilcox AJ, Baird DD. Reduced fecundability in women with prenatal exposure to cigarette smoking. Am J Epidemiol 1989;129(5):1072–8.
49. Gao YJ, Holloway AC, Zeng ZH, et al. Prenatal exposure to nicotine causes postnatal obesity and altered perivascular adipose tissue function. Obes Res 2005; 13(4):687–92.
50. Van Voorhis BJ, Dawson JD, Stovall DW, et al. The effects of smoking on ovarian function and fertility during assisted reproduction cycles. Obstet Gynecol 1996; 88(5):785–91.
51. Neal MS, Hughes EG, Holloway AC, et al. Sidestream smoking is equally as damaging as mainstream smoking on IVF outcomes. Hum Reprod 2005;20(9): 2531–5.

52. Maximovich A, Beyler SA. Cigarette smoking at time of in vitro fertilization cycle initiation has negative effect on in vitro fertilization-embryo transfer success rate. J Assist Reprod Genet 1995;12(2):75–7.

53. Waylen AL, Metwally M, Jones GL, et al. Effects of cigarette smoking upon clinical outcomes of assisted reproduction: a meta-analysis. Hum Reprod Update 2009; 15(1):31–44.

54. Howe G, Westhoff C, Vessey M, et al. Effects of age, cigarette smoking, and other factors on fertility: findings in a large prospective study. Br Med J (Clin Res Ed) 1985;290(6483):1697–700.

55. Vine MF, Tse CK, Hu P, et al. Cigarette smoking and semen quality. Fertil Steril 1996;65(4):835–42.

56. Jarrell JF, Villeneuve D, Franklin C, et al. Contamination of human ovarian follicular fluid and serum by chlorinated organic compounds in three Canadian cities. CMAJ 1993;148(8):1321–7.

57. Takeuchi T, Tsutsumi O, Ikezuki Y, et al. Positive relationship between androgen and the endocrine disruptor, bisphenol A, in normal women and women with ovarian dysfunction. Endocr J 2004;51(2):165–9.

58. Chedid S, Camus M, Smitz J, et al. Comparison among different ovarian stimulation regimens for assisted procreation procedures in patients with endometriosis. Hum Reprod 1995;10(9):2406–11.

59. Halme J, Hammond MG, Hulka JF, et al. Retrograde menstruation in healthy women and in patients with endometriosis. Obstet Gynecol 1984;64(2):151–4.

60. Rier S, Foster WG. Environmental dioxins and endometriosis. Toxicol Sci 2002; 70(2):161–70.

61. Foster WG, Agarwal SK. Environmental contaminants and dietary factors in endometriosis. Ann N Y Acad Sci 2002;955:213–29 [discussion: 230–2, 396–406].

62. Anger DL, Foster WG. The link between environmental toxicant exposure and endometriosis. Front Biosci 2008;13:1578–93.

Ketamine

A Cause of Urinary Tract Dysfunction

Frank Anthony Myers Jr, MD[a], Martin H. Bluth, MD, PhD[b,c],
Wellman W. Cheung, MD[a],*

KEYWORDS

- Ketamine • Urology • Urinary Tract Dysfunction • Inflammation • Bladder • Illicit

KEY POINTS

- Lower urinary tract symptoms such as urgency, frequency, dysuria, and hematuria are common urologic complaints in men and women and the differential remains broad.
- Illicit ketamine abuse is a growing problem and can lead to a cystitis symptom complex that mimics common genitourinary complaints.
- Ketamine abuse induces complex changes to the environment of the urinary tract, specifically the bladder, that can be observed clinically and at the molecular level.
- Currently, there is no standard for diagnosing and treating ketamine induced cystitis, however, treatment currently involves symptom management.
- More investigations should be done to develop standard and/or individually targeted diagnostic and treatment protocols for this emerging cause of cystitis.

INTRODUCTION

According to the 2014 national survey on drug use and health, approximately hundreds of thousands of people in the United States aged 12 and over have used illicit substances of varying types.[1] Drug addiction is a chronic relapsing disorder, and people who suffer with it tend to demonstrate binge use, intoxication, withdrawal associated with a negative emotional state, and anticipation of substance use that modifies the brain reward and stress systems.[2] The association between reward and stress has been demonstrated previously. For example, using a mouse model, Piazza and colleagues[3] found that when mice were injected with corticosterone, self-administration frequency increased, particularly at higher doses. Interestingly, in

Disclosures: Nothing to disclose.
[a] Department of Urology, State University of New York Downstate Medical Center, 450 Clarkson Avenue, Brooklyn, NY 11203, USA; [b] Department of Pathology, Wayne State University School of Medicine, 540 East Canfield, Detroit, MI 48201, USA; [c] Consolidated Laboratory Management Systems, 24555 Southfield Road, Southfield, MI 48075, USA
* Corresponding author.
E-mail address: Wellman.cheung@downstate.edu

Clin Lab Med 36 (2016) 721–744
http://dx.doi.org/10.1016/j.cll.2016.07.008
0272-2712/16/© 2016 Elsevier Inc. All rights reserved.

labmed.theclinics.com

this study, the investigators also found that different animals had different propensities to self-administer the steroids based on their individual sensitivities to drugs of abuse.

The neurobiological basis of addiction involves a complex array of circuitry and brain structures, and a detailed discussion of this topic is beyond the scope of this work. In brief, the mesocorticolimbic dopamine system involves forebrain structures like the nucleus accumbens, the midbrain's ventral tegmental area, and the amygdala, and is critical in modulating the reinforcing actions of many drugs of abuse (**Fig. 1**).

Aside from dopamine, other molecules like glutamate, dynorphin, corticotrophin-releasing factor, neuropeptide Y, and endocannabinoid also appear to be involved.[2,4-6]

It is estimated that the lifetime prevalence for any prescription opiate use disorder in treated patients with chronic pain is approximately 42%.[7] Other substances are also abused. For example, in a sample of 921 patients with prescriptions for opiates, a portion of these patients had promethazine- and benzodiazepine-positive urine. Of these individuals, only 50% had prescriptions for promethazine. In addition, the finding of benzodiazepine-positive urine without a prescription for it was associated with illicit promethazine use.[8] Because of these kinds of findings, clinicians must be conscious of the abuse of other classes of medications.

In the urologic setting, a commonly abused drug that is becoming more of a problem worldwide is ketamine (**Fig. 2**).

Ketamine is important to the urologist because it can adversely impact the lower urinary tract. In addition, the clinical and objective findings can mimic a commonly

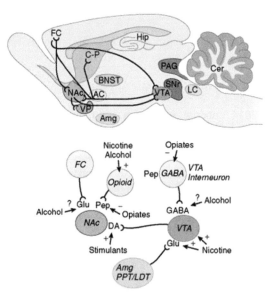

Fig. 1. Substances of abuse and complex interactions of brain neurocircuits. AC, anterior commissure; Amg, amygdala; BNST, bed nucleus stria terminalis; Cer, cerebellum; C-P, caudate-putamen; DA, dopamine; FC, cerebrofrontal cortex; Glu, glutamate; Hip, hippocampus; LC, locus ceruleus; NAc, nucleus accumbens; PAG, periaqueductal gray; Pep, opioid peptides; PPT/LDT, peduncular pontine tegmentum/lateral dorsal tegmentum; SNr, substantia nigra pars reticulata; VP, ventral pallidum; VTA, ventral tegmental area. (*From* Choi DS, Karpyak VM, Frye MA, et al. Drug addiction. In: Waldman SA, editor. Pharmacology and therapeutics: principles to practice. Philadelphia: Elsevier Saunders; 2009. p. 821; with permission.)

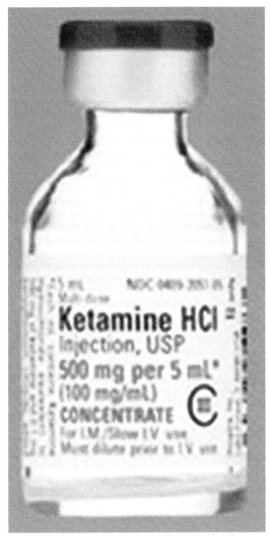

Fig. 2. Ketamine prescription. (*From* AccessMedicine Drug Monographs Online Database. Available at: www.accessmedicine.mhmedical.com/drugs.aspx. Accessed June 5, 2016; with permission.)

encountered urologic chronic pain syndrome called bladder pain syndrome/interstitial cystitis (BPS/IC). This presents a unique dilemma for the urologist or any clinician managing these kinds of urologic problems, which tend to be chronic in nature. In this work, the toxicology of ketamine, primarily from a urologic frame of reference, is discussed.

KETAMINE

Ketamine, also called "K," "Special K," "Vitamin K," or "Kiddy Smack" to name a few pseudonyms, is an *N*-methyl-ᴅ-aspartate (NMDA) receptor antagonist (**Fig. 3**).[9–13]

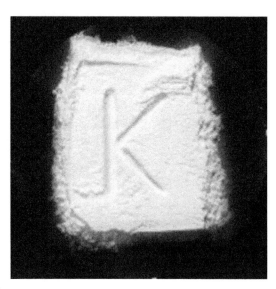

Fig. 3. Ketamine.

In the central nervous system (CNS), NMDA receptors reside on cation-gated channels that respond to the excitatory neurotransmitter glutamate, rendering these channels permeable to calcium and causing depolarization of neurons (**Fig. 4**).[11,14]

Other excitatory amino acids, such as glycine, are also thought to interact with the NMDA receptor. It is thought that NMDA receptors responding to glutamate influence some of these other neuronal circuits through GABAergic neurons and inhibit them.[11,12,15]

N-METHYL-D-ASPARTATE RECEPTORS AND KETAMINE

NMDA receptors are present throughout the CNS, including the cerebral cortex, cerebellum, brain stem, and spinal cord, and appear to be crucial in the processing of complex communication at the neuronal level. The limbic system, for example, is important in regulating memory, emotion, and subsequent integration with sensory input and becomes affected by the administration of ketamie.[11]

KETAMINE AS AN ILLICIT SUBSTANCE

According to the World Health Organization (WHO) in 2012, approximately 1.1% of the Australian population had abused ketamine at some point in their life and less than 2% of youths in Denmark had used ketamine. At that time, 19 countries worldwide reported illicit activities related to ketamine, with the United States and China reporting the largest seizures of the substance.[16] That same year, up to 1.5% of US high school students reported ketamine use.[17] Interestingly, as per the WHO, in some African countries, there were no reports of ketamine abuse.[16]

As per the US Drug Enforcement Agency (DEA), drugs, or chemicals used to make drugs, are classified into 5 categories (or schedules) depending on medical uses for the drug and the drug's potential for abuse or dependency. Essentially, the higher the schedule, the lower the potential for abuse.[18] Ketamine has been a schedule III drug in the United States since 1999 and has been associated with recreational drug abuse for more than 30 years.[17,19]

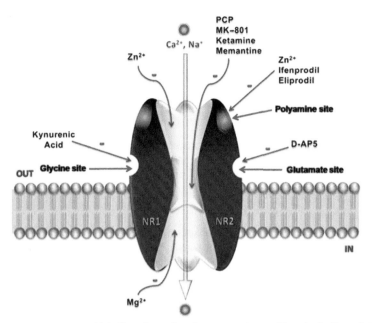

Fig. 4. NMDA receptor and binding sites of various neurotransmitters including glutamate. Mg^{2+}, MK-801, ketamine, PCP, and memantine act as noncompetitive antagonists whose binding sites are within the ion channel pore region. (*From* Ghasemi M, Schachter SC. The NMDA receptor complex as a therapeutic target in epilepsy: a review. Epilepsy Behav 2011;22(4):618; with permission.)

In certain Asian cities and countries, ketamine has had a huge impact. In Hong Kong for example, ketamine has become a common drug of abuse, surpassing opiates, which were formerly responsible for most of the problems associated with illegal drugs in that city.[20] In Taiwan, ketamine use is popular among high school students and is part of a popular drug sequence called "Trinity," which includes the use of MDMA/ecstasy, followed by ketamine and then marijuana.[21] Although several investigators have reported on ketamine abuse in Asian populations,[10,22–26] it is important to note that ketamine abuse is also seen in non-Asian populations. In a US cohort of 23 patients who reported chronic ketamine use, 57% were Caucasian/White, 22% were Latino/Hispanic, and 17% were biracial, compared with only 4% who were Asian.[27] This finding suggests that a ketamine use may not follow any ethnic predilections.

In nonclinical settings, ketamine has been obtained illegally typically from medical offices and has been sold in 10-mL bottles for as much as $200.[28] Ketamine can be snorted, mixed in drinks, injected, smoked, or inhaled as a powder; however, intramuscular (IM), rectal, and oral (PO) formulations also exist, and in these forms, the drug is absorbed relatively quickly.[9–11,17,28–32] Lankenau and Clatts[27] interviewed 40 young injection drug users from New York City, assessing their injection practices, and found that the route of administration varies with the individual.

When used in a recreational setting, the ketamine doses vary. According to the US National Highway Traffic Safety Administration, dosages for the IM, intranasal, and PO routes are 25 to 50 mg, 30 to 75 mg, and 75 to 300 mg, respectively.[31] According to the DEA, an average street dose is 100 mg.[17] In one case report, a 35-year-old woman reported 2 to 3 mL IM per day and gradually progressed to 10 to 20 mL IM per day.[33]

For illicit production of ketamine, which has a reputation of being laborious, the substances cyclohexanone, methylamine and chlorobenzene, o-chlorobenzonitrile, and cyclopentyl bromide are thought to be a few precursors with several other solvents used in the synthesis process.[20] The purity of "street" ketamine is questionable, and at least 2 analogues have been found on the black market with effects lasting longer than ketamine itself.[31,34]

KETAMINE PHARMOKINETICS AND METABOLISM: CONTROLLED SETTING

Although up to 30% is bound to plasma proteins, ketamine itself is highly lipid soluble and can quickly cross the blood-brain barrier to redistribute throughout body tissues.[13,29,35,36] Ketamine has a pK_a of 7.5, and under normal circumstances, can be administered as a racemic mixture, the active S isomer and inactive R isomer. The R isomer can inhibit the S isomer, and as such, formulations with only the S isomer exist (**Fig. 5**).[34,37]

The liver and the kidneys are sights of ketamine metabolism, and concurrent use of medications that rely on the same pathways impact ketamine processing.[11,13,37,38] For example, Lo and Cumming[38] demonstrated that the ketamine-induced sleep time in patients that were premedicated with diazepam, hydroxyzine, and secobarbital, all metabolized by liver, were approximately 137 ± 3.8 minutes, 138 ± 9.2 minutes, and 128 ± 4.7 minutes, respectively, in comparison to 98.5 ± 4.4 minutes in those not premedicated ($P<.05$). The plasma half-life of ketamine

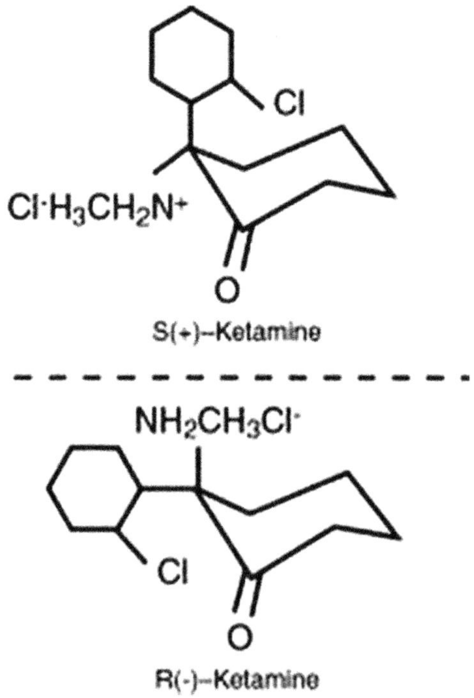

Fig. 5. Ketamine enantiomers (The molecular formula of ketamine hydrochloride, C13H16ClNOHCl). (*From* Blaise GA. Ketamine. In: Murray MJ, editor. Faust's anesthesiology review. Philadelphia: Elsevier Saunders; 2015. p. 166; with permission.)

was also increased in a statistically significant manner when coadministered with these same medications.

Approximately 80% of ketamine is metabolized to norketamine by microsomal enzymes. Norketamine is of particular importance, because this metabolite has been shown to have about 35% the biologic activity of ketamine itself. In addition, after intravenous (IV) administration, norketamine appears in blood approximately 2 to 3 minutes after administration and reaches peak concentrations in about half an hour. Other ketamine metabolites formed (to lesser degrees) include 4-OH-ketamine and 5-OH-ketamine.[37] These metabolites can be biologically active and contribute to lower urinary tract abnormality (**Fig. 6**).[39–41]

When used in the clinical setting, ketamine administration routes include IV, IM, rectal, PO, and intranasal.[11,35,37] Intranasal administrations can be dosed from 3 to 8 mg/kg/dose depending on age; rectal administration can be dosed 4 to 10 mg/kg/dose, and PO forms can be dosed at 6 to 8 mg/kg/dose. Of note, PO, rectal, and intranasal routes are commonly used in younger patients. For IV and IM formulations, dosages from 1 to 4.5 mg/kg and 5 to 13 mg/kg, respectively, have been used. Onsets of action for intranasal, PO, IM, and IV formulations are 5 to 8 minutes, within 30 minutes, 3 to 25 minutes, and immediate to 10 minutes, respectively. The bioavailability for ketamine for the IM route is about 93% with peak plasma concentration obtained in about 5 minutes. Because of hepatic metabolism, bioavailability for the PO route is around 20% to 30% with a plasma concentration peak in up to 30 minutes. Intrarectal ketamine administration demonstrates bioavailability of about 25% with peak concentrations achieved at about 45 minutes, and intranasal bioavailability is about 25% with peak concentrations in 20 minutes. The half-life of ketamine can be up to 3 hours depending on aroute.[35,37]

LABORATORY DETECTION OF KETAMINE

Ketamine and some of its derivatives have been detected in hair, urine, and blood,[29,42,43] however primarily in urine and blood. Ketamine and norketamine have been detected in urine for 5 and 6 days, respectively. Dehydronorketamine, another metabolite, has been detected for up to 10 days.[41] Examples of detection methods include gas and liquid chromatography and mass spectrometry (MS).[39,44] In a recent report by Moreno and colleagues[42] using gas chromatography-tandem mass spectrometry (GS-MS), the investigators were able to identify ketamine and norketamine in artificial laboratory–produced samples of 0.25 mL with high recoveries of the compounds. The investigators extracted the target compounds using a technique referred

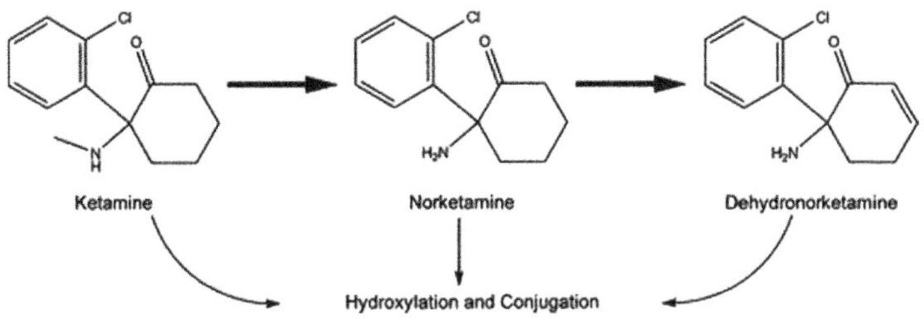

Fig. 6. Molecular structure of ketamine and its metabolites. (*From* Bairros AV, Lanaro R, Almeida RM, et al. Determination of ketamine, norketamine and dehydronorketamine in urine by hollow-fiber liquid-phase microextraction using an essential oil as supported liquid membrane. Forensic Sci Int 2014;243:48; with permission.)

to as microextraction by packed sorbent (MEPS). Of note, the researchers applied these same methods to samples of suspected ketamine abusers, and ketamine and norketamine were not detected. The investigators thought that the likely reason that these metabolites were not detected was because they were no longer present in the body at the time of sampling. The researchers then administered ketamine intraperitoneally at 50 mg/mg to one rat and obtained plasma and urine samples 1 hour following administration. The metabolites were identified in both samples and the investigators concluded that their method provides a quick and effective approach to detect ketamine and norketamine in biological fluid samples, with specific usefulness in the field of forensic toxicology.

EFFECTS

Along with phencyclidine, or PCP, which is commonly called "angel dust,"[23,30] ketamine belongs to a class of drugs called arylcyclohexylamines and is typically used as a dissociative anesthetic.[11,30,34,45,46] Several synthetic agents have emerged within this same drug class. Some of these agents include methoxetamine, 3-methoxy-PCP, 4-Meo-PCP, Diphendine, and methoxyphenidine and provide similar dissociative effects as PCP and ketamine.[46]

Ketamine also exhibits analgesic properties by binding mu opioid receptors and has proven beneficial in palliative care patients for analgesia.[11,17,47] Ketamine has agonist activity at α and β receptors, antagonist activity at muscarinic receptors in the CNS, and has been shown to prevent the uptake of catecholemines.[11,12] Research has also shown that ketamine may also have antidepressant properties; however, this indication has been questioned.[30]

Many potential side effects of ketamine have been described, including cardiopulmonary, neuropsychological, and neuromuscular symptoms.[11,15,30,48–50] Following ketamine infusions, elevated systolic and diastolic blood pressures and increased heart rate can be seen.[30,48] There has also been suggestion that ketamine causes arrhythmias; however, the evidence is somewhat controversial. Some investigators have proposed that the reason for the hemodynamic changes following ketamine administration may be secondary to a centrally acting mechanism, specifically, ketamine's demonstrated ability to block the reuptake of catecholemines.[11]

Ketamine appears to have respiratory effects as well.[11,49] Hamza and colleagues[49] demonstrated a statistically significant decrease in the CO_2 response curves (minute ventilation/end-tidal CO_2) of 9 children ages 6 to 10 years undergoing lower abdominal or minor reconstructive procedures treated with an IV bolus of ketamine followed by a continuous infusion compared with controls. The investigators state that the respiratory depressant effects of ketamine appear to be similar in their cohort of children as has been shown in adults. Care should also be taken when ketamine is coadministered with other agents because synergistic effects have been reported.[11,51]

Psychotropic effects, such as intense euphoria and dissociation, can be experienced with ketamine and are some of the most well-known side effects of the drug.[30] At lower doses, hallucinations can be experienced; however, at higher doses of greater than 150 mg, a severe dissociative state called the "K Hole" occurs.[9,50] The "K Hole" experience can be dampened with administration of certain medications like benzodiazepenes.[52]

As stated earlier, glutamate, acting through γ-aminobutyric acid (GABA)ergic NMDA receptors throughout the CNS, maintain the tonic inhibition of multiple excitatory neuronal circuits. It is thought that in certain individuals with hypofunctioning glutamate-mediated NMDA receptors, there is an inability to inhibit activity of neurons in the corticolimbic system, leading to psychosis. Olney and Farber[15] suggest that NMDA receptor antagonists like ketamine produce a similar situation. Furthermore, the investigators suggest that structural changes in the brains of rats with hypofunctioning NMDA receptors demonstrated structural changes similar to those with schizophrenia. In a separate review, Li and colleagues[50] state that the brains of chronic ketamine users demonstrate a reduced volume of gray matter in the frontal cortex bilaterally, similar to those with schizophrenia. These findings explain the psychosis-like effects of ketamine by highlighting similarities with a condition characterized by similar symptoms.

KETAMINE AND BLADDER PAIN SYNDROME/INTERSTITIAL CYSTITIS

Aside from the cardiopulmonary and neurologic effects, ketamine can cause genitourinary dysfunction, especially urothelial dysfunction. This dysfunction can mimic a common urologic condition known as BPS/IC (**Fig. 7**).[22]

BPS/IC has been defined as an unpleasant sensation (pain, pressure, discomfort) perceived to be related to the urinary bladder, associated with lower urinary tract symptoms of more than 6 weeks' duration, in the absence of infection or other identifiable causes.[53] BPS/IC can be associated with flares that have a physical and emotional impact on the patient. Different definitions have been used over the years for clinical and research purposes; however, depending on the definition used, one can see prevalence from 1% to almost 3%. Women tend to be affected more than men. Some studies quote incidence as high as almost 7% in women.[54] Those with a lower socioeconomic status are more impacted compared with their counterparts.[55]

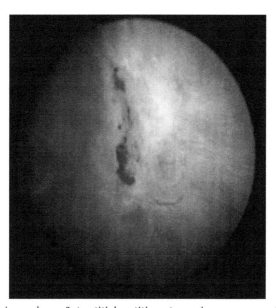

Fig. 7. Bladder pain syndrome/Interstitial cystitis cystoscopic appearance. (*From* Quillin RB, Erickson DR. Management of interstitial cystitis/bladder pain syndrome: a urology perspective. Urol Clin N Am 2012;39(3):391. © 2011, American Urological Association Education and Research, Inc; with permission.)

UROTHELIUM

The urothelium is usually composed of at least 3 to 6 layers of cells at different stages of differentiation.[56,57] From basal to superficial, these layers include basal cells, intermediate cells, and "umbrella" cells. The umbrella cells on the apical surface of the urothelium prevent the penetration of ions and toxins from the urine through bladder tissue with the aid of tight junction proteins and a cytoskeleton acting as scaffolding (**Fig. 8**).[58]

Some of these proteins include the cytoplasmic zonula occludens-1 and membrane proteins called claudins and occludins, which can also be decreased in bladders exposed to noxious substances like ketamine.[59–61] The superficial umbrella cells themselves are composed of proteins called uroplakins.[57,61,62]

Although relatively impermeable, normal urothelium is highly flexible, accommodating large changes in volume.[62,63] The urothelium as a whole contains a significant amount of glycosylation, with the luminal surface containing a matrix of sugars and proteins called glycocalyx.[57] Glycocalyx also contributes to its barrier function.

Exterior to the urothelium, the layers of the bladder include the lamina propria, muscularis mucosa, muscularis propria, and serosa.[58,64,65] The term "mucosa" generally refers to urothelium, lamina propria, and muscularis mucosa and contains both sensory and motor nerves within it that respond to various neurotransmitters.[56,64–67] It is thought that these nerve fibers work in conjunction with a nonselective ion channel called transient receptor potential vanilloid subfamily 1 (TRPV1), which has been shown to mediate noxious bladder stimuli and high-frequency bladder contractions occurring during pathologic conditions using an animal model (**Fig. 9**).[68]

KETAMINE AND THE LOWER URINARY TRACT

The impact of ketamine on the genitourinary tract has been documented clinically, and with objective measures like voiding diaries, imaging, histologic examinations, cystoscopy, video urodynamics, and even semen analyses (**Figs. 10–12**).[10,19,22–24,26,32,61,69–77]

Shahani and colleagues[36] provided what is thought to be one of the earliest descriptions of ketamine-associated lower urinary tract dysfunction in 2007. The investigators described the associated genitourinary symptoms of 9 ketamine users. Each patient had similar findings on cystoscopy, which typically demonstrated erythematous

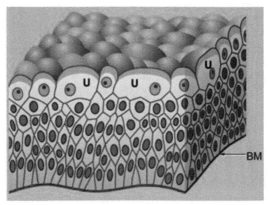

Fig. 8. Urothelium. U, umbrella cells; BM, basement membrane. (*From* Young B, O'Dowd G, Woodford P. Epithelial tissues. In: Wheater's functional histology. Elsevier Churchill Livingstone; 2014. p. 82–100; with permission.)

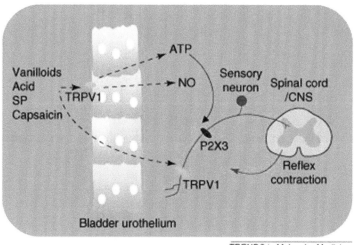

Fig. 9. TRPV1 receptor and neurogenic bladder. NO, nitric oxide; P2X3, a type of purine receptor; SP, substance P. (*From* Khairatkar-Joshi N, Szallasi A. TRPV1 antagonists: the challenges for therapeutic targeting. Trends Mol Med 2009;15(1):17; with permission.)

ulcerated patches. Four of the patients underwent bladder biopsies. In all of the specimens, the urothelial mucosa appeared to be denuded with evidence of a thin layer of reactive epithelium. With respect to the lamina propria, the superficial aspect was edematous with an abundance of inflammatory cells and granulation tissue. The deeper aspect of the lamina propria was fibrotic. In the stroma, many eosinophils were noted along with mast cells.

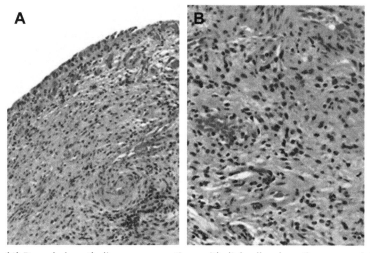

Fig. 10. (*A*) Denuded urothelium, regenerating epithelial cells, ulcerations, granulation tissue, and inflammatory cells (hematoxylin-eosin, original magnification ×10). (*B*) Stroma showing eosinophils, mast cells, and lymphocytes (hematoxylin-eosin, original magnification ×100).

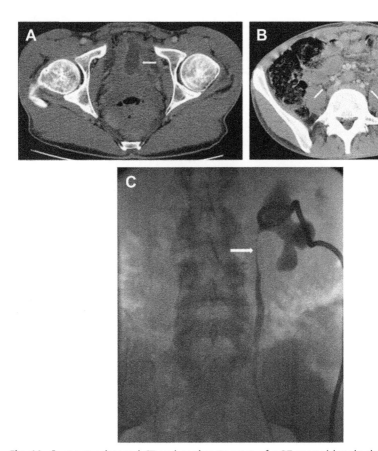

Fig. 11. Contrast-enhanced CT and nephrostogram of a 27-year-old male chronic ketamine abuser with (*A*) thickened bladder wall, (*B*) dilated ureters bilaterally, (*C*) nephrostogram demonstrating narrowing of proximal ureter and dilation of collecting system. Please see corresponding arrows. (*From* Mason K, Cottrell AM, Corrigan AG, et al. Ketamine-associated lower urinary tract destruction: a new radiological challenge. Clin Radiol 2010;65(10):799; with permission.)

All patients demonstrated some degree of irritative urinary symptoms and painful hematuria. Improvement with cessation of ketamine use was noted in only some subjects. Computed tomographic (CT) scans of the abdomen and pelvis demonstrated thickened and contracted bladders.

In a cohort of 10 patients from Hong Kong who abused ketamine chronically (1–4 years), urgency with and without incontinence, dysuria, frequency, and hematuria were noted in all patients. Each patient, aged 20 to 30 years, had total bladder capacities of 30 to 100 mL, and 7 patients had documented detrusor over activity on urodynamic studies.[10] In 2008, the same lead author retrospectively looked at 59 patients with moderate to severe lower urinary tract symptoms. They found that 71% of the cohort had cystoscopic examinations showing many different degrees of epithelial inflammation and neovascularization. Biopsies were performed on 12 patients, and histologic examinations generally revealed denuded epithelium and a lamina propria with granulation tissue and infiltrates of eosinophils and lymphocytes. The average bladder capacity was approximately 150 mL; however, 51% of the 59 patients had

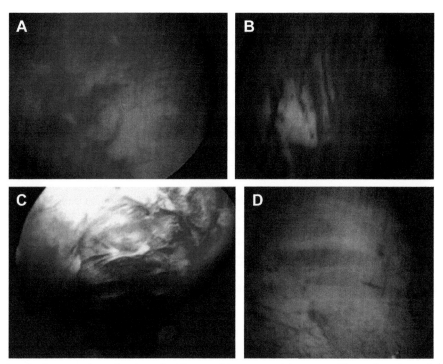

Fig. 12. Cystoscopic evaluation of a 23-year-old woman with 1 year of ketamine abuse: (*A*) erythematous lesions, (*B*) diffuse hemorrhage postdistention, (*C*) ulcerated mucosa, (*D*) bladder perforation. (*From* Chen CH, Lee MH, Chen YC, et al. Ketamine-snorting associated cystitis. J Formos Med Assoc 2011;110(12):788; with permission.)

bladder capacities less than 150 mL. The investigators noted that most of the participants had reduced bladder compliance and detrusor over activity at volumes as low as 14 mL. Approximately 50% of the study subjects had either unilateral or bilateral hydronephrosis on renal ultrasound; 7% had radiologic features suggestive of papillary necrosis, and 8 patients had elevated serum creatinine levels. The specific causes of ketamine-induced lower urinary tract dysfunction remain unknown. The investigators go on to surmise possible theories that could account for the lower urinary tract damage sustained from ketamine exposure. First, they state that ketamine's impact on the lower urinary tract may be secondary to direct toxic effects, causing significant edema and an inflammatory response, leading to some of the clinical and histopathological effects noted. Second, they suggested that ketamine exposure causes changes in the microvascular of the bladder and kidney, leading to endothelial cell dysfunction and compromised circulation. The findings of neovascularity and papillary necrosis support this idea. The investigators also suggest that the presence of ketamine or its metabolites in the urine may induce an autoimmune response and induce some of the findings noted in bladders exposed to ketamine.[22] Lai and colleagues[23] also demonstrated similar lower urinary tract symptoms and reduced bladder capacities, in addition to hydronephrosis.

Using a mouse model, Song and colleagues[75] also demonstrated ketamine's deleterious impact on the lower urinary tract. Forty-two rats were evenly distributed into 6 groups, 5 with increasing concentrations of IV ketamine chloride at 1, 5, 10, 25, and 50 mg/kg and one control group, wherein phosphate-buffered saline was used. The investigators compared various cystometric parameters, histology, and apoptotic changes 2 weeks following administration. With respect to cystometric parameters, the investigators found that the voiding intervals and the bladder capacities tended to decrease in a statistically significant manner as the ketamine concentration increased compared with the control group. Bladder compliance, maximum micturition pressure, and residual urine volume did not significantly differ between groups. Histologically, the thickness of fibrosis in the urothelium increased significantly directly proportional to the amount of ketamine that each mouse was exposed to. When staining for cytokeratin, an epithelium-specific protein, the bladders exposed to ketamine demonstrated less.

APOPTOSIS

Ketamine impacts the urothelium's ability to make new cells and has been shown to induce apoptosis. Apoptosis, a complex interplay of cellular functions that leads to programmed cell death, is typically mediated by a cascade of proteases called caspases.[78,79] Cytochrome C, a mitochondrial protein involved in the respiratory chain located on inner mitochondrial membrane,[61,80] is released and triggers some of these caspases.[78] On the contrary, the bcl-2 protein, located on the outer membrane of the mitochandria, has been implicated in the prevention of apoptosis through an unknown mechanism **(Fig. 13)**.[81,82]

Several studies have demonstrated ketamine's ability to induce apoptosis of urothelial cells by demonstrating high levels of caspase activity, decreased expression of bcl-2, by demonstrating reduced urothelial cell counts in bladders exposed to ketamine at different concentrations and for varying periods of time, and/or with special staining techniques.[61,73,75,83–85]

Using a human tissue engineered bladder model and cultured urothelial cells, Bureau and colleagues[85] examined the impact of ketamine on the bladder urothelium. Bladders were exposed to ketamine-soaked filter paper at increasing concentrations and incubated for 48 hours before being compared with controls. The investigators assessed the amount of caspase-3, a marker for apoptosis, using a fluorescence assay kit for the same single layer of urothelial cells. The concentrations of ketamine used were 1.5, 5, and 10 mM. Increasing amounts of caspase activity at higher

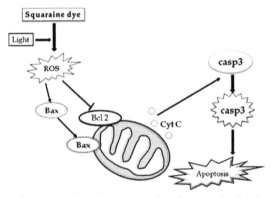

Fig. 13. Regulation of apoptosis. BAX, BCL2 associated X protein; BCL2, B-cell lymphoma 2; casp 3, caspase-3; Cyt c, cytochrome c; ROS, reactive oxygen species. (*From* Devi DG, Cibin TR, Abraham A. Bis(3,5-diiodo-2,4,6-trihydroxyphenyl) squaraine photodynamic therapy induces in vivo tumor ablation by triggering cytochrome c dependent mitochondria mediated apoptosis. Photodiagnosis Photodyn Ther 2013;10(4):516; with permission.)

concentrations of ketamine were noted. Of note, there was no difference in caspase activity at the highest concentration of ketamine used in the study, 10 mM. The investigators also noted a reduced amount of urothelial cells at higher ketamine concentrations with what appeared to be apoptotic bodies within the cells.

In their study, Song and colleagues[75] used terminal dUTP nick end-labeling staining to assess the level of apoptosis in ketamine-exposed bladders. The amount of apoptotic cells were increased compared with controls. The investigators also found that the BAX protein, indicative of apoptosis, and tumor necrosis factor-α, a marker for inflammation, were both upregulated in the bladders of the groups exposed to ketamine, and these findings were statistically significant.

Liu and colleagues[61] also demonstrated similar findings, in the urothelium, the detrusor muscle itself, and the bladder interstitium in subjects chronically exposed to ketamine. In their study, 48 rats were randomized to a control group that received either 0.5 mL normal saline intraperitoneally for either 2 or 4 weeks or study groups receiving 25 mg/kg/d of ketamine for either 2 or 4 weeks. Mitochondrial and endoplasmic reticulum (ER) –mediated apoptotic pathways were involved with the clinical findings associated with chronic ketamine use. Similar to the findings by Bureau and colleagues,[85] apoptotic urothelial cells in the groups exposed to ketamine were also noted using special staining techniques. The proapoptosis proteins cytochrome c and caspases 3, 8, and 9 were present at significantly higher concentrations in those study subjects exposed to ketamine for longer periods of time compared with controls. Furthermore, the ER chaperone protein Glucose Regulated Protein 78 (GRP78) and the ER protein C/EBP Homologous Protein (CHOP), associated with apoptosis, were significantly increased in those exposed to ketamine compared with controls.[61] GRP78 is an ER protein that regulates this organelle's ability to combat cell stress, such as the abnormal processing of misfolded proteins, in an adaptive process called the "Unfolded Protein Response." Although this mechanism is meant to promote cell survival, prolonged stress can lead to apoptosis through the CHOP protein.[86] The investigators also found that the antiapoptotic protein bcl-2 was significantly decreased in study subjects compared with controls.

NEUROPATHOLOGY

Pathologic neuroanatomy within the urothelium itself results from ketamine exposure. In 21 patients with ketamine-induced cystitis, prominent nerve fibers were noted within the lamina propria.[87] Approximately 95% of subjects had nerve fibers that stained positive for neurofilament protein compared with 3 of 21 patients in other BPSs. Peripheral nerve fascicle hyperplasia was also noted in 20 of 21 subjects with ketamine-induced cystitis compared with their counterparts. Jhang and colleagues[32] also demonstrated increased nerve tissue in bladder urothelium exposed to ketamine.

OXIDATION

It has been suggested that oxidation may a play a prime role in several types of bladder abnormalities. In a study by Abraham and colleagues,[88] rats treated with cyclophosphamide, a cause of hemorrhagic cystitis, demonstrated decreased activity of several antioxidant enzymes compared with those pretreated with the antioxidant aminoguanidin. As another example, with partial bladder obstruction, the levels of protein carbonylation and nitrotyrosine, both markers for oxidative stress, increase as these bladders move toward decompensation. It has also been shown that symptoms associated with hyperactive detrusor can be dampened with administration of reactive oxygen species scavengers.[89] The study by Liu and colleagues[61] addressed this idea and examined the impact that ketamine has on oxidative stress markers and mitochondrial reactive oxidative species in relation to the bladder's urothelium. In this study, the oxidative stress markers nitrotyrosine and 2,4-dinitriphenol were significantly higher in study subjects treated with ketamine. Of note, nitrotyrosine levels were seen even after shorter exposure times. The antioxidants superoxide dismutase (SOD), which catalyzes superoxide to peroxide, and catalase, which forms oxygen and water from peroxide after its generation by SOD, were decreased in bladders of the study participants after assessing messenger RNA (mRNA) expressions and polymerase chain reactions. In fact, expression levels of some of the antioxidants were as low as 40% less in those treated with ketamine for 1 month compared with controls. The investigators even reported significantly increased expressions of certain mitochondrial respiratory enzyme complexes that contribute to the generation of reactive oxygen species in those treated with ketamine, suggesting a potential role of the generation of these toxic molecules secondary to ketamine use.

INFLAMMATION

Treating ketamine's destruction of the lower urinary tract tends to be empiric and is usually similar to BPS/IC,[25,90,91] although some potential strategies do exist. For example, interest in anti-inflammatory therapies has surfaced given the inflammatory histologic and cystoscopic findings. In a retrospective study, Lin and colleagues[24] performed urothelial biopsies on 23 Taiwanese patients with a self-reported history of ketamine abuse and confirmed cystitis. The samples were then immunostained to assess for cyclo-oxygenase-2 (COX-2), inducible nitric oxide synthase (iNOS), matrix metallopeptidase-9, mammalian target of rapamycin, and phosphorylated 40s ribosomal protein S6 (Phos-S6). The investigators stratified the degree of inflammation as mild, moderate, or severe. The immunostains were all positive. The investigators also noted immunopositive stains in vessel walls and smooth muscle. Of note, the amount of COX-2 differed significantly between the different levels of inflammation, with the amount of COX-2 proportional to the degree of inflammation. The amount of iNOS staining differed significantly between the different degrees of inflammation in smooth muscle tissue only. There was also a positive correlation between the amount of inflammation and Phos-S6 ($P = .001$). Juan and colleagues[90] also found that COX-2 is upregulated in the tissue of lower urinary tracts exposed to ketamine and one of its metabolites norketamine, facilitated by the transcription factor nuclear factor kappa light chain enhancer of activated B cells (NF-kB). The investigators divided 36 rats into 3 groups, receiving saline, ketamine with the COX-2 inhibitor parecoxib, or ketamine alone, all intraperitoneally. The investigators found that in the group treated with ketamine alone, detrusor hyperactivity, reduced bladder capacity, and increased interstitial fibrosis, as well as increased mRNA and protein levels of NF-kB and COX-2, were higher compared with controls. These effects were not as pronounced in the group receiving ketamine with the COX-2 inhibitor. Because of the above findings, these investigators and others[22] have questioned the role that anti-inflammatory drugs may play in ketamine cystitis.

TREATMENT AND ABSTINENCE

Formal approaches to treatment (including abstinence[76]) of ketamine-associated lower urinary tract dysfunction have been explored in an attempt to halt or reverse the detrimental impact that ketamine has on the urinary tract. Yee and colleagues[25] examined a 4-tier treatment approach in 463 patients with ketamine lower urinary tract dysfunction who presented to their institution between December 2011 and June 2014. Follow-up data were present for approximately 68.9%. First-line therapy included nonsteroidal anti-inflammatory drugs (NSAIDs) and anticholinergics. Phenazopyridine and paracetamol were used for analgesia in this tier. Opiates and pregabalin were second-line treatments. Eight weeks of intravesical therapy with sodium hyaluronate was considered third-line therapy. If symptoms were still severe and patients could maintain ketamine abstinence for 6 months, surgical therapy to include hydrodistention or augmentation cystoplasty was considered the last line of therapy. On the first visit, serum creatinine, uroflowmetry, and urinalysis and culture were performed. Functional bladder capacity (FBC) was also calculated. The investigators assessed patient symptoms using the pelvic pain and urgency or frequency score (PUF) and EuroQol visual analog scale (EQ VAS). Ultrasonography of the urinary tract was used to assess for obstructive uropathy. The patients were further subdivided into 3 groups based on abstinence. Group 1 became abstinent before attending the clinic; group 2 patients became abstinent after attending the clinic, and patients in group 3 were active ketamine users at last follow-up. Mean follow-up was 10.7 ± 8.5 months. Two hundred ninety patients underwent first-line therapy, and 42 patients had second-line therapy with significant improvements in PUF, EQ VAS, and FBC. The amount of ketamine used and abstinence status were significant predictors of first-line treatment failure on multivariate analysis. A total of 17 patients required third-line therapy; however, only 8 completed the treatment. Of these patients, 5 were able to decrease the amount of PO medications taken. One patient underwent hydrodistention and another had an augmentation cystoplasty. Overall, the investigators reported 109 adverse effects, primarily secondary to anticholinergics. The investigators conclude that NSAIDs and anticholinergics in conjunction with abstinence from ketamine could potentially be an effective treatment for ketamine-associated urinary dysfunction.

STAGING

Some investigators have even postulated a clinical staging system to classify patients with ketamine-associated dysfunction of the urinary tract with implications for treatment. Wu and colleagues[91] retrospectively examined 81 hospitalized patients with ketamine-associated urinary dysfunction from January 2008 to June 2014. Patients were stratified into 3 stages based on history of ketamine use, approximate amount, renal and liver function, bladder wall thickening, decreased bladder capacity, ureteral wall thickening, ureteral dilation, and hydronephrosis. The 3 stages included I, inflammatory stimulation; II, initial bladder fibrosis; and III, end-stage bladder fibrosis and contracture. Voided volume, micturition interval, nocturnal void frequency, and symptom assessment scores were evaluated after treatment. Stage I patients received behavioral modification treatment to include cessation of ketamine, dietary restrictions, and bladder training. Medical therapy for patients in this stage included antibiotics, glucocorticoids, antihistamines, antioxidants, and anticholinergics. Stage II patients received intravesical hydrodistention with heparin, lidocaine, and sodium bicarbonate. Stage III patients received augmentation cystoplasty or cystectomy with urinary diversion if medical therapies and/or hydrodistention failed. Of note, stage II and III patients with ureteral strictures and hydronephrosis received ureteral stents. In total, there were 24, 47, and 10 patients in stages I, II, and III, respectively. All patients in each stage demonstrated statistically significant improvements in void volume, micturition interval, nocturnal void frequency, and symptom scores. The investigators conclude that their staging system may serve as a tool for assessing progression of ketamine-associated urinary tract dysfunction progression and stage-based treatment that could avoid inappropriate interventions.

PROPOSED INITIAL ASSESSMENT/LABORATORY ASSESSMENT OF KETAMINE

Although no specific algorithm for the assessment and management of ketamine abusers exists, the authors would like to propose a reasonable strategy based on the literature presented in this work. As with other medical conditions, management should start with a history and physical examination. With respect to the history, a thorough substance use and abuse history and psychiatric assessment should be obtained in a nonjudgmental manner. Clinicians should ascertain the formulation of ketamine used, duration of use, frequency, and any use of other illicit substances. Any lower urinary tract symptoms such as hematuria, dysuria, frequency, urgency, incomplete emptying, or other obstructive symptoms should be noted. Any abnormal weight loss or other constitutional symptoms, especially in the setting of a tobacco use history, should be part of the assessment because urothelial cancer may also present with similar lower urinary tract symptoms. A validated symptom assessment may be helpful in characterizing the patient's symptoms. For the physical examination, a thorough skin assessment to identify any needle tracks, a focused abdominal examination (to assess suprapubic tenderness and distention and costovertebral tenderness) and genitourinary examination should be performed.

Clinicians should also obtain serum and urine studies to include comprehensive metabolic panel, human immunodeficiency virus testing (with patient consent), urinalysis with microscopy, and urine culture, and should strongly consider urine cytology. In addition, detecting ketamine or its metabolites in biologic fluid specimens can be an important part of the workup, especially in facilities with the capabilities to do so and with patients who endorse recent use. Many techniques for detection of ketamine and its metabolites have been used; however, they can be expensive, labor intense, and time consuming. These techniques also require organic solvents that can have an adverse impact on the environment. Moreno and colleagues[42] provide a validated, accurate, and precise method of detection using a combination of MEPS and GS-MS to detect ketamine and norketamine in blood and urine from small quantities with high recoveries. The methods outlined in their paper can serve as a method for the detection of ketamine and/or its metabolite(s) in suspected users. Please refer to the referenced paper for specific details of the procedure.

Mid and upper tract imaging is likely to be helpful, so the treating health care provider can consider obtaining an imaging study when no recent one is available (renal/bladder ultrasound or CT scan, preferably a CT urogram, especially if the patient has gross hematuria or >3 red blood cells per high power field on urinalysis; if patient has an iodinated contrast allergy or other contraindication to obtaining a CT scan, an MR urogram can be considered). Once the above steps are taken, the patient should then be referred to a urologist for a cystoscopic evaluation and urodynamics evaluation (to include uroflowmetry).

If the patient has any evidence of chronic kidney disease, clinicians should consider involving a nephrologist. Mental health counseling should be considered for addiction and substance abuse, and patients should be offered abstinence resources. A pain specialist may also play a role in the management of these patients. For symptomatic relief, clinicians can consider oxybutynin or mirabegron (consider prescribing after urodynamics evaluation), pain control with NSAIDs, COX-2 inhibitors, pregabalin, phenazopyridine, and/or opiates assuming no contraindications. For more refractory cases, urologists can consider intravesical therapies such as lidocaine and hydrodistention (similar to that recommended for BPS as per the American Urological Association guidelines). In rare cases, the urologist can consider augmentation cystoplasty.

SUMMARY

In conclusion, the abuse of the anesthetic ketamine is becoming more prevalent recreationally. The inappropriate use of ketamine presents a great dilemma to the urologist because of its negative impact on the urinary tract. From a clinical standpoint, the symptoms produced as a result of ketamine-associated lower urinary tract dysfunction mimic the common chronic pain syndrome called BPS/IC. BPS/IC is a very complex disease, and ketamine abuse is also complex. As a result, the treating physician must effectively integrate multiple aspects of the patient to ensure that the patient is being appropriately treated. Ketamine causes severe destruction to the urinary tract, specifically the bladder, ureters, and kidneys. Most patients are young and go on to develop debilitating changes to the urinary tract that can be demonstrated clinically through symptom score instruments, radiographically, and on cystoscopic and videourodynamic studies. Inflammatory and apoptotic changes can also be seen histologically. End-stage renal disease from upper tract obstruction is another very real threat to chronic ketamine users.

The literature regarding ketamine's impact on the urinary tract is relatively new, so it is likely that a more accurate characterization of long-term effects will become elucidated with time, and although unfortunate, as illicit ketamine use increases. One would presume that fibrosis is generally a permanent anatomic and functional alteration; however, ketamine abstinence does seem to have promising results with respect to prevention of progressive dysfunction. Whether abstinence can induce total reversal of the signs and symptoms of ketamine-associated lower urinary tract changes remains to be seen. What is clear is that ketamine use should be assessed and remain on the list of differential diagnoses in any patient presenting with lower urinary tract symptoms, cystometric findings suggestive of bladder dysfunction, and suspicious mid and upper tract radiographic findings.

Ketamine's deleterious impact of the urinary tract is a serious matter with an end result of poor quality of life, chronic pain, and even end-stage renal disease. By keeping this entity at the forefront of clinical suspicion in the appropriate situation, ketamine-associated urinary tract dysfunction can be identified, and it is hoped, halted in its tracks. Ketamine abuse as a cause of urinary dysfunction requires a multidisciplinary effort, because the psychosocial aspects of drug abuse and addiction need to be addressed along with the urologic aspects. More work needs to be done to better understand the natural history of the lower urinary tract dysfunction, progression, treatment, and prevention of ketamine-induced cystitis.

REFERENCES

1. 2014 National Survey on Drug Use and Health: Detailed Tables. 2015. Available at: http://www.samhsa.gov/data/s ites/default/files/NSDUH-DetTabs2014/NSDUH-DetTabs2014.pdf. Accessed June 5, 2016.
2. Koob GF, Mason BJ. Existing and future drugs for the treatment of the dark side of addiction. Annu Rev Pharmacol Toxicol 2016;56:299–322.
3. Piazza PV, Deroche V, Deminière JM, et al. Corticosterone in the range of stress-induced levels possesses reinforcing properties: implications for sensation-seeking behaviors. Proc Natl Acad Sci U S A 1993;90(24):11738–42.

4. Valdez GR, Koob GF. Allostasis and dysregulation of corticotropin-releasing factor and neuropeptide Y systems: implications for the development of alcoholism. Pharmacol Biochem Behav 2004;79(4):671–89.
5. Koob GF. Addiction is a reward deficit and stress surfeit disorder. Front Psychiatry 2013;4:72.
6. D'Souza MS. Glutamatergic transmission in drug reward: implications for drug addiction. Front Neurosci 2015;9:404.
7. Boscarino JA, Hoffman SN, Han JJ. Opioid-use disorder among patients on long-term opioid therapy: impact of final DSM-5 diagnostic criteria on prevalence and correlates. Subst Abuse Rehabil 2015;6:83–91.
8. Lynch KL, Shapiro BJ, Coffa D, et al. Promethazine use among chronic pain patients. Drug Alcohol Depend 2015;150:92–7.
9. Muetzelfeldt L, Kamboj SK, Rees H, et al. Journey through the K-hole: phenomenological aspects of ketamine use. Drug Alcohol Depend 2008;95(3):219–29.
10. Chu PS, Kwok SC, Lam KM, et al. 'Street ketamine'-associated bladder dysfunction: a report of ten cases. Hong Kong Med J 2007;13(4):311–3.
11. Bergman SA. Ketamine: review of its pharmacology and its use in pediatric anesthesia. Anesth Prog 1999;46(1):10–20.
12. Anis NA, Berry SC, Burton NR, et al. The dissociative anaesthetics, ketamine and phencyclidine, selectively reduce excitation of central mammalian neurones by N-methyl-aspartate. Br J Pharmacol 1983;79(2):565–75.
13. Ketamine (INN): update review report. Geneva. 2015.
14. Gu X, Zhou L, Lu W. An NMDA receptor-dependent mechanism underlies inhibitory synapse development. Cell Rep 2016;14(3):471–8.
15. Olney JW, Farber NB. Glutamate receptor dysfunction and schizophrenia. Arch Gen Psychiatry 1995;52(12):998–1007.
16. 35th Expert Committee on Drug Dependence, W.H.O. Ketamine: Expert peer review on critical review report (2). 2012. Available at: http://www.who.int/medicines/areas/quality_safety/4.2.2ExpertreviewKetaminecriticalreview.pdf. Accessed June 5, 2016.
17. Ketamine (Street names: Special K, "K", Kit Kat, Cat Valium). 2013. Available at: http://www.deadiversion.usdoj.gov/drug_chem_info/ketamine.pdf. Accessed June 5, 2016.
18. United States Drug Enforcement Administration, U.S.D.o.J. Available from: Available at: http://www.dea.gov/druginfo/ds.shtml. Accessed June 5, 2016.
19. Ho CC, Pezhman H, Praveen S, et al. Ketamine-associated ulcerative cystitis: a case report and literature review. Malays J Med Sci 2010;17(2):61–5.
20. Joe Laidler KA. The rise of club drugs in a heroin society: the case of Hong Kong. Subst Use Misuse 2005;40(9–10):1257–78.
21. Leung KS, Li JH, Tsay WI, et al. Dinosaur girls, candy girls, and Trinity: voices of Taiwanese club drug users. J Ethn Subst Abuse 2008;7(3):237–57.
22. Chu PS, Ma WK, Wong SC, et al. The destruction of the lower urinary tract by ketamine abuse: a new syndrome? BJU Int 2008;102(11):1616–22.
23. Lai Y, Wu S, Ni L, et al. Ketamine-associated urinary tract dysfunction: an under-recognized clinical entity. Urol Int 2012;89(1):93–6.
24. Lin HC, Lee HS, Chiueh TS, et al. Histopathological assessment of inflammation and expression of inflammatory markers in patients with ketamine-induced cystitis. Mol Med Rep 2015;11(4):2421–8.
25. Yee CH, Lai PT, Lee WM, et al. Clinical outcome of a prospective case series of patients with ketamine cystitis who underwent standardized treatment protocol. Urology 2015;86(2):236–43.

26. Yek J, Sundaram P, Aydin H, et al. The clinical presentation and diagnosis of ketamine-associated urinary tract dysfunction in Singapore. Singapore Med J 2015;56(12):660–5.

27. Lankenau SE, Clatts MC. Drug injection practices among high-risk youths: the first shot of ketamine. J Urban Health 2004;81(2):232–48.

28. Lankenau SE, Clatts MC. Ketamine injection among high risk youth: preliminary findings from New York City. J Drug Issues 2002;32(3):893–905.

29. Adamowicz P, Kala M. Urinary excretion rates of ketamine and norketamine following therapeutic ketamine administration: method and detection window considerations. J Anal Toxicol 2005;29(5):376–82.

30. Zhang MW, Harris KM, Ho RC. Is off-label repeat prescription of ketamine as a rapid antidepressant safe? Controversies, ethical concerns, and legal implications. BMC Med Ethics 2016;17(1):4.

31. Drugs and Human Performance Fact Sheet. Available at: http://www.nhtsa.gov/people/injury/research/job185drugs/ketamine.htm. Accessed June 5, 2016.

32. Jhang JF, Hsu YH, Kuo HC. Possible pathophysiology of ketamine-related cystitis and associated treatment strategies. Int J Urol 2015;22(9):816–25.

33. Avinash De Sousa AP, Macheswalla Y. Ketamine dependence: case report and review. J Pak Psychiatr Soc 2010;7(2):1.

34. Critical Review of Ketamine. 2006.

35. Ketamine, in AccessMedicine: Drug Monographs.

36. Shahani R, Streutker C, Dickson B, et al. Ketamine-associated ulcerative cystitis: a new clinical entity. Urology 2007;69(5):810–2.

37. Mion G, Villevieille T. Ketamine pharmacology: an update (pharmacodynamics and molecular aspects, recent findings). CNS Neurosci Ther 2013;19(6):370–80.

38. Lo JN, Cumming JF. Interaction between sedative premedicants and ketamine in man in isolated perfused rat livers. Anesthesiology 1975;43(3):307–12.

39. Chen CY, Lee MR, Cheng FC, et al. Determination of ketamine and metabolites in urine by liquid chromatography-mass spectrometry. Talanta 2007;72(3):1217–22.

40. Moore KA, Sklerov J, Levine B, et al. Urine concentrations of ketamine and norketamine following illegal consumption. J Anal Toxicol 2001;25(7):583–8.

41. Parkin MC, Turfus SC, Smith NW, et al. Detection of ketamine and its metabolites in urine by ultra high pressure liquid chromatography-tandem mass spectrometry. J Chromatogr B Analyt Technol Biomed Life Sci 2008;876(1):137–42.

42. Moreno I, Barroso M, Martinho A, et al. Determination of ketamine and its major metabolite, norketamine, in urine and plasma samples using microextraction by packed sorbent and gas chromatography-tandem mass spectrometry. J Chromatogr B Analyt Technol Biomed Life Sci 2015;1004:67–78.

43. Favretto D, Vogliardi S, Tucci M, et al. Occupational exposure to ketamine detected by hair analysis: a retrospective and prospective toxicological study. Forensic Sci Int 2016;265:193–9.

44. Lian K, Zhang P, Niu L, et al. A novel derivatization approach for determination of ketamine in urine and plasma by gas chromatography-mass spectrometry. J Chromatogr A 2012;1264:104–9.

45. Halberstadt AL, Slepak N, Hyun J, et al. The novel ketamine analog methoxetamine produces dissociative-like behavioral effects in rodents. Psychopharmacology (Berl) 2016;233(7):1215–25.

46. Backberg M, Beck O, Helander A. Phencyclidine analog use in Sweden–intoxication cases involving 3-MeO-PCP and 4-MeO-PCP from the STRIDA project. Clin Toxicol (Phila) 2015;53(9):856–64.

47. Storr TM, Quibell R. Can ketamine prescribed for pain cause damage to the urinary tract? Palliat Med 2009;23(7):670–2.

48. Geisslinger G, Hering W, Thomann P, et al. Pharmacokinetics and pharmacodynamics of ketamine enantiomers in surgical patients using a stereoselective analytical method. Br J Anaesth 1993;70(6):666–71.

49. Hamza J, Ecoffey C, Gross JB. Ventilatory response to CO2 following intravenous ketamine in children. Anesthesiology 1989;70(3):422–5.

50. Li JH, Vicknasingam B, Cheung YW, et al. To use or not to use: an update on licit and illicit ketamine use. Subst Abuse Rehabil 2011;2:11–20.

51. Roelofse JA, Roelofse PG. Oxygen desaturation in a child receiving a combination of ketamine and midazolam for dental extractions. Anesth Prog 1997;44(2): 68–70.

52. Mattila MA, Larni HM, Nummi SE, et al. Effect of diazepam on emergence from ketamine anaesthesia. A double-blind study. Anaesthesist 1979;28(1):20–3.

53. Hanno P, Dmochowski R. Status of international consensus on interstitial cystitis/bladder pain syndrome/painful bladder syndrome: 2008 snapshot. Neurourol Urodyn 2009;28(4):274–86.

54. Berry SH, Elliott MN, Suttorp M, et al. Prevalence of symptoms of bladder pain syndrome/interstitial cystitis among adult females in the United States. J Urol 2011;186(2):540–4.

55. Clemens JQ, Link CL, Eggers PW, et al. Prevalence of painful bladder symptoms and effect on quality of life in black, Hispanic and white men and women. J Urol 2007;177(4):1390–4.

56. Birder LA, Andersson KE, Kanai AJ, et al. Urothelial mucosal signaling and the overactive bladder-ICI-RS 2013. Neurourol Urodyn 2014;33(5):597–601.

57. Katnik-Prastowska I, Lis J, Matejuk A. Glycosylation of uroplakins. Implications for bladder physiopathology. Glycoconj J 2014;31(9):623–36.

58. Lazzeri M. The physiological function of the urothelium–more than a simple barrier. Urol Int 2006;76(4):289–95.

59. Langbein L, Grund C, Kuhn C, et al. Tight junctions and compositionally related junctional structures in mammalian stratified epithelia and cell cultures derived therefrom. Eur J Cell Biol 2002;81(8):419–35.

60. Acharya P, Beckel J, Ruiz WG, et al. Distribution of the tight junction proteins ZO-1, occludin, and claudin-4, -8, and -12 in bladder epithelium. Am J Physiol Renal Physiol 2004;287(2):F305–18.

61. Liu KM, Chuang SM, Long CY, et al. Ketamine-induced ulcerative cystitis and bladder apoptosis involve oxidative stress mediated by mitochondria and the endoplasmic reticulum. Am J Physiol Renal Physiol 2015;309(4):F318–31.

62. Wu XR, Kong XP, Pellicer A, et al. Uroplakins in urothelial biology, function, and disease. Kidney Int 2009;75(11):1153–65.

63. Smith NJ, Hinley J, Varley CL, et al. The human urothelial tight junction: claudin 3 and the ZO-1alpha switch. Bladder (San Franc) 2015;2(1):e9.

64. de Groat WC, Yoshimura N. Afferent nerve regulation of bladder function in health and disease. Handb Exp Pharmacol 2009;(194):91–138.

65. Chai TC, Russo A, Yu S, et al. Mucosal signaling in the bladder. Auton Neurosci 2015. [Epub ahead of print].

66. Kanai A, Andersson KE. Bladder afferent signaling: recent findings. J Urol 2010; 183(4):1288–95.

67. Hill WG. Control of urinary drainage and voiding. Clin J Am Soc Nephrol 2015; 10(3):480–92.

68. Charrua A, Cruz CD, Cruz F, et al. Transient receptor potential vanilloid subfamily 1 is essential for the generation of noxious bladder input and bladder overactivity in cystitis. J Urol 2007;177(4):1537–41.
69. Colebunders B, Van Erps P. Cystitis due to the use of ketamine as a recreational drug: a case report. J Med Case Rep 2008;2:219.
70. Chen CH, Lee MH, Chen YC, et al. Ketamine-snorting associated cystitis. J Formos Med Assoc 2011;110(12):787–91.
71. Mason K, Cottrell AM, Corrigan AG, et al. Ketamine-associated lower urinary tract destruction: a new radiological challenge. Clin Radiol 2010;65(10):795–800.
72. Tan S, Chan WM, Wai MS, et al. Ketamine effects on the urogenital system–changes in the urinary bladder and sperm motility. Microsc Res Tech 2011; 74(12):1192–8.
73. Lee CL, Jiang YH, Kuo HC. Increased apoptosis and suburothelial inflammation in patients with ketamine-related cystitis: a comparison with non-ulcerative interstitial cystitis and controls. BJU Int 2013;112(8):1156–62.
74. Gu D, Huang J, Yin Y, et al. Long-term ketamine abuse induces cystitis in rats by impairing the bladder epithelial barrier. Mol Biol Rep 2014;41(11):7313–22.
75. Song M, Yu HY, Chun JY, et al. The fibrosis of ketamine, a noncompetitive N-methyl-d-aspartic acid receptor antagonist dose-dependent change in a ketamine-induced cystitis rat model. Drug Chem Toxicol 2016;39(2):206–12.
76. Zeng M, Huang L, Tang Z, et al. A preliminary study on mechanisms for urinary system disorders before and after ketamine withdrawal in rats. Zhong Nan Da Xue Xue Bao Yi Xue Ban 2015;40(3):269–75 [in Chinese].
77. Yong GL, Kong CY, Ooi MW, et al. Resonance metallic ureteric stent in a case of ketamine bladder induced bilateral ureteric obstruction with one year follow up. Int J Surg Case Rep 2015;8c:49–51.
78. Kluck RM, Bossy-Wetzel E, Green DR, et al. The release of cytochrome c from mitochondria: a primary site for Bcl-2 regulation of apoptosis. Science 1997; 275(5303):1132–6.
79. Budd SL, Tenneti L, Lishnak T, et al. Mitochondrial and extramitochondrial apoptotic signaling pathways in cerebrocortical neurons. Proc Natl Acad Sci U S A 2000;97(11):6161–6.
80. DiMauro S, Schon EA. Mitochondrial respiratory-chain diseases. N Engl J Med 2003;348(26):2656–68.
81. Susin SA, Zamzami N, Castedo M, et al. Bcl-2 inhibits the mitochondrial release of an apoptogenic protease. J Exp Med 1996;184(4):1331–41.
82. Yang J, Liu X, Bhalla K, et al. Prevention of apoptosis by Bcl-2: release of cytochrome c from mitochondria blocked. Science 1997;275(5303):1129–32.
83. Wu P, Shan Z, Wang Q, et al. Involvement of mitochondrial pathway of apoptosis in urothelium in ketamine-associated urinary dysfunction. Am J Med Sci 2015; 349(4):344–51.
84. Huang L, Tang Z, Li D, et al. Ketamine induces apoptosis of human uroepithelial SV-HUC-1 cells. Zhong Nan Da Xue Xue Bao Yi Xue Ban 2014;39(7):703–7 [in Chinese].
85. Bureau M, Pelletier J, Rousseau A, et al. Demonstration of the direct impact of ketamine on urothelium using a tissue engineered bladder model. Can Urol Assoc J 2015;9(9–10):E613–7.
86. Flodby P, Li C, Liu Y, et al. GRP78 regulates ER homeostasis and distal epithelial cell survival during lung development. Am J Respir Cell Mol Biol 2016;55(1): 135–49.

87. Baker SC, Stahlschmidt J, Oxley J, et al. Nerve hyperplasia: a unique feature of ketamine cystitis. Acta Neuropathol Commun 2013;1:64.
88. Abraham P, Rabi S, Selvakumar D. Protective effect of aminoguanidine against oxidative stress and bladder injury in cyclophosphamide-induced hemorrhagic cystitis in rat. Cell Biochem Funct 2009;27(1):56–62.
89. Chien CT, Yu HJ, Lin TB, et al. Substance P via NK1 receptor facilitates hyperactive bladder afferent signaling via action of ROS. Am J Physiol Renal Physiol 2003;284(4):F840–51.
90. Juan YS, Lee YL, Long CY, et al. Translocation of NF-kappaB and expression of cyclooxygenase-2 are enhanced by ketamine-induced ulcerative cystitis in rat bladder. Am J Pathol 2015;185(8):2269–85.
91. Wu P, Wang Q, Huang Z, et al. Clinical staging of ketamine-associated urinary dysfunction: a strategy for assessment and treatment. World J Urol 2016;34: 1329–36.

Otolaryngology Concerns for Illicit and Prescription Drug Use

Nathan J. Gonik, MD, MHSA[a],*, Martin H. Bluth, MD, PhD[b,c]

KEYWORDS

- Otolaryngology • Codeine • Narcotic • Cocaine • Sinonasal • Black box

KEY POINTS

- Illicit drug use is common in patients presenting with routine otolaryngology complaints in the inpatient and outpatient settings.
- Medically recalcitrant sinonasal complaints may be related to illicit drug use and drug testing should include illegal drugs and commonly abused prescription narcotics.
- Routine drug testing should be considered for patients with septal perforation or necrosis of midline nasal and palatal structures.
- The FDA warning regarding codeine after pediatric adenotonsillectomy is related to variable codeine metabolism and concern for airway compromise.
- In cases of suspected codeine overdose, testing for the ratio of codeine:morphine metabolites and CYP2D6 allelic variations may identify an ultrametabolizer phenotype as the etiology.

INTRODUCTION

Concern for illicit and restricted drug use in otolaryngology is similar to other surgical specialties with a few notable exceptions. First, many illicit drugs are consumed transnasally. Repeated nasal exposure to stimulants or narcotics can cause local tissue destruction that can present as chronic rhinosinusitis or nasoseptal perforation. Care must be taken to ensure exposure to offending agents has ceased before attempting repair and consequently, otolaryngologists may insist on drug testing before proceeding to surgery. Second, the US Food and Drug Administration (FDA) has taken a stance against the use of certain prescription narcotics in pediatric

The author has nothing to disclose.
[a] Department of Otolaryngology Head and Neck Surgery, ENT Clinic, Children's Hospital of Michigan, Wayne State University School of Medicine, 3rd Floor Carl's Building, 3901 Beaubien Avenue, Detroit, MI 48201, USA; [b] Department of Pathology, Wayne State University School of Medicine, 540 East Canfield, Detroit, MI 48201, USA; [c] Consolidated Laboratory Management Systems, 24555 Southfield Road, Southfield, MI 48075, USA
* Corresponding author.
E-mail address: ngonik@dmc.org

Clin Lab Med 36 (2016) 745–752
http://dx.doi.org/10.1016/j.cll.2016.07.012   labmed.theclinics.com
0272-2712/16/© 2016 Elsevier Inc. All rights reserved.

patients undergoing adenotonsillectomy (AT). A black box warning has been issued on all codeine products, prohibiting their use in tonsillectomies under the age of 18. They have identified an increased risk of death postoperatively with these medications owing to pharmacogenomic properties. Because codeine has traditionally been the most commonly prescribed narcotic, this dramatic stance has shifted the standard practice. Pharmacogenomic testing has been advocated by many, but may not be an economical option.

SINONASAL MANIFESTATIONS OF ILLICIT DRUG USE

Sinus disease is often a disabling chronic condition manifested by nasal obstruction, recurrent infections, nasal discharge, and facial pain. Quality of life can be significantly impacted and patients seek frequent medical care. If medical management fails, which generally includes antibiotics, topical nasal steroids, and saline irrigations, surgery is indicated. Most patients have drastic improvement in sinonasal complaints after endoscopic sinus surgery. Several subsets of patients are predisposed to poor outcomes, including those with nasal manifestations of rheumatologic disease, immunocompromise, sinonasal polyposis, and those actively using illicit intranasal drugs. Before considering surgery in patients with possible drug-related pathology, it is helpful to understand the mechanism of injury and whether the insult is historical or ongoing. Thus, many surgeons require negative drug tests before proceeding with surgery.

Most surgeons underestimate the prevalence of illicit drug use in patients presenting for surgery. A study investigating drug use in patients sustaining maxillofacial trauma found that 47% of urine drug screens were positive despite few patients admitting to the activity.[1] The same researchers tested urine samples from the general population and found 2.5% tested positive for cocaine or amphetamines. Although surgery on patients with recent drug use can be performed, it requires careful anesthetic titrations and awareness by the entire surgical team.[2] Cocaine and amphetamines can cause cardiac arrhythmias owing to their sodium channel blockade. Prolonged QT, ventricular tachycardia, and torsade de pointes are common concerns. Benzodiazepine and narcotic use may potentiate the effects of analgesics administered at routine doses. Given the frequency of abuse in the general population, otolaryngologists should be aware of common manifestations of illicit drug use in patients with head and neck complaints.

Sinusitis and septal perforation related to illicit drugs were initially described in cases of cocaine abuse. Cocaine use is relatively common with 5% of 15- to 34-year-olds using cocaine recreationally; it is the fourth most common illegal drug used after marijuana, heroin, and ecstasy.[3] Its anesthetic properties derive from its ability to block sodium channels similar to amine local anesthetics.[4] Cocaine also has vasoconstrictive effects owing to blockage of catecholamine reuptake and metabolism. Intranasally, vasoconstriction can lead to thinning and ulceration of the nasal mucosa. The bony and cartilaginous septae of the sinonasal tract rely on the mucosal blood supply for oxygenation and nourishment. Prolonged exposure to vasoconstrictors leads to necrosis and degradation of these structures (**Figs. 1** and **2**). Cocaine additives, often including baking soda, ammonia, lidocaine, or other chemicals, cause inflammatory reactions that can lead to granulation and erosion. Cocaine also impairs ciliary function by reducing beat frequency and ciliary harmony.[5] Cilia are needed to clear debris and secretions from the sinus tracts. If debris stagnates, it can become trapped in sinus cavities leading to inflammation that mimics routine bacterial chronic sinusitis.

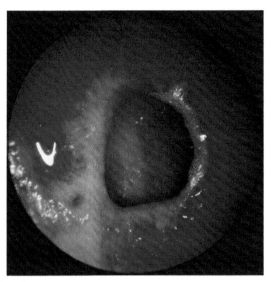

Fig. 1. Septal perforation.

After chronic topical use of short-acting vasoconstrictors, like cocaine, nasal mucosa becomes resistant to topical adrenergics. Rhinitis medicamentosa describes a clinical scenario in which mucosal blood vessels are desensitized to normal adrenergic levels and dilate and engorge at rest. The vessels return to normal caliber only when exposed again to concentrated adrenergics, and the effects are generally short lived. Patients then become dependent on topical vasoconstrictors for rhinitis recalcitrant to normal medical management. Because patients may not always see the true effects of their drug abuse, many will seek surgery to alleviate symptoms. However,

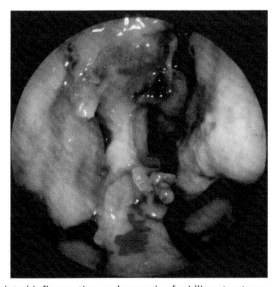

Fig. 2. Cocaine-related inflammation and necrosis of midline structures.

during endonasal surgery, short-acting vasoconstrictors are necessary to limit blood loss and facilitate a clean endoscopic approach. Chronic cocaine and amphetamine exposure cause resistance to local application of adrenergics, which can lead to increased operative blood loss and surgical misadventure.[6] Patients actively using drugs are also likely have poor healing and persistence of symptoms after surgery.

Recently, prescription narcotics have become more prevalent in illicit drug use. To hasten the effects of these narcotics, many users crush and inhale tablets of commonly prescribed pain medications including oxycodone, hydrocodone, and codeine. Despite the lack of inherent vasoconstrictive properties, this type of drug use causes similar nasal and sinus complications. Many authors have noted midline ulceration, chronic sinusitis, hyposmia, palatal necrosis, and other associated complaints.[7,8] Intranasal prescription narcotic use seems to cause pathologic changes to the nasal mucosa not dissimilar to cocaine. Tablet binders that solidify the powder before it is crushed for inhalation can cause an inflammation similar to talc.[9] There also seems to be local immunosuppression in exposed mucosa that allows for colonization and infection of opportunistic fungal species. Repeated and persistent abuse and chronic exposure inevitably leads to irreversible damage to the sinonasal tract. Successful management requires abstention from illicit drug use and frequent operative debridement of inflamed tissue. When illicit drug use is suspected as a source of sinonasal pathology, the surgeon should screen for illegal stimulants and narcotics as well as prescription medication that has been used for recreational purposes.

NARCOTICS AFTER TONSILLECTOMY

Tonsillectomy with or without adenoidectomy, or AT is one of the most common surgeries performed in the United States with more than 500,000 cases annually.[10] It has also been performed, in some iteration, since its first description by Cornelio Celsius in the first century. Historically, AT was predominantly performed for recurrent or severe pharyngeal infections. More recently, there has been a dramatic shift toward surgery for sleep disordered breathing or obstructive sleep apnea (OSA). Although the surgical technique is the same, conceptually and practically, these are different etiologies and should be managed differently in the postoperative setting. AT is the first line therapy for sleep disordered breathing and OSA, especially in younger, preschool-aged children.

OSA is a diagnosis that can only be made on polysomnography (PSG) or a sleep study. During PSG, monitors are attached to a sleeping patient to measure arousals from sleep, airflow through the nose and mouth, and oxygen saturation, among other parameters. The most useful metric derived from this study is the apnea-hypopnea index. Apneas refer to cessation of breathing for at least 10 seconds that lead to desaturations and arousals. Hypopneas refer to a 50% reduction in airflow for the same time period. The apnea-hypopnea index represents the number of times per hour that one of these events occur. In children, an apnea-hypopnea index of greater than 10 or oxygen desaturation below 85% are considered severe OSA.[11] Rosen and colleagues,[12] in their landmark paper, document several risk factors predisposing children to complications after tonsillectomy. Of those, age younger than 3, morbid obesity, and severe sleep apnea significantly increase the risk of morbidity after AT. Children with these risk factors are more likely to have respiratory complications after surgery; many of these complications can be attributable to postoperative narcotic administration.

To better understand the risk of respiratory compromise in the postoperative setting and how it relates to narcotic administration, we have to consider factors unique to OSA patients and the analgesic options available for administration. OSA is a chronic condition that significantly alters respiratory physiology on a nightly basis. While asleep, restricted airflow exposes these children to prolonged and repeated episodes of hypercarbia. This blunts respiratory response curves and desensitizes the respiratory drive in response to chemoreceptor triggers.[13] OSA patients are also more sensitive to the effects of narcotics. Children with oxygen desaturations of less than 85% on PSG require one-half the analgesic dose of patients without OSA.[14] Additionally, severe OSA alters the distribution of central mu-opioid and neurokinin receptors, further increasing the respiratory suppressant activity of narcotics.

Obesity, frequent in this patient population, leads to fat deposition in the chest wall and pharynx that adds to airway resistance and work of breathing. Postoperatively, pharyngeal edema is expected and further narrows the upper airway. Coupled with the respiratory suppression caused by anesthesia and analgesia, these children are truly set up for respiratory compromise and hypoxia postoperatively. Studies looking at PSG the night after surgery routinely show worsening sleep parameters after surgery.[15] Identifying patients at risk for respiratory compromise and selecting an appropriate analgesic regimen are key to minimizing risk after tonsillectomy.

A Case Against Codeine

The FDA targeted codeine in its 2012 black box warning, prohibiting its use in the United States for AT in children under the age of 18.[16] Leading up to this declaration, between 1969 and 2011 only 10 deaths and 3 morbidities related to codeine administration were reported in the FDA Adverse Events Database.[17] However, this likely underrepresented the impact of its use. In a survey of more than 2300 pediatric anesthesiologists, Cote and colleagues[18] identified 129 cases of morbidity or mortality in the postoperative setting, most related to the administration of narcotics. A similar survey of otolaryngologists cataloged 51 mortalities in the postoperative period. Thirty-one percent were of unknown etiology and 22% were directly attributable to narcotic administration. At least 1 case was linked to a genetic predisposition to altered codeine metabolism.

Codeine has historically been used as a safe alternative to morphine and other narcotics. It has an equianalgesic dose of 6 to 10:1 compared with oral morphine and a similar length of action with slower onset.[19] Although this led to its expansive use for acute and chronic pain management in all medical applications, its efficacy as an analgesic has often been scrutinized. Several studies comparing codeine with nonsteroidal antiinflammatory pain medication have shown mixed results, some demonstrating better pain control with the nonnarcotic medications.[20] Codeine itself is a weak opiate with little activity on opioid receptors. Its metabolites are far more active. Codeine is metabolized via 3 separate pathways: glucuronidation to codeine-6-glucuronide, O-demethylation to morphine via cytochrome P450 2D6 (CYP2D6), and N-demethylation to norcodeine via cytochrome P450 3A4 (CYP3A4)[21] (**Fig. 3**). Fifty to 70% of codeine will form codeine-6-glucuronide and 10% will be converted to norcodeine. Both of these metabolites have similar

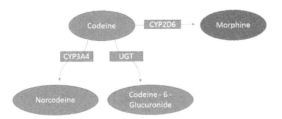

Fig. 3. Codeine metabolism pathways.

affinity to mu-opioid receptors as codeine. Morphine and its metabolites, morphine-6-glucuronide and morphine-3-glucuronide have up to a 200-fold greater mu-opioid affinity and significantly more analgesic and respiratory effects. Codeine's variable efficacy and higher risk profile is attributed to variations in CYP2D6 metabolism, shifting the ratio of codeine and morphine metabolites. There are more than 50 known allelic variants of CYP2D6, each with its own metabolic efficiency.[22] Patients with 2 highly functional alleles produce significantly more morphine and morphine-6-glucuronide for a standard dose of codeine. These patients are often called rapid or ultrarapid metabolizers (UM). Conversely, those with 2 poorly functioning alleles are slow or poor metabolizers and produce less morphine. Owing to the allelic heterogeneity, it is hard to predict how particular patients will respond to the administration of codeine. Studies estimate that close to 20% to 50% of the United States population may be poor metabolizers and produce little to no morphine.[23] Less common, but more concerning, UM individuals may produce 50% more morphine than intermediate metabolizers, with no more than 1 highly functioning allele.[24] In several cases of death after tonsillectomy, UM patients have been identified; however, this association is neither constant nor dependable.

Alternatives to Codeine

Some had advocated for genetic testing before surgery to assess metabolism and tailor narcotic doses for the individual. Although this is a logical approach, focusing on genetic or genomic testing alone would discount the effects of age, diet, activity, comorbidities, and polypharmacy on CYP activity.[25] Additionally, a good corollary for the narcotic dosing dilemma has been described in oncology literature. Oncologic medications like tamoxifen are subject to similar CYP metabolism. Genomic testing to determine therapeutic doses for oncologic effects is only cost effective in medications that have no adequate alternatives.[26] Morphine and oxycodone are examples of narcotics that have more reproducible analgesic effects and are generally preferred to codeine. It is thus hard to argue for preemptive genetic testing in this setting. However, in patients with respiratory suppression or narcotic toxicity after normal codeine dosing, laboratory testing to determine the proportion of codeine and morphine byproducts and genetic testing of CYP2D6 alleles may identify an underlying UM/rapid metabolizer genotype.

SUMMARY

The field of otolaryngology, both adult and pediatric, is subject to unique symptomatology and anatomic changes resulting from patients who are ingesting or administering narcotic analgesic as well as illicit drugs. Furthermore, transnasal administration, in particular, of both prescribed and illicit drugs can pose unique challenges to the otolaryngologist. Clinical laboratory toxicology testing via blood or genetic specimen procurement can provide objective insight into select disease etiologies and alert the clinician to inappropriate drug use as well as provide management support for choice of analgesia toward optimal patient care.

REFERENCES

1. McAllister P, Jenner S, Laverick S. Toxicology screening in oral and maxillofacial trauma patients. Br J Oral Maxillofac Surg 2013;51(8):773–8.
2. Hill GE, Ogunnaike BO, Johnson ER. General anaesthesia for the cocaine abusing patient. Is it safe? Br J Anaesth 2006;97(5):654–7.

3. United Nations Office on Drugs an Crime (UNDOC). World drug report. Geneva (Switzerland): UNODC; 2015. Available at. https://www.unodc.org/documents/wdr2015/World_Drug_Report_2015.pdf.

4. Harper SJ, Jones NS. Cocaine: what role does it have in current ENT practice? A review of the current literature. J Laryngol Otol 2006;120(10):808–11.

5. Ingels KJ, Nijziel MR, Graamans K, et al. Influence of cocaine and lidocaine on human nasal cilia - beat frequency and harmony in vitro. Arch Otolaryngol Head Neck Surg 1994;120(2):197–201.

6. Robison JG, Pant H, Ferguson BJ. Rhinitis medicamentosa as a cause of increased intraoperative bleeding. Laryngoscope 2010;120(10):2106–7.

7. Alexander D, Alexander K, Valentino J. Intranasal hydrocodone-acetaminophen abuse induced necrosis of the nasal cavity and pharynx. Laryngoscope 2012; 122(11):2378–81.

8. Yewell J, Haydon R, Archer S, et al. Complications of intranasal prescription narcotic abuse. Ann Otol Rhinol Laryngol 2002;111(2):174–7.

9. Vosler PS, Ferguson BJ, Contreras JI, et al. Clinical and pathologic characteristics of intranasal abuse of combined opioid-acetaminophen medications. Int Forum Allergy Rhinol 2014;4(10):839–44.

10. Baugh RF, Archer SM, Mitchell RB, et al. Clinical practice guideline: tonsillectomy in children. Otolaryngol Head Neck Surg 2011;144(1 Suppl):S1–30.

11. Marcus CL, Brooks LJ, Draper KA, et al. Diagnosis and management of childhood obstructive sleep apnea syndrome. Pediatrics 2012;130(3):e714–55.

12. Rosen GM, Muckle RP, Mahowald MW, et al. Postoperative respiratory compromise in children with obstructive sleep apnea syndrome: can it be anticipated? Pediatrics 1994;93(5):784–8.

13. Strauss SG, Lynn AM, Bratton SL, et al. Ventilatory response to CO2 in children with obstructive sleep apnea from adenotonsillar hypertrophy. Anesth Analg 1999;89:328–32.

14. Brown KA, Laferrière A, Lakheeram I, et al. Recurrent hypoxemia in children is associated with increased analgesic sensitivity to opiates. Anesthesiology 2006;105:665–9.

15. Nixon GM, Kermack AS, McGregor CD, et al. Sleep and breathing on the first night after adenotonsillectomy for obstructive sleep apnea. Pediatr Pulmonol 2005;39:332–8.

16. Lauder G, Emmott A. Confronting the challenges of effective pain management in children following tonsillectomy. Int J Pediatr Otorhinolaryngol 2014;78(11): 1813–27.

17. Subramanyam R, Varughese A, Willging JP, et al. Future of pediatric tonsillectomy and perioperative outcomes. Int J Pediatr Otorhinolaryngol 2013;77(2):194–9.

18. Cote CJ, Posner KL, Domino KB. Death or neurologic injury after tonsillectomy in children with a focus on obstructive sleep apnea: Houston, we have a problem! Anesth Analg 2014;118:1276–83.

19. Brownstein MJ. A brief history of opiates, opioid peptides and opioid receptors. Proc Natl Acad Sci 1993;90:5391–3.

20. Moir MS, Bair E, Shinnick P, et al. Acetaminophen versus acetaminophen with codeine after pediatric tonsillectomy. Laryngoscope 2000;110(11):1824–7.

21. Madadi P, Koren G. Pharmacogenetic insights into codeine analgesia: implications to pediatric codeine use. Pharmacogenomics 2008;9:1267–84.

22. Bernard S, Neville KA, Nguyen AT, et al. Interethnic differences in genetic polymorphisms of CYP2D6 in the U.S. population: clinical implications. Oncologist 2006;11(2):126–35.

23. Williams DG, Patel A, Howard RF. Pharmacogenetics of codeine metabolism in an urban population of children and its implications for analgesic reliability. Br J Anaesth 2002;89(6):839–45.
24. Smith HS. Opioid metabolism. Mayo Clin Proc 2009;84(7):613–24.
25. Brown KA, Brouillette RT. The elephant in the room: lethal apnea at home after adenotonsillectomy. Anesth Analg 2014;118:1157–9.
26. Rodriguez-Antona C, Gomez A, Karlgren M, et al. Molecular genetics and epigenetics of the cytochrome P450 gene family and its relevance for cancer risk and treatment. Hum Genet 2010;127(1):1–17.

Forensic Toxicology

An Introduction

Michael P. Smith, PhD[a,b],*, Martin H. Bluth, MD, PhD[c,d]

KEYWORDS

- Forensic toxicology • Workplace drug testing • Postmortem toxicology
- Human performance toxicology

KEY POINTS

- The difference in the science behind the fields of forensic toxicology and clinical toxicology is minimal, if any.
- Providing toxicology results to the legal system requires the use of terms and language used in that field, as opposed to strictly medical language.
- There are 3 components of forensic toxicology: workplace drug testing, postmortem toxicology, and human performance toxicology.

Forensics, by definition, is the use of science within the legal system. Forensic toxicology is no different. The difference between clinical toxicology and forensic toxicology is not in the science or the methods. Those are exactly the same. The difference lies in the end use of the results. In clinical toxicology, the end user is a physician who is using the results to treat and care for a patient. In forensic toxicology, the end user can be a physician, or a nonmedical professional such as a lawyer, a human resources employee, or probation officer who is using the results to determine a cause of death, employment eligibility, or compliance with terms of parole.

Forensic toxicology can be generally divided into 3 areas:
- Workplace or preemployment testing
- Human performance
- Postmortem

Workplace toxicology deals with preemployment drug screens or drug screens required by the Department of Transportation. Human performance deals with correlating a person's actions with a drug(s) they ingested. This could be driving under the

The author has no commercial or financial conflict of interest.

[a] Oakland University William Beaumont School of Medicine, Rochester, MI, USA; [b] Toxicology and Therapeutic Drug Monitoring Laboratory, Beaumont Laboratories, Beaumont Hospital-Royal Oak, 3601 West 13 Mile Road, Royal Oak, MI 48073, USA; [c] Department of Pathology, Wayne State University School of Medicine, 540 East Canfield, Detroit, MI 48201, USA; [d] Consolidated Laboratory Management Systems, 24555 Southfield Road, Southfield, MI 48075, USA
* Corresponding author. Oakland University William Beaumont School of Medicine, Rochester, MI.
E-mail address: michaelp.smith@beaumont.org

influence of alcohol or drugs, committing a crime while on a drug, or having a crime committed against an individal such as a sexual assault. Postmortem toxicology deals with the toxicology testing on deceased individuals and is a routine part of the autopsy process.

WORKPLACE DRUG TESTING

Workplace drug testing is divided into two areas, regulated and nonregulated testing. Regulated testing is testing that is mandated by the federal government via the Department of Health and Human Services, and is overseen by Substance Abuse and Mental Health Services Administration (SAMHSA). This testing is mandatory for truck drivers who cross state lines, all federal employees, military employees, and for those with many other federal jobs. Nonregulated Workplace drug testing is any testing that is required of a new employee to start a job. The guidelines are not as stringent as regulated testing, although the basic tenants are still adhered to.[1]

Accreditation

Regulated workplace drug testing laboratories are accredited by SAMHSA through the National Laboratory Certification Program. Laboratories are inspected twice a year. They are challenged with proficiency samples 4 times per year, 25 samples per challenge. As of 2016, there were 30 accredited laboratories in the country. It is a very difficult, but prestigious, accreditation to obtain, hence the low number of accredited laboratories. To qualify as a federal drug testing laboratory, the laboratory has to demonstrate and adhere to the most stringent protocols in the world for drug testing. The goal of the National Laboratory Certification Program is to ensure consistency among all certified laboratories. So that regardless of the location where the sample is tested, the same result would be produced. It also creates an environment where split-sample testing can be instituted, and the comparison of results of "A" and "B" samples are made easier. At the time of collection, the specimen is split into 2 separate containers, "A" and "B." Each container is sealed and sent to the testing laboratory. The "A" sample is tested and the results are reported. If those results are disputed by the donor, they have the option to have the "B" sample reconfirmed at a separate laboratory. Additionally, the guidelines that are imposed are designed to protect the laboratory in litigation.

Nonregulated laboratories are accredited by the Collage of American Pathology's Forensic Drug Testing program. Although not as stringent as the SAMHSA program, the same forensic principles are adhered to.

Specimen

The specimen for regulated workplace testing is always urine. It must be collected under direct observation or with measures in place so that tampering with the collection are eliminated. Once a sample is collected, it is split into 2 containers ("A" and "B"). A tamper-evident seal is placed across each lid and is signed by both the donor and collector. A paper requisition must be presented by the donor to the collector before sample collection. This is known as the Custody Control Form. This paperwork will accompany the specimen from the time it is collected until final results are recorded.

The specimen for nonregulated workplace testing is also urine. The collection may or may not be observed, and the use of a tamper-evident seal is also optional, although many establishments do use it. There is usually a paper requisition that accompanies the specimen; however, the results are usually not reported on it.

The Department of Health and Human Services has proposed guidelines as to the use of oral fluid and hair as acceptable samples for regulated testing.[2] Oral fluid is becoming more routine as a testing specimen. The ease of collection makes this an ideal specimen to collect where a restroom is not available, such as at the scene of a traffic accident. Because oral fluid is a hyperfiltrate of blood, parent compounds are detected opposed to metabolites. Detection lengths are thus shorter than urine, 1 to 2 days compared with 2 to 5 days with urine.[3,4] Hair is also another sample type that can be used for drug testing. The main advantage is the length of detection in hair is 3 months. However, environmental contamination is a significant concern with hair testing, so laboratories must take special concern during the specimen preparation steps to ensure as much environmental contamination is removed.[3,4]

Testing

Initial testing

Initial testing of the specimen, also known as screening or screen testing, is done by immunoassay. For regulated testing, the cutoffs to determine negative from nonnegative are established by SAMHSA. Nonregulated testing can have any cutoff, although many laboratories use SAMHSA values. Any value greater than or equal to the cutoff is considered "nonnegative" (note that the term *positive* can only be used with the confirmatory testing because of the possibility of false-positive screening test). Screening is for a specific class of drugs as shown in **Table 1**.

If all screening tests are negative, the results are released and there is no additional testing. If any of the results are greater than or equal to the cutoff value, a new aliquot

Table 1
Screening for a specific class of drugs

Initial Test Analyte	Initial Test Cutoff (ng/mL)	Confirmatory Test Analyte	Confirmatory Test Cutoff (ng/mL)
Marijuana (THCA)	50	THCA	15
Benzolecogonine	150	Benzoylecgonine	100
Codeine/morphine	2000[a]	Codeine	2000
		Morphine	2000
Hydrocodone/ hydromorphone[b]	300[a]	Hydrocodone	100
		Hydromorphone	100
Oxycodone/ oxymorphone[b]	100[a]	Oxycodone	50
		Oxymorphone	50
6-Acetylmorphine	10	6-Acetylmorphine	10
Phencyclidine	25	Phencyclidine	25
Amphetamine/ methamphetamine	500[a]	Amphetamine	250
		Methamphetamine	250
MDMA/MDA/MDEA	500[a]	MDMA	250
		MDA	250
		MDEA	250

Abbreviations: MDA, methylenedioxyamphetamine; MDEA, methylenedioxyethylamphetamine; MDMA, methylenedioxymethamphetamine; THCA, Δ-9-tetrahydrocannabinol-9-carboxylic acid.

[a] *Immunoassay:* The test must be calibrated with one analyte from the group identified as the target analyte. The cross-reactivity of the immunoassay to the other analyte(s) within the group must be ≥80%. If not, separate immunoassays must be used for the analytes within the group.
[b] Proposed analytes source.

Data from Drug Enforcement Administration, Department of Justice. Schedules of controlled substances: extension of temporary placement of UR-144, XLR11, and AKB48 in schedule I of the Controlled Substances Act. Final order. Fed Reg 2015;80(94)27854–6.

is taken from the original specimen and is subjected to confirmatory testing. Results are not released until all testing is complete.

Another part of the screening process is specimen validity testing. This portion of the testing determines if the specimen has been tampered with in any way. The specimen is tested for creatinine, specific gravity, pH, and oxidants (nitrites). When specimen validity testing falls out of the specified ranges of what is considered normal, it is labeled with 1 of 4 categories: dilute, substituted, adulterated, or invalid.

Dilute A specimen will be reported as dilute when:

- The creatinine concentration is greater than 5 mg/dL and less than 20 mg/dL; and
- The specific gravity is greater than 1.0010 and less than 1.0030.

Substituted Substituted means the donor has submitted a nonhuman specimen for testing. A specimen will be reported as substituted when:

- The creatinine concentration is less than 2 mg/dL; and
- The specific gravity is less than or equal to 1.0010 or greater than or equal to 1.0200.

Adulterated Adulterated indicates that the donor has added a substance to the specimen after it has been collected. A specimen will be reported as adulterated when 1 of the following criteria is met:

- pH of less than 3
- pH of 11 or greater
- Nitrite of 500 µg/mL or greater
- Chromium (VI) is present
- A halogen (eg, bleach, iodine, fluoride) is present
- Glutaraldehyde is present
- Pryidine is present
- A surfactant is present

Invalid A specimen will be reported as invalid when 1 of the following criteria is met:

1. Creatinine concentration and specific gravity results are discrepant:
   - Creatinine of less than 2 mg/dL and specific gravity of greater than 1.0010 and less than 1.0200
   - Creatinine is 2 mg/dL or greater and specific gravity is 1.0010 or less.
2. pH is outside the acceptable range:
   - pH of 3 or greater and less than 4.5
   - pH of 9 or greater and less than 11
3. Nitrite is 200 µg/mL or greater and less than 500 µg/mL.

Urine that falls into 1 of these 4 categories is considered to have failed the drug test, even if the tests for drugs are all negative.[5]

Confirmatory testing

Confirmation testing is performed by mass spectrometry, coupled either to gas chromatography or liquid chromatography. Confirmatory testing is specific to a unique drug analyte. The testing occurs on a fresh aliquot from the original sample, just in case there was a mix up with the initial screening aliquot. There are specific confirmation tests for each of the classes of drugs that are screened. The confirmatory testing result is definitive, and when performed correctly, is indisputable. Part of this assurance is based in the fact that the confirmed analyte is defined by multiple parameters.

When confirming using mass spectrometry–gas chromatography operating in single ion monitoring mode, the analyte is defined by the retention time compared with the calibrators, and the ratios of multiple ions within the ionic spectra that are unique to the specific analyte. Typically, the most abundant ion is called the "quantitation ion." The next 2 most abundant ions are called the first and second "qualifier ions". The ratios of the quantitation ion to the first and second qualifiers are used to positively identify the analyte. If they fall within a specified range of the same ratios from the calibrators, the analyte is identified positively. When using mass spectrometry–liquid chromatography, the use of 2 separate ion transitions is considered unique and is sufficient for identification, where the first and most abundant transition is called the quantitation transition, and the second transition is the qualifier transition.[2] The quantitation of the drug is greater than or equal to the confirmation cutoff value. This cutoff value is less than the screening cutoff but greater than the limit of quantitation. If developed correctly and properly maintained through proficiency testing, the confirmation test is considered to be definitive and unquestionable.

Resulting

Reporting of the results occurs after a second review of all results by someone within the laboratory that was not part of the testing process. If all results are in order, the results are certified and released either to the client or to a medical review officer. A medical review officer is a physician who acts an intermediary between the testing facility and the client who requested the test. The medical review officer is trained specifically to explain to the client and/or donor the results of the testing. They are often required to confront a donor whose specimen is positive and determine if the confirmed drug was taken in accordance to a physician's orders or recreationally. If the donor feels there is compelling evidence that a possible mistake was made in the laboratory, they can request the "B" sample be retested. In this case, the original testing laboratory sends the unopened "B" sample to another certified laboratory for testing of the contested analyte.

POSTMORTEM TESTING

Toxicology testing is a routine component of the autopsy process. When death occurs, metabolism of drugs and other substances stop. If an autopsy is performed within a reasonable amount of time, and the body has not been exposed to harsh environmental conditions, the results of toxicology testing are a snapshot of what was in the body at the time of death. Quantitation of these drugs can indicate if an overdose occurred, a subtherapeutic level of drug was present, or a combination of multiple substances contributed to the cause of death.[6]

Accreditation

With the National Academy of Sciences report on the State of Forensic Sciences, laboratory accreditation was one of the recommendations to standardize the field.[7] This can be overseen by the American Board of Forensic Toxicology, which also has testing programs for individuals to become certified.

Specimen

Postmortem testing is not limited to only urine. Specimens can be blood, urine, vitreous humor, gastric contents, liver tissue, hair, fingernails, or bile. This is not a comprehensive list. In addition to testing specimens collected at autopsy, the forensic pathologist may be interested to know the status of the decedent, particularly if they were seen at a medical facility. Specimens that may have been collected by the hospital or health care facility before death (antemortem specimens) are often tested as well. Last, it is not uncommon for nonhuman items to be found at the time of death, which may have contributed to the death. Items such as unmarked pills, powders, syringes, or liquids may be submitted for analysis as well.

It is important that an accurate description of the sample type and the location of the collection be noted and sent to the laboratory with the samples. Blood can be taken from many different parts of the body, and each area can have a very different concentration of drugs. For example, blood can be taken from the heart, jugular, subclavian, and femoral veins. Blood from the heart is called "central blood," and blood from other sites is called peripheral.[6] Ideally, blood is collected from the central and at least 1 peripheral site, in case one of the sites is contaminated owing to the manner of death. Blood is collected into tubes with sodium oxalate preservative. This is important because specimens are often stored for extended amounts of time. Also, the state of the specimens can be compromised by bacteria. Depending on the manner of death, certain specimens may become contaminated with bacteria, either through exposure to the normal flora or from outside contamination, such as in the example of a body with open wounds that is not found for an extended amount of time and microorganisms have entered the body. The collection of specimens as well as the testing of these samples is always performed under chain of custody.

Testing

Instrumentation ranging from automated chemistry analyzers to manual enzyme-linked immunosorbent assay systems are used routinely for the initial screening. Because of the variety of specimens, both sample type and sample quality, enzyme-linked immunosorbent assay is the most widely used screening methodology. Postmortem blood is difficult to work with as a result of coagulation and/or degradation, and because of the state of the specimen at the time of testing, the small sample probes on automated chemistry analyzers are often unable to aspirate the blood. Enzyme-linked immunosorbent assay also allows the laboratory to institute different cutoffs for the same tests when analyzing different sample types. Confirmation testing is performed by gas chromatography/mass spectrometry or liquid chromatography/mass spectrometry.

HUMAN PERFORMANCE

Human performance testing relates how a person acts when under the influence of a substance or drug. Examples of this type of testing are blood alcohol and drug testing from a suspected drunk/drugged driver, blood testing for drugs from a possible drug facilitated sexual assault, or for cause testing of a worker who is exhibiting strange behavior while at work.[8]

Specimen

The specimen of choice is blood, although oral fluid may begin to be used in the future. Testing of a blood specimen is critical because if a substance is confirmed, it is possible to establish a window as to when the substance was ingested. This is unfortunately not possible if urine is used, because drugs have a longer detection window in urine. Being able to definitively prove the timeframe of when a substance is ingested is critical in human performance testing.

Testing

The testing panel is widely different, and depends on the situation that the specimen is being tested for. An alcohol only panel may be requested when a subject agrees to a field breath alcohol test and the result is positive. If a drug-facilitated sexual assault is suspected, a panel that would include alcohol, benzodiazepines, barbiturates, opiates, Δ-9-Tetrahydrocannabinol-9-carboxylic acid, gamma-hydroxybutyrate, zolpidem, and other depressants would be appropriate.

SUMMARY

Although forensic toxicology and clinical toxicology are defined as separate fields, the difference in the science behind these fields is minimal, if any. However, the differences are with the use of the results, and who is the recipient of those results. Providing toxicology results to the legal system requires the use of terms and language used in that field, as opposed to strictly medical language. For example, a common set of qualitative terms used are "positive" and "negative." However, these terms do not provide any room for the situation of false-positive or false-negative results. More accurate terms instead of *positive* are *presumptive positive* and *confirmed positive*. The results are often an integral part of the case and if one does not use the correct terminology and leaves ambiguity in the report, the many hours of work to generate those results could be for naught.

REFERENCES

1. Jenkins AJ. Forensic drug testing. In: Levine B, editor. Principles of forensic toxicology. 3rd edition. Washington, DC: AACC Press; 2009. p. 31–45.
2. Drug Enforcement Administration, Department of Justice. Schedules of controlled substances: extension of temporary placement of UR-144, XLR11, and AKB48 in schedule I of the Controlled Substances Act. Final order. Fed Reg 2015;80(94): 27854–6.
3. Jones JT. Advances in drug testing for substance abuse alternative programs. J Nurs Regul 2016;6(4):62–7.
4. Skopp G. Preanalytical aspects in postmortem toxicology. Forensic Sci Int 2004; 142(2–3):75–100.
5. US Department of Health and Human Services, Substance Abuse and Mental Health Services Administration. Medical review officer manual for federal agency workplace drug testing programs. Rockville (MD): Substance Abuse and Mental Health Services Administration; 2010.
6. Levine B. Postmortem forensic toxicology. In: Levine B, editor. Principles of forensic toxicology. 3rd edition. Washington, DC: AACC Press; 2009. p. 3–13.
7. Committee on Identifying the Needs of the Forensic Sciences Community, National Research Council. Strengthening forensic science in the United States: a path forward. Washington (DC): National Academies Press; 2009.
8. Kunsman GW. Human performance toxicology. In: Levine B, editor. Principles of forensic toxicology. 3rd edition. Washington, DC: AACC Press; 2009. p. 15–29.

Drug Toxicities of Common Analgesic Medications in the Emergency Department

Mateusz Ciejka, MD[a], Khoa Nguyen, MD[a],
Martin H. Bluth, MD, PhD[b,c], Elizabeth Dubey, MD[a,*]

KEYWORDS

- Toxicity • Acetaminophen • Opioid • Narcotic • Aspirin • Salicylate
- Emergency department

KEY POINTS

- Acute acetaminophen toxicity is commonly associated with hepatic dysfunction that may not manifest until 24 hours after ingestion; the modified Rumack-Matthews nomogram is used to determine whether treatment with N-acetylcysteine is indicated and is based on the serum acetaminophen level beginning at 4 hours after ingestion.
- Acute opioid toxicity is classically characterized by central nervous system depression, respiratory depression, and pupillary constriction; naloxone should be administered to achieve adequate respiration rather than a normal level of consciousness.
- Many opioids have a longer duration of action than naloxone; thus, patients who respond to naloxone should continue to be observed for persistent opioid toxicity.
- Acute aspirin toxicity can present with hyperthermia, altered mental status, coma, pulmonary edema, and shock, which require prompt recognition and initiation of therapy with hydration, sodium bicarbonate administration, electrolyte replacement, and dialysis when indicated.

ACETAMINOPHEN TOXICITY

Background

Acetaminophen was first clinically used in 1955 and since then has become the most commonly used antipyretic and analgesic medication in the United States. Acetaminophen is available as an isolated agent and is a component of prescription and over-the-counter medications used throughout the world. Acetaminophen is safe to administer at standard therapeutic doses, although it has been shown that prolonged use and overdosing of the drug can lead to nonfatal or fatal hepatic injury.[1] In fact,

[a] Department of Emergency Medicine, Wayne State University School of Medicine, 4201 St. Antoine, 6F UHC, Detroit, MI 48201, USA; [b] Department of Pathology, Wayne State University School of Medicine, 540 East Canfield, Detroit, MI 48201, USA; [c] Consolidated Laboratory Management Systems, 24555 Southfield Road, Southfield, MI 48075, USA
* Corresponding author.
E-mail address: edube@med.wayne.edu

Clin Lab Med 36 (2016) 761–776
http://dx.doi.org/10.1016/j.cll.2016.07.003
0272-2712/16/© 2016 Elsevier Inc. All rights reserved.
labmed.theclinics.com

acetaminophen toxicity is the most common cause of acute hepatic failure in the United States.[2]

Pathophysiology

Acetaminophen is typically used for its antipyretic and analgesic properties, although it also has mild anti-inflammatory and antiplatelet functions, which are induced by inhibiting prostaglandin synthesis. Contrary to the mechanism of action of nonsteroidal anti-inflammatory drugs, which inhibit peripheral prostaglandin synthesis through the direct inhibition of prostaglandin E_2 (PGE_2) synthase enzymatic activity via the cyclo-oxygenase (COX) binding site, acetaminophen acts on the peroxidase binding site on PGE_2 and indirectly inhibits COX activation.[3,4]

At therapeutic levels, most circulating acetaminophen is metabolized through conjugation with glucuronide or sulfate moieties, converting it into nontoxic products that are renally excreted.[4–6] However, 5% to 15% of acetaminophen is metabolized by cytochrome (CYP) P450 enzymes into N-acetyl-p-benzoquinone imine (NAPQI), a hepatotoxic highly reactive metabolite. NAPQI has a short half-life and is rapidly conjugated into nontoxic metabolites with glutathione and other moieties before being renally excreted. At therapeutic doses of acetaminophen, there are sufficient glutathione stores to maintain NAPQI metabolism at an adequate rate, and its nontoxic metabolites are renally excreted.

With excessive NAPQI production or with depletion of glutathione stores, such as in acetaminophen overdose or repeated supratherapeutic dosing, the glucuronidation and sulfation metabolizing pathways are saturated. In turn, additional acetaminophen is metabolized by CYP enzymes to NAPQI. It has been demonstrated that when hepatic glutathione stores are reduced by approximately 70% or more, unmetabolized NAPQI causes hepatotoxicity.[7,8] The reactive molecule covalently binds to hepatic cellular proteins, which leads to hepatocyte necrosis within hours of the drug ingestion.[9]

The current US Food and Drug Administration (FDA)-recommended maximum daily dose of acetaminophen is 4 g in individuals 50 kg and greater and 75 mg/kg in individuals less than 50 kg.[10] According to the FDA, exceeding the maximum recommended daily dose of acetaminophen can cause acute hepatotoxicity, particularly in those individuals with underling liver disease, chronic alcohol use, concomitant treatment with medications that induce CYP enzymes, such as phenytoin and isoniazid, malnutrition, and advanced age.[10–13] Such individuals with increased susceptibility can develop hepatotoxicity at lower doses.

Manifestations of Drug Toxicity

Within the first 24 hours of acetaminophen overdose, most patients will be asymptomatic or have mild nonspecific symptoms, such as nausea, vomiting, and malaise.[14] Laboratory studies are usually normal, and elevated anion gap metabolic acidosis (AGMA) is rare at this stage in massive overdoses.[15] Hepatotoxicity usually will not manifest until 24 hours after ingestion, at which point there may be elevations in transaminase levels (**Table 1**), which may be accompanied by other clinical signs of liver injury, including right upper quadrant abdominal pain or tenderness, liver enlargement, and jaundice. There may also be elevations in prothrombin time (PT) and bilirubin as well as signs of renal function abnormalities. Although with severe toxicity, elevations in transaminases may be seen within the first 24 hours.[6,16] The most severe cases of toxicity involve fulminant liver failure, which can manifest as renal injury, coagulopathy leading to hemorrhage, AGMA, cerebral edema, hepatic encephalopathy, sepsis, and multiorgan failure.[14] Patients who survive this phase generally have resolution of hepatic sequelae, although full histologic resolution may take months.[14]

Table 1
Acetaminophen-induced hepatotoxicity without treatment may be conceptualized as occurring in various stages with different manifestations depending on the time since ingestion

Stage	Time After Ingestion (d)	Clinical Signs	Laboratory Markers
1	0–1	Asymptomatic or mild nausea, vomiting, malaise	Normal or increased AST in severe cases
2	1–3	RUQ abdominal pain, nausea, vomiting, lethargy	Increased AST, ALT, PT, bilirubin, and lactic acid
3	3–5	Jaundice, coagulopathy, hypoglycemia, renal dysfunction, hepatic encephalopathy, multiorgan failure	AGMA, increased serum creatinine and ammonia
4	5+	Resolution of hepatotoxicity	Normalization

The first stage may involve mild or no associated symptoms, except in severe toxicity. The fourth stage represents the recovery period and involves the resolution of hepatic injury, which may take months.

Abbreviations: ALT, alanine aminotransferase; RUQ, right upper quadrant.

Data from Defendi GL. Acetaminophen toxicity in children: diagnosis, clinical assessment, and treatment of acute overingestion. Cons Pediat 2013;12(7):301.

Diagnostic Evaluations in Suspected Toxicity

Acetaminophen toxicity risk is most reliably established by correlating the serum concentration level to the time since ingestion. In suspected overdose, a serum concentration level at 4 hours after ingestion should ideally be obtained, although levels drawn before 4 hours may not be representative of peak serum levels due to incomplete absorption and should not be used in the assessment of toxicity. The ingested dose should not be used to predict the risk of hepatotoxicity or need for therapy, because a serum concentration level is a more reliable predictor than ingested dose.[17] Because of its effectiveness and safety profile, the modified Rumack-Matthew nomogram (**Fig. 1**) is the preferred tool to assess the need for treatment with N-acetylcysteine (NAC) in those presenting within 24 hours of a single ingestion with a known time of the ingestion.[18] The treatment line indicates serum levels corresponding to hourly time points after ingestion at which NAC should be administered. The initial level is 150 μg/mL at 4 hours, and the final level is 4.7 μg/mL at 24 hours. It is not necessary to treat patients with NAC before the 6-hour mark after ingestion because those treated up to 6 hours afterward, regardless of the initial level or amount ingested, do not have an increased risk of hepatotoxicity.[14] However, even with treatment, the incidence of hepatotoxicity (aspartate aminotransferase [AST] >1000 IU/L) in patients presenting 8 hours after ingestion is approximately 30%.[14] Administering a loading dose of NAC should be considered in cases where a level cannot be obtained before 8 hours after ingestion. Patients with a level below the treatment line can be discharged if otherwise medically cleared. Those with signs of severe toxicity, including AGMA, coagulopathy, hepatic failure, or encephalopathy, should be treated and managed in an intensive care setting.

Management of Toxicity

Appropriate initial care in acute toxicity involves assessment of airway, breathing, and circulatory status as well as assessment of other possible life-threatening coingestions.

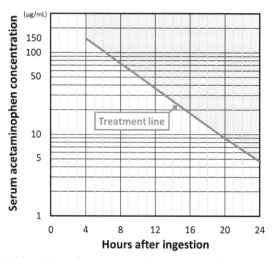

Fig. 1. Modified Matthew-Rumack nomogram demonstrating the treatment line, which indicates the serum acetaminophen level at which NAC should be administered based on the time after ingestion. The 4-hour mark corresponds to 150 µg/mL and the 24-hour mark corresponds to 4.7 µg/mL. (*Adapted from* Smilkstein MJ, Knapp GL, Kulig KW, et al. Efficacy of oral N-acetylcysteine in the treatment of acetaminophen overdose. Analysis of the national multicenter study (1976–1985). N Engl J Med 1988;319(24):1558.)

If a patient presents with stable mental status within 1 hour of ingestion, activated charcoal can be administered, because it effectively adsorbs acetaminophen, although there is ongoing debate regarding its efficacy in improving clinical outcomes.[19,20] It is universally accepted that early administration of NAC is the ideal currently available treatment.[18] NAC acts as a precursor for glutathione synthesis and thus provides more substrate for the conjugation of NAPQI, which leads to detoxification of this reactive metabolite.[21,22] If administered within 8 hours of acetaminophen ingestion, NAC has nearly 100% efficacy in preventing hepatotoxicity, and death is extremely rare regardless of the initial plasma concentration.[18,23] However, there is a significantly higher rate of hepatotoxicity if NAC is administered after 8 hours after ingestion.[14] NAC may be administered via an oral or intravenous route, and both formulations are effective when administered up to 24 hours after ingestion.[14] However, if hepatotoxicity is evident, such as with the onset of coagulopathy or encephalopathy, the intravenous formulation should be administered and is the only formulation that has been studied in such cases.[14] Common side effects of oral NAC include nausea and vomiting in approximately 23% of individuals, which may be attributable to its very unpleasant taste and odor.[24] Severe side effects of the oral formulation such as major anaphylactoid reactions are rare. Side effects of intravenous NAC include mild anaphylactoid reactions, such as rash, pruritus, and vomiting, which are seen in 2% to 6% of individuals.[14] Severe anaphylactoid reactions, such as angioedema, bronchospasm, and hypotension, have been reported with a less than 1% incidence.[14]

Two used NAC administration protocols include a 21-hour intravenous protocol and a 72-hour oral protocol.[25] It remains controversial which treatment protocol is preferable and whether it is essential to complete the full treatment course.[25,26] NAC may be discontinued once the administration protocol is completed, provided that serum acetaminophen has been metabolized (level <10 µg/mL) and there is no sign of ongoing hepatic injury (normal AST level). If acetaminophen metabolism has not completed (level >10 μg/mL) or there is ongoing liver injury, NAC administration should continue until there are no further signs of liver injury.[14]

OPIOID TOXICITY

Background

Many medications in various drug classes are available for management of acute and chronic pain, with opioids being the most potent and among the most commonly prescribed. The opioid drug class includes natural, synthetic, and semisynthetic drugs, whereas "opiates" specifically include natural agents. Furthermore, the term "narcotic" refers specifically to any substance that blunts the senses, induces coma, or relieves pain and may erroneously be used to refer to any illicit psychotropic substance.

Opioids, which are directly derived from opium, have been used for medicinal and recreational purposes since approximately 3400 BC when opium is known to have first been cultivated.[27] Opium itself is an extract derived from the dried sap of the poppy plant, *Papaver somniferum*. The natural extract contains the opioid alkaloids morphine, codeine, and other nonanalgesic alkaloids.[28] Today opioids and its many derivatives are used predominantly for pain control, although they are frequently abused because of their highly addictive potential.

Pharmacoepidemiology

Opioids are the mainstay treatment of moderate or severe pain and improve quality of life for many individuals despite their potential for misuse and the increase of deaths related to overdose. Opioids, mainly heroin and prescription pain medications, are the drugs most commonly associated with overdose deaths.[29] In 2014, opioid drugs were involved in more than 28,000 deaths, or 61% of all drug overdose deaths.[29] Acute or chronic pain is the chief complaint in more than half of emergency department (ED) visits in the United States, and ED physicians are among the top 5 most prescribing physicians of opioids to patients with chronic noncancer pain.[30,31] As opioid use becomes more common, the risk for dependence and the incidence of overdoses continue to increase. Between 2001 and 2010, the percentage of ED visits during which opioids were prescribed increased from 21% to 31%.[31] The current prevalence of opioid dependence is almost 5 million people in the United States.

Mechanism of Action

Analogous to endogenous opioidlike molecules, including endorphins, dynorphins, and enkephalins, exogenous opioids primarily bind to 3 receptor types to impede neuronal transmission within the central nervous system (CNS) and peripheral nervous system to mediate brain- and spinal-level analgesia, sedation, euphoria, gastrointestinal secretion and motility, respiration, and other functions.[32,33] The 3 primary receptor types, mu (μ), kappa (κ), and delta (δ), are structurally similar transmembrane G protein–coupled receptors that are distributed in various locations, including in sensory neurons, vascular endothelial cells, neurologic respiratory centers, and the gastrointestinal tract.[14,34] Activation of these receptors results in modulating the release of neurotransmitters at the target sites. Opioid receptor antagonists, such as naloxone and naltrexone, competitively inhibit these receptors and reverse the opioid-mediated actions.[14]

Pharmacokinetics

The various types of opioids have different pharmacokinetic properties and varying rates of metabolism. Opioids are generally well absorbed through oral, nasal, and gastrointestinal mucosal surfaces as well as subcutaneous and intramuscular routes. Synthetic opioids such as fentanyl are also routinely administered through a transdermal patch. Opioids absorbed through the gastrointestinal tract may have reduced bioavailability because of first-pass metabolism in the liver and intestinal wall.[35] Most opioids have relatively large volumes of distribution ranging from 1 to 10 L/kg and consequently are poorly dialyzable.[36] Opioids traverse the placenta, and when administered before delivery, may induce respiratory depression in the infant.[37,38] All opioids are metabolized through hepatic conjugation, and the resultant active or inactive metabolites are renally excreted.[14,39] Thus, opioids have an extended duration of action in the setting of hepatic dysfunction because of decreased hepatic metabolism, which can further potentiate opioid toxicity.[39] Furthermore, renal dysfunction can reduce the excretion of active metabolites, potentiating their effects. Such is the case with morphine, which is conjugated into the active metabolites morphine-3-glucoronide and morphine-6-gluconoride, which are both normally renally excreted.[36,40]

Opioids vary significantly in their serum half-life, which can further be influenced by dose, individual tolerance level, extent of active metabolite presence, and drug distribution (**Table 2**). In opioid-naïve individuals, the serum half-life of a single administered dose varies from approximately 2 to 3 hours with morphine to potentially 150 hours with methadone.[41] Opioids also vary in lipid solubility, which is significant as high lipid solubility promotes more rapid molecule absorption and confers a higher propensity to cross lipid barriers and enter the CNS, providing a more rapid onset and shorter duration of efficacy.[42] Consequently, fentanyl, a highly lipid-soluble opioid, has quick onset and short duration of action when administered intravenously, in contrast to morphine, which is approximately 40 times less lipid soluble and has a longer time of onset and longer duration of action.[42,43]

Table 2
Opioid analgesics vary widely in terms of half-life and duration of action

Opioid	Onset (min)	Duration (h)	Half-Life (h)
Morphine IR	PO 15–60 IM 15–30 IV <5	3–6	2–3
Morphine CR (PO)	20–40	8–12	2–3
Oxycodone IR (PO)	15–30	3–6	2–3.5
Oxycodone CR (PO)	15–30	8–12	2–3
Hydromorphone	PO 15–30 IM 15–30 IV <5	3–6	2–3
Codeine (PO)	30–60	4–6	2.5–3.5
Hydrocodone (PO)	20–30	3–6	2–4.5
Methadone (PO)	30–90	24–48	12–150
Fentanyl (IV)	<1	0.5–1	3.7
Fentanyl (transdermal)	8–12 h	48–72	16–24

Various formulations of routinely used opioid analgesics are shown.
Abbreviations: CR, controlled-release; IM, intramuscular; IR, immediate-release; IV, intravenous; PO, oral.
Data from Smith HS. Current therapy in pain. Philadelphia: Saunders Elsevier; 2009.

Manifestations of Drug Toxicity

Opioid toxicity generally involves, among other symptoms, CNS depression, respiratory depression, pupillary constriction, and decreased gastrointestinal motility. Direct CNS depression is common and can further be complicated by disturbances such as seizures or acute psychosis.[14] Meperidine is known to produce an active metabolite with CNS excitatory function, which has the ability to induce seizures, particularly in individuals with hepatic or renal dysfunction.[44] Parkinsonian symptoms have been identified in intravenous drug users who had injected MPTP (1-methyl-4-phenyl-1,2,3,6-tetrahydropyridine), a product in the illicit synthesis of MPP (1-methyl-4-phenylpyridinium), a meperidine analogue, which has been shown to damage dopamine-producing cells in the substantia nigra.[45,46] Serotonin syndrome has been associated with opioids that inhibit serotonin reuptake, including meperidine, dextromethorphan, methadone, and buprenorphine.[14,47]

Respiratory depression, secondary to reduction in respiratory rate or tidal volume, is induced by reducing the sensitivity of chemoreceptors in the medulla to hypercapnia.[48] Acute opioid toxicity has been implicated as a cause of acute lung injury, clinically indistinguishable from acute respiratory distress syndrome. The exact involved mechanisms are unclear but presumably involve increased pulmonary capillary leakage from hypoxemia and histamine release.[49] Opioids induce arterial and venous dilation, causing mild hypotension, which may be advantageous in the setting of acute cardiogenic pulmonary edema by transiently reducing preload in addition to their anxiolytic effects.[50] Common gastrointestinal effects of opioid toxicity include nausea and vomiting, which occur secondary to reduced gastric emptying, increased vestibular sensitivity, and direct stimulation of the medullary chemoreceptor trigger zone.[51] Decreased gastrointestinal motility occurs commonly and in severe cases may progress to intestinal ileus.[52]

Diagnostic Evaluations in Suspected Toxicity

Overdoses of opioids are especially important to identify because of the high morbidity and mortality when left untreated and the ease with which their effects can be reversed. Identifying opioid toxicity is predominantly dependent on elements of the history and physical examination. History should be obtained from Emergency Medical Services providers, family, friends, or bystanders, including any information regarding possible access to medications or drug paraphernalia, and if known, time since ingestion, amount of substance ingested, and presence of other coingested substances. In addition to the aforementioned clinical findings, patients may have needle track marks from repeated intravenous or subcutaneous ("skin-popping") injections. Patients should be inspected for the presence of transdermal opioid patches. Patients should be screened for hypoglycemia, although other laboratory abnormalities are not seen consistently. Oxygen saturation and capnography may help to identify hypoxia and respiratory depression. A plain abdominal radiograph may be helpful in cases of suspected body packers, also known as "mules," because ingested packets of paraphernalia such as opioids have a reported detection sensitivity of 85% to 90%.[53] Serum acetaminophen and aspirin concentrations should be obtained in cases where the formulation of the ingested opioid is unknown. Most urine toxicology screening (immunoassays) assays will detect opioids, and the presence and specificity of such analytes can be verified through confirmatory testing modalities, such as gas chromatography-mass spectrometry or liquid chromatography-mass spectrometry. However, routine urine toxicology screens are not recommended, because a false positive test can result from the detection of nonspecific analytes. Furthermore, a positive screen may not necessarily indicate acute toxicity because a urine test can remain positive for several days after last intake, depending on the half-life of the specific substance.[54] The ingestion of poppy seeds can produce a urine test that is positive for morphine and codeine.[55]

Management of Toxicity

Initial management of patients with opioid toxicity involves aggressive airway control. Emergent intubation may be necessary in patients who are not able to protect their airway despite treatment. Naloxone is a rapid-onset μ-receptor antagonist that should be administered in the presence of severe CNS or respiratory depression. The goal of naloxone administration is adequate respiration rather than a normal level of consciousness. Intravenous administration is preferred due to a faster onset of action of 1 to 2 minutes, although obtaining intravenous access may be time consuming and difficult, particularly in chronic intravenous drug abusers.[56–58] Alternatively, intramuscular, subcutaneous, endotracheal, intraosseous, and intranasal routes may be used. Intranasal delivery of naloxone using an atomizer spray is frequently practiced in the prehospital setting because of the relative ease of administration as well as its rapid onset and effectiveness.[59,60] Regardless of the route, naloxone should be administered judiciously because it may precipitate withdrawal symptoms in some patients, particularly in long-term opioid users. With severe CNS or respiratory depression, an intravenous dose of 0.4 to 2 mg should be administered. With the presence of spontaneous respirations, an initial intravenous dose of 0.04 mg is appropriate and may be titrated up to achieve adequate spontaneous ventilation.[61] Acute withdrawal symptoms may involve nausea, vomiting, and agitation with the potential for aspiration of gastric contents. Additional opioids should not be administered to counter withdrawal symptoms, because intravenous naloxone has a short duration of action of 30 to 60 minutes, and further sedation may occur once its effect dissipates.[56,62]

Because of the short duration of action of naloxone and the long duration of many opioids, it may be necessary to administer additional doses of naloxone, depending on the duration of efficacy of the opioid involved. In this situation, a continuous naloxone infusion may be considered in lieu of repeated bolus administration. A proposed nomogram for naloxone infusion dosing suggests administering at every hour a continuous infusion of two-thirds of the bolus dose that resulted in opioid action reversal.[63] The infusion should be discontinued with the onset of withdrawal symptoms.

Gastrointestinal decontamination using gastric lavage or activated charcoal administration is not appropriate in most cases of opioid toxicity, because there is no available clinical evidence demonstrating benefit. The theoretic benefits of extracting undissolved pill fragments or allowing activated charcoal to bind unabsorbed drugs are outweighed by the risk of aspiration, particularly in patients with CNS depression. Whole-bowel irrigation is occasionally performed in the setting of body stuffing with opioid-containing packets, although there is no convincing evidence from clinical studies that it improves patient outcomes.[64,65]

Opioid withdrawal symptoms that are not precipitated by naloxone administration are not life-threatening and can be managed conservatively. However, administration of naloxone may induce a catecholamine surge with resultant hemodynamic instability and in some cases may cause pulmonary edema.[66,67] Supportive care in the ED is appropriate in the management of most cases of opioid toxicity that required treatment with naloxone. As the effective duration of action of naloxone is 30 to 60 minutes, observing patients for 2 hours to assess symptom resolution and clinical improvement is appropriate.[68] Overdoses of long-acting opioids such as methadone may require prolonged monitoring and possible hospital admission.

ASPIRIN TOXICITY
Background

Aspirin, also known as acetylsalicylic acid, is a commonly used salicylate drug due to its analgesic, antipyretic, and anti-inflammatory properties through the inhibition of COX isozymes.[69] It is used as an isolated compound in the long-term prevention of cardiovascular diseases or in combination, as seen with drugs such as Fioritol and Excedrin to treat headache.[69–71] Clinicians need to know the signs and symptoms of salicylate toxicity, which can occur in patients who unintentionally take aspirin or cold medication preparations that also contain aspirin.[4] Fortunately, safety packaging and the use of alternatives to aspirin have decreased the incidence of accidental salicylate toxicity.[4,14]

Pathophysiology

Salts of salicylic acid are rapidly absorbed intact from the gastrointestinal tract, and serum concentrations increase within 30 minutes after ingestion; however, large ingestions or ingestions of enteric capsules can prolong absorption.[4,14] Aspirin is hydrolyzed to free salicylic acid in the intestinal wall, liver, and red blood cells.[14] In turn, salicylate is conjugated with glucuronic acid and glycine, whereas a small percentage is oxidized (**Fig. 2**).[4,14] Free salicylate and its conjugates are renally excreted, which follows first-order kinetics at therapeutic concentrations. However, when the concentration is greater than 30 mg/dL, the elimination follows zero-order kinetics.[4,14]

Effects of Aspirin on Aerobic Metabolism

Salicylate stimulates the respiratory center, which causes respiratory alkalosis but depresses the respiratory center at prolonged high serum concentrations.[4,14,69]

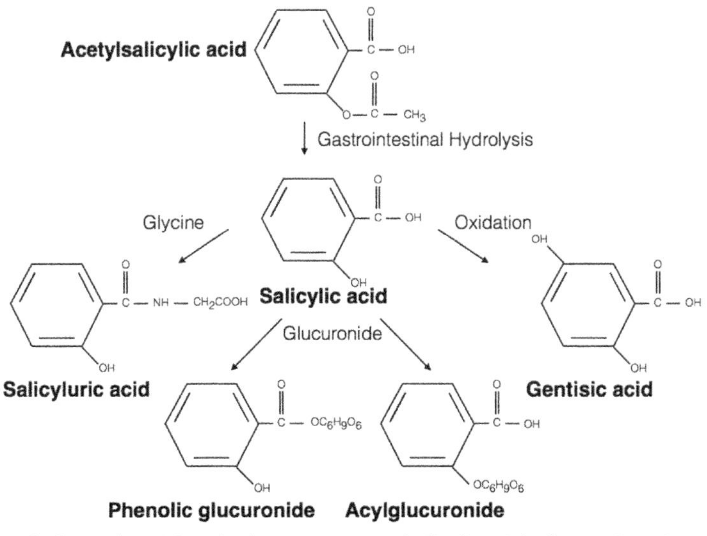

Fig. 2. Metabolism of aspirin, also known as acetylsalicylic acid. The conjugation or oxidation of salicylic acid produces its metabolites, which can be renally excreted. (*Adapted from* Nelson LS, Lewin NA, Howland MA, et al. Goldfrank's toxicologic emergencies. New York: McGraw-Hill; 2011.)

Toxicity of salicylate is caused by its interference with aerobic metabolism.[4] For instance, aspirin inhibits the Krebs cycle and delivery of the metabolites needed by the electron transport chain,[4,14,72] thus reducing the mitochondrial fuel supply and energy flux needed for adenosine triphosphate (ATP) synthesis (**Fig. 3**).[72] On the other hand, salicylate induces the mitochondrial permeability transition, which uncouples mitochondrial oxidative phosphorylation.[72,73] Uncoupling of mitochondrial oxidative phosphorylation and inhibition of the Krebs cycle lead to accumulation of pyruvate and lactic acid. The production of ketone bodies increases due to increased lipid metabolism. Moreover, salicylate toxicity is prone to hypoglycemia due to the increase in tissue glycolysis. The net outcome of these metabolic processes is AGMA.[4,14]

Manifestations of Drug Toxicity

Patients with aspirin toxicity can develop symptoms ranging from vomiting to altered mental status and seizures. These symptoms cause metabolic derangements associated with aspirin toxicity. For example, vomiting due to local gastric irritation at lower doses and stimulation of the medullary chemoreceptor trigger zone at higher doses of aspirin can lead to hypokalemia and metabolic alkalosis. Vomiting and insensible fluid loss from hyperventilation can lead to dehydration, which causes acute kidney insufficiency. The uncoupling of oxidative phosphorylation can lead to decreases in hepatic glycogen storage secondary to increased glycogenolysis and glycolysis. As the salicylate level increases in the CNS, neuronal energy depletion occurs, resulting in cerebral edema. Acute lung injury occurs in the setting of salicylate toxicity due to increased pulmonary capillary permeability and exudation of protein edema fluid into the interstitial or alveolar space.

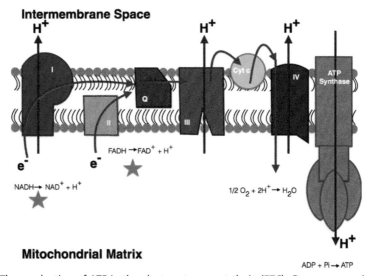

Fig. 3. The production of ATP in the electron transport chain (ETC). Green arrows depict the transfer of electrons from Krebs cycle substrates, whereas the blue arrows depict the movement of protons through the complexes. Blue stars represent the lack of substrates needed for the ETC secondary to inhibition of Krebs cycle by aspirin. (*Adapted from* Fosslien E. Mitochondrial medicine—molecular pathology of defective oxidative phosphorylation. Ann Clin Lab Sci 2001;31(1):46.)

Bleeding can occur secondary to platelet dysfunction from irreversible inhibition of COX-1 and COX-2 isozymes, which prevents the formation of thromboxane A2. However, it is important to realize that the number and morphology of platelets are normal.[4,14]

Diagnostic Evaluations in Suspected Toxicity

The laboratory evaluation in the setting of aspirin toxicity includes a basic metabolic panel, initial serum salicylate level, a repeat serum salicylate level at 2 hours to determine if the concentration is increasing or decreasing, venous or arterial blood pH, and a serum drug screen to evaluate for coingestions, such as acetaminophen and tricyclic antidepressants.[4,14,74] Aspirin uncouples mitochondria and stimulates the respiratory center; this leads to a mixed acid-base disorder with AGMA and respiratory alkalosis (**Table 3**). The bicarbonate is used to neutralize the acid while the body is losing carbon dioxide gas from hyperventilation. The ferric chloride test, Ames Phenistix test, and Trinder spot test have been previously used as bedside salicylate screening tests.[74] However, these tests are not permissible outside of a certified laboratory according to the federal Clinical Laboratory Improvement Amendments in the United States.[4] Spectrophotometry is now used to determine salicylate concentration, which relies on chemical reactions to form a light-absorbing substance. The spectrophotometer takes multiple absorbance measurements in order to determine the rate of change in light absorbance as the reaction proceeds. The rate is constant and proportional to the initial concentration of the analyte at the beginning of the reaction. Unfortunately, spectrophotometry is subjected to interferences by substances that produce light-absorbing products or by substances that consume reagents without producing light-absorbing products. In order to improve the selectivity of the assay, enzymes are often used to catalyze highly selective reactions.[4] The concentration of salicylates in a sample is determined by using salicylate hydroxylase to convert salicylate and NADH to catechol and NAD^+. The change in absorbance at 340 nm is directly proportional to the concentration of salicylate in the sample.[69]

Management of Toxicity

When patients present with clinical findings of salicylate toxicity, it is imperative to initiate treatment as soon as possible (**Box 1**). Activated charcoal has been used

Table 3
The signs and symptoms, laboratory results, and the effects of aspirin toxicity at the cellular level

Symptoms/Signs	Laboratory Results	Cellular Level Effects
Convulsions	AGMA (decreased HCO_3^{2-})	Uncoupling of mitochondrial oxidative phosphorylation
Hyperpnea	Respiratory alkalosis (decreased CO_2)	Increased glycolysis/glycogenolysis
Cerebral edema	Lactic acidosis	Increased ketone production
Pulmonary edema	Hypokalemia	Inefficient ATP production
Dehydration	Elevated creatinine	Inhibition of Krebs cycle

Abbreviations: CO_2, carbon dioxide; HCO_3^{2-}, bicarbonate.
Adapted from Marx JA, Hockberger RS, Walls RM. Rosen's emergency medicine concepts and clinical practice. Philadelphia: Elsevier Saunders; 2014; with permission.

Box 1
Management of patients with aspirin toxicity

Therapy

- Gastrointestinal decontamination with activated charcoal
- Enhance elimination via urine alkalinization
- Hemodialysis
- Fluid replacement
- Correct hypokalemia
- Mechanical ventilation

Adapted from Marx JA, Hockberger RS, Walls RM. Rosen's emergency medicine concepts and clinical practice. Philadelphia: Elsevier Saunders; 2014; with permission.

---

for treatment of many drug ingestions, including aspirin. Studies have shown that activated charcoal reduces absorption of salicylates by 50% to 80%, and it is recommended that a 10:1 ratio of activated charcoal to ingested salicylate be used in treating salicylate poisoning.[4] Dehydration is a known complication of aspirin toxicity secondary to vomiting, insensible fluid loss, and a hypermetabolic state, which requires careful repletion with intravenous fluid because excessive fluid replacement can worsen cerebral and pulmonary edema.[14] It is recommended that fluid contains dextrose because aspirin toxicity is also associated with hypoglycemia. The administration of intravenous sodium bicarbonate (1–2 mEq/kg) has been recommended as part of the management of salicylate toxicity. Alkalinization of serum reduces the percentage of salicylate in the nonionized form and increases the pH gradient with cerebrospinal fluid, both of which prevent entry and removal of salicylates from the CNS.[4] Furthermore, alkalinization with a target urine pH of 7.5 to 8.0 increases excretion of aspirin from the kidney.[14] It is important to correct hypokalemia to maintain alkaline urine. Hemodialysis should be initiated sooner rather than later in certain patients **(Box 2)**.[4,14]

Box 2
Indications to initiate hemodialysis in aspirin toxicity

Indications for hemodialysis

- Renal failure
- Altered mental status
- Hepatic failure
- Pulmonary edema
- Severe acid-based disturbance
- Salicylate concentration greater than 100 mg/dL (acute) or greater than 50 mg/dL (chronic)
- Failure to respond to conservative management

Adapted from Marx JA, Hockberger RS, Walls RM. Rosen's emergency medicine concepts and clinical practice. Philadelphia: Elsevier Saunders; 2014; with permission.

SUMMARY

About 75% of patients present to the ED with a complaint of pain, making it the most common chief complaint[75,76] and leading to the Joint Commission on Accreditation of Hospitals Organization recommending in 2000 that pain be assessed as a fifth vital sign and mandating effective treatment of pain.[76] There are multiple prescribed and over-the-counter medications that are available for the treatment of pain. Aspirin, acetaminophen, and opioids are commonly used agents that are available as single agents or in combination with other medications. However, all of these agents are susceptible to toxic overdose, which requires prompt recognition and initiation of therapy to reduce the risk of morbidity and mortality.

REFERENCES

1. Zimmerman HJ, Maddrey WC. Acetaminophen (paracetamol) hepatotoxicity with regular intake of alcohol: analysis of instances of therapeutic misadventure. Hepatology 1995;22(3):767–73.
2. Lee WM. Acetaminophen and the U.S. Acute Liver Failure Study Group: lowering the risks of hepatic failure. Hepatology 2004;40(1):6–9.
3. Vane JR, Botting RM. Mechanism of action of nonsteroidal anti-inflammatory drugs. Am J Med 1998;104(3):2S–8S.
4. Nelson LS, Lewin NA, Howland MA, et al. Goldfrank's toxicologic emergencies. New York: McGraw-Hill; 2011.
5. Schenker S, Speeg KV Jr, Perez A, et al. The effects of food restriction in man on hepatic metabolism of acetaminophen. Clin Nutr 2001;20(2):145–50.
6. Defendi GL. Acetaminophen toxicity in children: diagnosis, clinical assessment, and treatment of acute overingestion. Cons Pediat 2013;12(7):299–306. Available at: http://www.pediatricsconsultant360.com/article/acetaminophen-toxicity-children-diagnosis-clinical-assessment-and-treatment-acute. Accessed May 13, 2016.
7. Taylor RB, David AK, Johnson TA Jr, et al. Family medicine principles & practice. New York: Springer; 1998.
8. Linden CH, Rumack BH. Acetaminophen overdose. Emerg Med Clin North Am 1984;2(1):103–19.
9. Birge RB, Bartolone JB, Hart SG, et al. Acetaminophen hepatotoxicity: correspondence of selective protein arylation in human and mouse liver in vitro, in culture, and in vivo. Toxicol Appl Pharmacol 1990;105(3):472–82.
10. Ganley C, Dal Pan G, Rappaport B. Acetaminophen overdose and liver injury—background and options for reducing injury. Silver Spring (MD): Department of Health and Human Services: Food and Drug Administration; 2009. Available at: http://www.fda.gov/downloads/AdvisoryCommittees/CommitteesMeetingMaterials/Drugs/DrugSafetyandRiskManagementAdvisoryCommittee/UCM164897.pdf. Accessed April 15, 2016.
11. Lee MW. Drug-induced hepatotoxicity. N Engl J Med 2003;349(5):474–85.
12. Schmidt LE, Dalhoff K, Poulsen HE. Acute versus chronic alcohol consumption in acetaminophen-induced hepatotoxicity. Hepatology 2002;35(4):876–82.
13. Whitcomb DC, Block GD. Association of acetaminophen hepatotoxicity with fasting and ethanol use. JAMA 1994;272(23):1845–50.
14. Marx JA, Hockberger RS, Walls RM. Rosen's emergency medicine concepts and clinical practice. Philadelphia: Elsevier Saunders; 2014.
15. Zein JG, Wallace DJ, Kinasewitz G, et al. Early anion gap metabolic acidosis in acetaminophen overdose. Am J Emerg Med 2010;28(7):798–802.

16. Green TJ, Sivilotti ML, Langmann C, et al. When do the aminotransferases rise after acute acetaminophen overdose? Clin Toxicol (Phila) 2010;48(8):787–92.

17. Ambre J, Alexander M. Liver toxicity after acetaminophen ingestion. Inadequacy of the dose estimate as an index of risk. JAMA 1977;238(6):500–1.

18. Smilkstein MJ, Knapp GL, Kulig KW, et al. Efficacy of oral N-acetylcysteine in the treatment of acetaminophen overdose. Analysis of the national multicenter study (1976 to 1985). N Engl J Med 1988;319(24):1557–62.

19. Chamberlain JM, Gorman RL, Oderda GM, et al. Use of activated charcoal in a simulated poisoning with acetaminophen: a new loading dose for N-acetylcysteine? Ann Emerg Med 1993;22(9):1398–402.

20. Lapus RM. Activated charcoal for pediatric poisonings: the universal antidote? Curr Opin Pediatr 2007;19(2):216–22.

21. Lauterburg BH, Corcoran GB, Mitchell JR. Mechanism of action of N-acetylcysteine in the protection against the hepatotoxicity of acetaminophen in rats in vivo. J Clin Invest 1983;71(4):980–91.

22. Pratt S, Ioannides C. Mechanism of the protective action of N-acetylcysteine and methionine against paracetamol toxicity in the hamster. Arch Toxicol 1985;57(3): 173–7.

23. Smilkstein MJ, Bronstein AC, Linden C, et al. Acetaminophen overdose: a 48-hour intravenous N-acetylcysteine treatment protocol. Ann Emerg Med 1991; 20(10):1058–63.

24. Bebarta VS, Kao L, Froberg B, et al. A multicenter comparison of the safety of oral versus intravenous acetylcysteine for treatment of acetaminophen overdose. Clin Toxicol (Phila) 2010;48(5):424–30.

25. Woodhead JL, Howell BA, Yang Y, et al. An analysis of N-acetylcysteine treatment for acetaminophen overdose using a systems model of drug-induced liver injury. J Pharmacol Exp Ther 2012;342(2):529–40.

26. Green JL, Heard KJ, Reynolds KM, et al. Oral and intravenous acetylcysteine for treatment of acetaminophen toxicity: a systematic review and meta-analysis. West J Emerg Med 2013;14(3):218–26.

27. Aggrawal A. Textbook of forensic medicine and toxicology. New Delhi: Avichal Publishing Company; 2014.

28. Martinez MA, Ballesteros S, Almarza E, et al. Death in a legal poppy field in Spain. Forensic Sci Int 2015;265:34–40.

29. Rudd RA, Aleshire N, Zibbell JE, et al. Increases in drug and opioid overdose deaths—United States, 2000–2014. MMWR Morb Mortal Wkly Rep 2016; 64(50–51):1378–82.

30. Cordwell WH, Keene KK, Giles BK, et al. The high prevalence of pain in emergency medical care. Am J Emerg Med 2002;20(3):165–9.

31. Ringwalt C, Gugelmann H, Garrettson M, et al. Differential prescribing of opioid analgesics according to physician specialty for Medicaid patients with chronic noncancer pain diagnoses. Pain Res Manag 2014;19(4):179–85.

32. Waldhoer M, Bartlett SE, Whistler JL. Opioid receptors. Annu Rev Biochem 2004; 73:953–90.

33. Dhawan BN, Cesselin F, Raghubir R, et al. International union of pharmacology XII classification of opioid receptors. Pharmacol Rev 1996;48(4):567–92.

34. Butelman ER, France CP, Woods JH, et al. Apparent pA2 analysis on the respiratory depressant effects of alfentanil, etonitazene, ethylketocyclazocine (EKC) and Mr2033 in rhesus monkeys. J Pharmacol Exp Ther 1993;264(1):145–51.

35. Trivedi M, Shaikh S, Gwinnutt C, et al. Pharmacology of opioids II. Anaesthesia United Kingdom; 2007. Available at: http://www.frca.co.uk/article.aspx?articleid=100946. Accessed May 10, 2016.
36. Dean M. Opioids in renal failure and dialysis patients. J Pain Symptom Manage 2014;28(5):497–504.
37. Malek A. Drugs and medicines in pregnancy: the placental disposition of opioids. Curr Pharm Biotechnol 2011;12(5):797–803.
38. Kumar A, Paes B. Epidural opioid analgesia and neonatal respiratory depression. J Perinatol 2003;23(5):425–7.
39. Smith HS. Opioid metabolism. Mayo Clin Proc 2009;84(7):613–24.
40. Pauli-Magnus C, Hofmann U, Mikus G, et al. Pharmacokinetics of morphine and its glucuronides following intravenous administration of morphine in patients undergoing continuous ambulatory peritoneal dialysis. Nephrol Dial Transplant 1999;14(4):903–9.
41. Smith HS. Current therapy in pain. Philadelphia: Saunders Elsevier; 2009.
42. Urman RD, Vadivelu N. Perioperative pain management. New York: Oxford University Press; 2013.
43. Jeremias A, Brown DL. Cardiac intensive care. Philadelphia: Saunders Elsevier; 2010.
44. Marinella MA. Meperidine-induced generalized seizures with normal renal function. South Med J 1997;90(5):556–8.
45. Langston JW, Ballard P, Tetrud JW, et al. Chronic Parkinsonism in humans due to a product of meperidine-analog synthesis. Science 1983;219(4587):979–80.
46. Ballard PA, Tetrud JW, Langston JW. Permanent human parkinsonism due to 1-methyl-4-phenyl-1,2,3,6-tetrahydropyridine (MPTP): seven cases. Neurology 1985;35(7):949–56.
47. Isenberg D, Wong SC, Curtis JA. Serotonin syndrome triggered by a single dose of suboxone. Am J Emerg Med 2008;26(7):840.e3-5.
48. Pattinson KTS. Opioids and the control of respiration. Br J Anaesth 2008;100(6):747–58.
49. Bhardwaj H, Bhardwaj B, Awab A. Revisiting opioid overdose induced acute respiratory distress syndrome. Indian J Crit Care Med 2014;18(2):119–20.
50. Millane T, Jackson G, Gibbs CR, et al. ABC of heart failure. Acute and chronic management strategies. BMJ 2000;320(7234):559–62.
51. Smith HS, Smith JM, Seidner P, et al. Opioid-induced nausea and vomiting. Ann Palliat Med 2012;1(2):121–9.
52. Kurz A, Sessler DI. Opioid-induced bowel dysfunction: pathophysiology and potential new therapies. Drugs 2003;63(7):649–71.
53. Traub SJ, Hoffman RS, Nelson LS. Body packing—the internal concealment of illicit drugs. N Engl J Med 2003;349(26):2519–26.
54. Standridge JB, Adams SM, Zotos AP. Urine drug screening: a valuable office procedure. Am Fam Physician 2010;81(5):635–40.
55. Rohrig TP, Moore C. The determination of morphine in urine and oral fluid following ingestion of poppy seeds. J Anal Toxicol 2003;27(7):449–52.
56. Miller RD. Miller's anesthesia. Philadelphia: Saunders Elsevier; 2015. Print.
57. Wermeling DP. A response to the opioid overdose epidemic: naloxone nasal spray. Drug Deliv Transl Res 2014;3(1):63–74.
58. Wanger K, Brough L, Macmillan I, et al. Intravenous vs subcutaneous naloxone for out-of-hospital management of presumed opioid overdose. Acad Emerg Med 1998;5(4):293–9.

59. Barton ED, Ramos J, Colwell C, et al. Intranasal administration of naloxone by paramedics. Prehosp Emerg Care 2002;6(1):54–8.
60. Kelly AM, Kerr D, Dietze P, et al. Randomised trial of intranasal versus intramuscular naloxone in prehospital treatment for suspected opioid overdose. Med J Aust 2005;182(1):24–7.
61. Osterwalder JJ. Naloxone—for intoxications with intravenous heroin and heroin mixtures—harmless or hazardous? A prospective clinical study. J Toxicol Clin Toxicol 1996;34(4):409–16.
62. Agasti TK. Textbook of anaesthesia for postgraduates. New Delhi (India): Jaypee Brothers Medical Publishers; 2011. Print.
63. Goldfrank L, Weisman RS, Errick JK, et al. A dosing nomogram for continuous infusion intravenous naloxone. Ann Emerg Med 1986;15(5):566–70.
64. Position paper: whole bowel irrigation. J Toxicol Clin Toxicol 2004;42:843–54.
65. Thanacoody R, Caravati EM, Troutman B, et al. Position paper update: whole bowel irrigation for gastrointestinal decontamination of overdose patients. J Toxicol Clin Toxicol 2015;53(1):5–12.
66. Schwartz JA, Koenigsberg MD. Naloxone-induced pulmonary edema. Ann Emerg Med 1987;16(11):1294–6.
67. Horng HC, Ho MT, Huang CH, et al. Negative pressure pulmonary edema following naloxone administration in a patient with fentanyl-induced respiratory depression. Acta Anaesthesiol Taiwan 2010;48(3):155–7.
68. Etherington J, Christenson J, Innes G, et al. Is early discharge safe after naloxone reversal of presumed opioid overdose? CJEM 2000;2(3):156–62.
69. Salicylate (SALY). Therapeutic drug monitoring. Brea, CA: Beckman Coulter, Inc; 2003. Available at: https://www.beckmancoulter.com/wsrportal/bibliography?docname=9282%20e9%20SALY.pdf. Accessed May 14, 2016.
70. Nulton-Persson A, Szweda LI, Sadek HA. Inhibition of cardiac mitochondrial respiration by salicylic acid and acetylsalicylate. J Cardiovasc Pharmacol 2004;44(5):591–5.
71. Paikin JS, Eikelboom JW. Cardiology patient page: aspirin. Circulation 2012;125:439–42.
72. Fosslien E. Mitochondrial medicine—molecular pathology of defective oxidative phosphorylation. Ann Clin Lab Sci 2001;31(1):25–67.
73. Trost LC, Lemasters JJ. The mitochondrial permeability transition: a new pathophysiological mechanism for Reye's syndrome and toxic liver injury. J Pharmacol Exp Ther 1996;278(3):1000–5.
74. Dart RC. Medical toxicology. Philadelphia: Lippincott Williams & Wilkins; 2004.
75. Tanabe P, Buschmann M. A prospective study of ED pain management practices and the patient's perspective. J Emerg Nurs 1999;25(3):171–7.
76. Downey LV, Zun LS. Pain management in the emergency department and its relationship to patient satisfaction. J Emerg Trauma Shock 2010;3(4):326–30.

Use of the Clinical Laboratory in Psychiatric Practice

Christopher Aloezos, MD[a], Jonathan M. Wai, MD[a],*,
Martin H. Bluth, MD, PhD[b,c], Howard Forman, MD[a]

KEYWORDS

- Clinical laboratory • Psychotropic prescribing practices
- Therapeutic drug monitoring • Urine drug testing • Substance abuse
- Blood drug levels • Urine drug levels

KEY POINTS

- The clinical laboratory is an invaluable tool for guiding prescribing practices of psychiatric medications. Laboratory results should always be correlated with a clinical examination and are rarely useful on their own.
- Care must be taken when testing patients for medication levels that the results of such testing can be useful and will affect treatment.
- There is much literature but still inconclusive evidence for the usefulness of medication levels in blood and other fluids for many psychotropic agents.
- For psychiatric care, medication levels may be best used when ordered with a specific clinical question as opposed to as a general screening battery for all patients.

INTRODUCTION

The clinical laboratory can be a useful tool in psychiatry, but is not always clinically indicated. Advances in laboratory testing technology can sometimes outpace clinical scientific advances of how to use this technology. When ordering a drug level or toxicology assessment in the discipline of psychiatry, one must think of the clinical setting, the potential significance of the results, the class of medication being tested, and most importantly whether the information will have an impact on treatment or expected treatment outcomes. Although the laboratory toxicology workup is used in pain, addiction, and other fields of medicine, psychiatric evaluation and assessment is unique in certain

All authors have no financial disclosures.
[a] Department of Psychiatry and Behavioral Sciences, Montefiore Medical Center, The University Hospital for Albert Einstein College of Medicine, 111 East 210th Street, Bronx, NY 10467, USA; [b] Deparment of Pathology, Wayne State University School of Medicine, 540 East Canfield, Detroit, MI 48201, USA; [c] Consolidated Laboratory Management Systems, 24555 Southfield Road, Southfield, MI 48075, USA
* Corresponding author.
E-mail address: jwai@montefiore.org

Clin Lab Med 36 (2016) 777–793
http://dx.doi.org/10.1016/j.cll.2016.07.004   labmed.theclinics.com

respects. Although the ability exists in our modern era to test for almost everything, the situations where one should test are far more limited. In this review, we address treatment considerations in different psychiatric settings and discuss how the clinical laboratory can be effectively used in each of these settings. We also review each of the major psychiatric medication classes and discuss how the clinical laboratory can be used to guide prescribing practices. Although substance use and addiction are closely intertwined with regular psychiatric care, therapeutic drug monitoring (TDM) and its role in psychiatric treatment are the primary focus of this review. Where applicable, we comment on the nonmedical use of psychiatric medication as well.

TREATMENT CONSIDERATIONS DEPENDING ON SETTING

The goals of treatment in psychiatry differ based on the clinical setting. The basic treatment settings are the emergency setting, inpatient setting (either psychiatrically or medically hospitalized), and the outpatient setting. Each setting will have slightly different considerations.

Emergency

In the emergency setting, the primary goal is stabilization of acute issues, some of which may be life threatening, and evaluation to determine if the patient can be treated as an outpatient or inpatient. In this setting, one can usually assume psychiatric treatment failure because many patients presenting to the psychiatric emergency room are in distress. Discharge planning is usually done in this setting to ensure continuity of care, but is not as involved as in the inpatient setting.

Contact between the clinician and patient is limited in this setting, with treatment often lasting less than 1 day. Patients sometimes present without records or collateral information, and their histories may be unknown, especially if a patient is unable to cooperate with a diagnostic interview. Safety is also always a concern in the emergency setting, and a thorough clinical interview and examination can be hindered by an aggressive or psychiatrically unstable patient.

In this setting, screening tests are invaluable sources of information, and clinicians will often order batteries of tests for every patient with minor adjustments when clinically indicated. Laboratory tests such as urine toxicology screens for drugs of abuse, thyroid-stimulating hormone levels, and computed tomography play an invaluable role in the evaluation of a patient in the emergency setting and play a large role in the decision-making process. In general, drug testing of urine may only be useful qualitatively, whereas drug testing in serum may be either qualitatively or quantitatively useful for therapeutic levels.

Checking for blood levels of therapeutic drugs with well-defined therapeutic windows, such as lithium or clozapine, can indicate whether treatment failure occurred when the patient was at a therapeutic level of a drug, or if low blood levels may have impacted a patient's psychiatric stability. It can also inform decision making when suspecting lithium toxicity, although this must also be correlated with a thorough clinical examination.[1] Specific medications where blood levels are more useful are discussed in the class-specific sections.

Although some studies have found routine drug screening to be helpful in the detection of substance use,[2,3] others have found that they did not affect disposition or duration of inpatient stays,[4] management,[5] or diagnosis.[6] There is little evidence for the usefulness of routine urine drug screening in the emergency setting for patients without clinical suspicion of substance use or intoxication.[7] Testing for substances in an acute intoxication or overdose are discussed elsewhere.

We could not find any literature on how to use urine drug testing to assess the therapeutic effect of psychotropic medications in the emergency setting. However, the literature on urine drug screens for drugs of abuse suggests that routine screening for psychotropic medications, in particular, does not significantly affect the treatment outcomes of patients in the emergency setting, and that such tests should only be used to confirm a clinical suspicion when it would affect clinical decision making.

In summary, there is little evidence that routine drug screening of all psychiatric patients in the emergency setting guides clinical care, and a thorough history and clinical examination may sometimes be sufficient in this setting. However, with clinical suspicion and in certain situations where a medication presence and/or level would affect care, then we would recommend ordering a medication level or urine drug test.

Inpatient

In the inpatient psychiatric setting, immediate life-threatening problems are ideally already managed in the emergency room or inpatient medical unit, and a basic laboratory workup has already been completed. Patients are generally more stable at this time; however, the same acute issues that present initially in the emergency room may occasionally arise. Patient care still is time limited, and unless it is in a long-term psychiatric inpatient unit, management is still in the acute phase of the illness. The care of patients under long-term hospitalization (such as patients in state hospitals) has similar treatment implications as in the outpatient setting, except that these patients will have more supervision and closer access to medical and psychiatric care.

Inpatient psychiatric hospitalization often has the goal of stabilizing patients so that they can be managed appropriately in the outpatient setting. The evaluation of a patient is more in depth than in the emergency setting, with a greater emphasis on psychosocial factors as well as long-term considerations for treatment. Patients are often started and titrated on new medications on the inpatient units. There is often an emphasis on quick stabilization and discharge, with a decreasing duration of stay as reimbursement for longer hospitalizations declines.

TDM can be invaluable in medications that have well-established therapeutic windows. Medications such as mood stabilizers should be titrated to achieve a therapeutic blood level, and if symptoms persist despite a therapeutic level, adjunctive medications can be considered. In medications with less well-established therapeutic windows, drug monitoring can be used to check if a patient has been taking a medication, or to indicate if a patient is possibly an ultrafast or ultraslow metabolizer. Because there is a range of therapeutic levels even for the well-established therapeutic windows of mood stabilizers, clinical response should be considered when deciding if a patient has an acceptable medication dose. As always, blood levels must be correlated with clinical judgment and is of little value in the absence of a clinical examination.

Outpatient

Since the dehospitalization of psychiatry in the late 20th century, there has been a major shift of services for the mentally ill from the inpatient to the outpatient setting.[8] The move brought with it many ethical and treatment implications that come with increased patient autonomy.

In contrast with the emergency and inpatient settings, decision making in the outpatient setting must take into account both immediate concerns as well as issues that may arise after years or decades of treatment. In addition, in the outpatient setting patients are volunteering themselves to be in treatment (except for cases of court-mandated treatment), and therefore have the right to adhere to or refuse treatment recommendations. Successful treatment in this setting must be more collaborative than in the emergency or inpatient treatment settings and highlights the importance of therapeutic alliance. Time and time again, evidence has shown that the quality of the therapeutic alliance between the doctor and patient is a reliable predictor of positive clinical outcome, independent of the type of psychotherapy modality and outcome measure.[9]

Many present-day outpatient mental health services are composed of a multidisciplinary team that provide both psychotherapy and medication management, if indicated. Various modalities of psychotherapy are usually conducted by either a psychiatrist, clinical psychologist, or a licensed social worker, and the vast majority of medication management is provided by psychiatrists, primary care physicians, and nurse practitioners.

For a significant number of patients with mental illness, treatment includes taking psychiatric medication for the long term. Some of these medications have significant side effect profiles and well-defined therapeutic windows. For these medications, such as clozapine, lithium, and valproic acid, routine TDM is required for the entire duration of treatment to prevent side effects and toxicity. Patients taking medications like these, with well-established therapeutic ranges, should undergo blood level monitoring as standard of care.

Unless patients are in crisis and require a more restrictive treatment setting, patients' symptoms are generally less acute in the outpatient setting. As such, when medications are started, titrated, augmented, tapered, or discontinued, they are typically done so at a slower pace to prevent inducing avoidable side effects, dosing medications too high, inciting withdrawal symptoms, and to ensure treatment adherence. Accordingly, TDM for medications without clearly established therapeutic windows may be considered when there is treatment nonresponse or failure that is not better explained through a sound history and examination. In the outpatient setting, treatment failure is often owing to medication nonadherence. A systematic review showed that the mean rate of treatment adherence was 58% among patients with psychoses and 65% among patients with depression,[10] leaving a significant percentage of patients nonadherent to medications. Another cause of treatment failure in the outpatient setting is medication diversion. TDM and urine drug testing may help the clinician to assess for possible treatment nonadherence when suspected.[11] Similar to the emergency and inpatient settings, drug testing of urine may only be useful qualitatively, to assess for the presence or absence of a medication.

In summary, psychiatric treatment in the outpatient setting is longitudinal, voluntary, and is often provided by various members of a multidisciplinary treatment team. These factors help to determine whether TDM should be a part of treatment. In the outpatient setting, for medications with a well-established therapeutic range, blood level monitoring should be the standard of care. For patients with treatment nonresponse or failure checking blood or other body fluids as appropriate may help to guide care.

HOW PSYCHIATRISTS PRESCRIBE

Many psychotropic medications are unique in their usage in that patients are often started on them at a relatively young age and continue to take them throughout their lifetime. Many psychiatric illnesses have their first presentation when patients are in their late teens to early 30s. Because of the lengthy duration of treatment, important consideration of side effects as well as efficacy are essential parts of the decision-making process. Because many side effects are dose related, the goal is always to maintain a patient on the lowest possible effective dose.

In general, psychotropic medications are started at a low therapeutic dose, and after a significant trial, titrated up for response. Sometimes medications are started at subtherapeutic doses when there are tolerability concerns. Medications should generally be titrated up to their maximum dose approved by the US Food and Drug Administration (FDA) if there is not a full remission of targeted symptoms. The length of time a clinician waits to increase the medication is determined by the pharmacodynamic and pharmacokinetic properties of the medication. Because of individual differences in these properties, the American Psychiatric Association practice guidelines recommends sometimes going above FDA-approved dosages for antidepressant medications to achieve adequate blood levels.[12] When checking blood levels, laboratory tests are usually drawn at the trough and care must be taken when ordering laboratory tests for a patient to have them drawn at the appropriate time to avoid misinterpretation of laboratory values.

For some medications, there are clearly defined therapeutic windows for blood levels. For these medications, too low of a blood level will not have therapeutic efficacy and too high of a level may either not be efficacious, or will unnecessarily increase the risk of side effects.

However, for a vast majority of psychiatric medications, there is not a clearly defined therapeutic window that is supported by scientific evidence. For these medications, we propose the following approach (**Fig. 1**). Proper medication administration must always be assessed, and a scrupulous assessment of how a patient is taking their medication must be performed whenever there is concern for improper medication usage. When a clinical assessment is either unrevealing or unreliable, then blood levels can help to guide treatment by grossly approximating whether or not the patient has too little or too much of a medication in their system.

For urine drug testing, there is no good evidence that urine medication levels can inform clinical efficacy of a medication. Urine drug testing for therapeutic medications (as opposed to medications being misused) may only be useful if the medication is not detected, which would indicate medication nonadherence. A positive value does not guarantee sufficient dosing or long-term and regular medication adherence, which are both important for medications to be effective. If the medication is absent from the

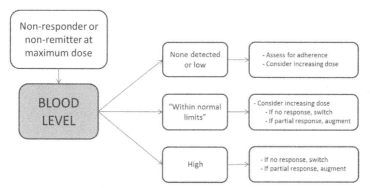

Fig. 1. General approach of using therapeutic drug monitoring for medications without well-established therapeutic windows. Blood levels are rarely useful alone and should always be correlated with a clinical assessment of variables such as medication adherence, drug–drug interactions, therapeutic response, and side effects. Considerations of individual medications should be taken into account when deciding dose adjustments, augmentation strategies, or switching between medications.

urine altogether, then the clinician can be reasonably certain that there is some degree of temporary medication nonadherence at the minimum, although this again does not inform long-term or regular nonadherence. Individual considerations of each medication by class are discussed in the sections herein.

ANTIDEPRESSANT MEDICATIONS

Antidepressant medications contain a heterogeneous group of medications that are used to treat not only depressive disorders, but also a variety of other psychiatric and pain disorders. Many psychiatric medications have a variety of FDA-approved indications, and antidepressant medications are perhaps the best exemplar of this. For example, fluoxetine, the oldest of the widely used selective serotonin reuptake inhibitors (SSRIs), is FDA approved for the treatment of major depressive disorder, obsessive–compulsive disorder, premenstrual dysphoric disorder, bulimia nervosa, panic disorder, and bipolar depression (when combined with olanzapine).[13] Antidepressant medications are implemented regularly in the treatment of anxiety and obsessive compulsive disorder. Indeed, the term "antidepressant" is a misnomer now, because the scope of these medications extends far beyond depression.

Antidepressant medications are used as first-line treatments for depression and anxiety, with treatment often being chronic. Medication is usually continued for at least 1 year, and patients with more severe symptomatology often require lifelong pharmacotherapy for maintenance, even in the absence of symptoms. Antidepressant medications are only one of several treatment modalities for the treatment of depression, with psychotherapy, psychosocial interventions, and electroconvulsive therapy being other effective options. The nature of therapy indicated is determined in part by the severity of the depression, with more aggressive interventions recommended for a more severe illness.

Because many psychiatric medications are taken chronically, and the effects of missing doses or even discontinuing some medications are not felt acutely, medication adherence is an important issue to address in treatment. Some antidepressant medications can cause withdrawal symptoms if discontinued abruptly, with the medications with shorter half-lives being more likely to do so.

Mechanism of Action

All antidepressant medications interact with the monoamine receptor system in the brain and have actions at the synapse. They all act to increase the amount of monoamines in the synapse.[14] Antidepressant medications have antidepressant therapeutic effects that occur within a matter of weeks, much longer than it takes to increase the amount of monoamines in the synapse. The exact mechanism that makes these medications cause their clinical effects remains unknown.

Among the available classes of antidepressant medications are SSRIs, serotonin-norepinephrine reuptake inhibitors (SNRIs), norepinephrine reuptake inhibitors, serotonin receptor antagonists and agonists, norepinephrine-dopamine reuptake inhibitors, alpha-2–adrenergic receptor antagonists, tricyclic antidepressants (TCAs), and monoamine oxidase inhibitors (MAOIs).[14] The different classes of antidepressant medications work on different parts of the synapse and on different variations of monoamines.

Antidepressant medications are almost all metabolized by the cytochrome P450 enzyme system and their blood levels are subsequently determined by both the dose of medication and level of enzyme activity. Pharmacogenomics can inform medication dosing, but known genotype differences that affect medication dosing often reflect differences in hepatic metabolism.[15]

Antidepressant medications almost all affect serotonin levels in the brain, with some antidepressant medications also affecting norepinephrine and/or dopamine. These medications likely do not have an immediate therapeutic effect through their known mechanisms of action[16] and there is generally a lag time for response, usually taking 2 to 4 weeks.[17] Consequently, patients do not feel an immediate improvement in their targeted symptoms as they would when taking an analgesic or a benzodiazepine. This lack of immediate efficacy can sometimes lead to cessation of medications, either because a patient may believe that they are not working, or that they no longer require the medication anymore because they are feeling better. Response monitoring is an important part of treatment, and can be monitored using scales or clinically assessing any improvement in symptoms or function.

The newer antidepressant medications (SSRIs, SNRIs, etc) all have more favorable side effect profiles over the older TCAs and MAOIs, and have consequently become the first-line treatment for depression. Because of the relatively safe side effect profiles of these newer medications, monitoring blood levels is no longer a necessary part of treatment like with the TCAs, which could cause cardiac toxicity and seizures at toxic levels.[18] In the absence of significant toxicity from high blood levels, it is difficult to determine definitively what an optimal therapeutic window should be. Although there is some evidence for an optimal therapeutic blood level for some of the SSRIs and SNRIs,[19,20] there are conflicting data on what that blood level should be and if blood levels are correlated with treatment response.[21]

Therapeutic Drug Monitoring

Although there has been evidence of a therapeutic window for some antidepressant medications, the literature remains inconclusive and following blood levels for most antidepressant medications is not a routine part of care when there is a good response to treatment.

Only plasma level monitoring of TCAs has been recommended specifically by the American Psychiatric Association.[12] Additionally, blood levels can be checked when using MAOIs to ensure that there are no drug interactions with other antidepressant medications that were being used before starting the MAOI, or after the MAOI has been discontinued. MAOIs used concomitantly with other antidepressant medications have a significant risk of serotonin syndrome, so greater care must be taken to ensure safety.

The literature on the usefulness of TDM for antidepressant medications has been inconclusive, with the exception of TCAs, for example, nortriptyline, amitriptyline, imipramine, and desipramine. Serum drug levels are useful for TCAs because there is a relatively well-established therapeutic window for these medications,[22] but also, unlike the newer SSRIs and SNRIs, high levels can lead to serious toxicities, such as cardiac conduction abnormalities.[23]

Several studies have demonstrated that for many antidepressant medications, there is a linear or curvilinear correlation between dose and plasma concentrations.[24] There is some evidence that using TDM early in treatment can help to lower medication dosages.[25]

There are limited reasons to check serum drug levels, and it should not be a part of routine care when a patient is showing a good response to a medication and is without significant side effects. Wide recommended therapeutic ranges for most of the antidepressant medications and low toxicity for many make interpretation of serum drug levels difficult.[26] TDM may be considered in medication-sensitive populations such as patients with complicated medical issues, pediatric patients, older patients, or patients on extensive medication regimens. At this stage, owing to a lack of well-established evidence of an optimal serum range for most antidepressant medications, TDM is of limited usefulness. The role of TDM for heterogenic antidepressant medications is further complicated by the fact that depression is a heterogenic illness, both in its symptomatology and neurobiology.[27]

At this time, there is no literature on urine levels of antidepressant medications that can be used to guide drug therapy. If urine drug levels are to be used, we recommend checking random urine drug levels, similar to the use of random drug screens for substance abuse. Urine drug levels may be used to check medication adherence, although it does not inform long-term adherence or if the patient is on a significantly high dose. Although there is much literature on detection methods of various antidepressant medications in urine,[28] there is yet to be any evidence of what a therapeutic urine level would be. Thus, the usefulness of urine toxicology for antidepressant medications would be similar to that of when checking for drugs of abuse—to inform the clinician simply if a patient has taken the substance at all within a given amount of time that depends on the specific assay, half-life, and metabolites.

MOOD STABILIZERS

Mood stabilizers are another heterogeneous group of medications used to treat bipolar disorder. For treatment of bipolar disorder, clinicians must consider both the acute and maintenance phases for both depression and mania. Mood stabilizers should be used both in the treatment of acute mania, and also as long-term maintenance therapy for prophylaxis against further manic or depressive episodes. The mood stabilizers can be classified into 2 main groups: lithium and the anticonvulsants. Lithium was the first drug to demonstrate antimanic effects and was discovered when Cade[29] noticed its ability to pacify animals in 1949 and then tried it on manic patients with profound effect. Antipsychotic medications and benzodiazepines also have a major role in the treatment of bipolar disorder; their properties are discussed in their respective sections.

Mechanisms of Action and Therapeutic Drug Monitoring

Lithium is the most established medication for treatment of bipolar disorder, being the oldest medication and the most efficacious for treatment and prevention of mania. The exact mechanism of action responsible for lithium's therapeutic effect remains unclear, although there are several hypotheses. The most researched is the inositol depletion hypothesis, which hypothesizes that lithium acts to decrease the amount of inositol in neurons by inhibiting inositol monophosphatase to block inositol synthesis, dampening neurotransmission that depends on the phosphatidylinositol 4,5-biphosphate second messenger system.[30] Another hypothesis is that lithium inhibits glycogen synthase kinase 3β activity, an enzyme that may play a role in signal transduction in the brain.[31]

Because lithium has a narrow therapeutic window, monitoring blood levels of lithium is an essential part of therapy. Additionally, its clinical efficacy has been correlated with blood levels and not the oral dose, with higher levels within the therapeutic window being more efficacious.[32] Because of its potential toxicity (cardiac, renal, and neurologic, among others), clinicians must ensure that a patient's lithium dose is not in the toxic range. Additionally, side effects and toxicity from lithium increase as blood levels increase.[1] Because lithium is excreted almost entirely by the kidneys, a patient's lithium level must be closely monitored when changing any medications that may affect renal clearance.

The 3 main anticonvulsants with the most evidence for efficacy as mood stabilizers are valproic acid, carbamazepine, and lamotrigine.[33–35] Valproic acid and carbamazepine are more effective in treating and preventing manic episodes, whereas lamotrigine has shown better efficacy for the treatment and prevention of bipolar depression.

The mechanism of action of valproic acid for the treatment of bipolar disorder remains unknown, but it is known to increase synaptic levels of the inhibitory neurotransmitter, gamma-aminobutyric acid (GABA). Although valproic acid has a variety of side effects and toxicities, and in an overdose severe neurologic symptoms such as sedation and ataxia may occur, death from an overdose is uncommon, unlike lithium.

Carbamazepine is thought to work by binding to the inactivated state of sodium channels to decrease repetitive action potentials and also block presynaptic sodium channels to inhibit depolarization of the presynaptic terminal. Like valproic acid, although this drug may have serious side effects, it is often not lethal in overdose, with the major concerns being atrioventricular block and excess sedation. Because carbamazepine induces its own metabolism through the cytochrome P450 system, periodic TDM is important to ensure that this medication is dosed sufficiently.

Lamotrigine is more effective for the treatment and prevention of bipolar depression than mania. Its mechanism of action for bipolar disorder remains unknown, but lamotrigine inhibits the release of glutamine, an excitatory amino acid, to decrease excitation in the central nervous system. It also blocks voltage-sensitive sodium channels. Therapeutic blood levels have not been clearly established for lamotrigine. An important side effect to be wary of is Stevens–Johnson syndrome, which may be fatal. This side effect is more likely to occur when dosages are increased rapidly, so a slow and gradual titration in lamotrigine is necessary.

Although there is evidence for therapeutic windows for valproic acid and carbamazepine, the ranges are wide and there is a poor correlation between blood levels and efficacy for mania. Blood levels of all of these medications are useful in assessing treatment adherence and for informing whether persistent symptoms are because of nonadherence or because of lack of efficacy of a medication. The presence of each of these mood stabilizers is testable in the urine, but there is no literature on what a therapeutic level would be. Thus, testing for these drugs in the urine will only inform the clinician if the patient has taken this medication at all within a given amount of time dependent on excretion rates.

In summary, mood stabilizers are a mainstay of treatment for patients with bipolar disorder. For many of the mood stabilizers there is evidence for maintaining blood levels within an established therapeutic window. Lithium has the most well-defined therapeutic window and, because of efficacy and toxicity concerns, it is imperative that the blood level be monitored and within the acceptable range. For other mood stabilizers, there is a wider range of therapeutic levels and less toxicity with overdose. TDM is important for correct dosing of these long-term medications to ensure that a patient is properly both treated and prophylaxed against any further mood episodes.

ANTIPSYCHOTIC MEDICATIONS

Antipsychotic medications have been in clinical use since the 1950s and are used primarily to treat severe mental illnesses like schizophrenia, schizoaffective disorder, and other psychotic disorders. Since then, many antipsychotic medications have been developed and their use has expanded to treat other psychiatric disorders as well. Certain antipsychotic medications have since been FDA approved to treat mood disorders such as major depressive disorder and bipolar disorder, both as monotherapy and as adjunctive treatment. In clinical practice, antipsychotic medications are also used off-label, for example, to treat behavioral manifestations of neurocognitive disorders and to treat symptoms of severe personality disorders, among others. Some commonly used first-generation antipsychotic medications are haloperidol, perphenazine, and fluphenazine. Commonly used second-generation antipsychotic medications are risperidone, quetiapine, clozapine, olanzapine, and aripiprazole, to name a few.

Mechanism of Action

Antipsychotic medications have complex binding properties, and accordingly it has been difficult to isolate the exact mechanism that confers antipsychotic properties. In general, antipsychotic medications are thought to treat psychosis primarily by blocking the dopamine D2 receptor in the mesolimbic and mesocortical dopamine tracts in the brain. However, they also block D2 receptors elsewhere, adding risk for causing extrapyramidal symptoms (EPS). As such, in general D2 receptor antagonism correlates both with efficacy and EPS, whereas serotonin 2A receptor blockade seems to diminish the risk of EPS.

The first antipsychotic medications developed have an increased risk for causing EPS and are thus called first-generation antipsychotic medications. They have been in use for more than one-half of a century. Additional antipsychotic medications were later developed in an effort to diminish the risk of EPS, and this was accomplished by developing medications with different receptor binding properties. For example, the newer antipsychotic medications antagonize the serotonin 2A receptor to a greater degree, thus lessening the risk of EPS. These antipsychotic medications that have a lower risk of EPS are called second-generation antipsychotic medications. First-generation antipsychotic medications in general tend to have a lesser affinity for antagonizing cholinergic, histaminic, and adrenergic receptors. This confers fewer metabolic side effects as compared with second-generation antipsychotic medications.[36] Both first- and second-generation antipsychotic medications have various options for routes of administration, including orally (as a pill or liquid), sublingually, intramuscularly, and intravenously. The intramuscular forms exist both in short-acting and long-acting forms for certain antipsychotic medications. Similar to antidepressant medications, full therapeutic effects take several weeks to accumulate, much slower than the time to dopamine blockade and steady state. This suggests that there potentially exists a secondary change in receptor blockade through receptor regulation.

Most antipsychotic medications are metabolized in the liver, where they are made more water soluble and thus more readily excreted. Liver metabolism is affected by several factors, including but not limited to age, intrinsic metabolic rates, and the presence of other hepatically metabolized medications, resulting in widely varying blood levels. Additionally, for certain antipsychotic medications, active metabolites exist following liver metabolism, which can confer additional antipsychotic properties.

Therapeutic Drug Monitoring

Because there are great individual differences in the metabolism of antipsychotic medications and nonadherence confers poor outcomes in patients with severe mental illness, it would be clinically useful to have an objective measure to assess for efficacy and adherence to these medications. Aside from clozapine, therapeutic drug level monitoring is not currently a routine part of care.

For clozapine, there is consistent evidence that there exists a therapeutic range that confers clinical efficacy. Studies have also shown that levels as low as 200 ng/mL can be therapeutic, whereas levels of greater than 600 ng/mL are associated with increased risk of side effects, most notably seizures.[37] As such, routine blood level monitoring should be a mainstay, because there is strong evidence for its therapeutic window. Also, patients taking clozapine are already subject to routine blood draws owing to risk of agranulocytosis, making the task of blood level testing less cumbersome for the patient. TDM should be used when there are significant dose adjustments, when there is a worsening of symptoms, or if there is concern for toxicity.

For other antipsychotic medications, including both first generation and second generation, there is no clear consensus whether TDM has a role in clinical care, but there are differences among the classes. For both first- and second-generation antipsychotic medications, some studies indicate possible usefulness of drug level monitoring, whereas others show a clear inconsistency of drug levels between individuals and within the same individual on the same medication. Still, although there is an overall lack of consensus, there seems to be more consistent evidence for potential TDM for first-generation antipsychotic medications. For example, for haloperidol, perphenazine, and fluphenazine, there is evidence showing that blood levels can be indicative of clinical response,[38,39] and others show a worsening in clinical response for haloperidol owing to EPS at levels of greater than 10 ng/mL.[40] This was similarly found for fluphenazine. For perphenazine, there is concern for EPS at blood level concentrations of greater than 5 ng/mL.[41] There is less consistent evidence for the remainder of the first-generation antipsychotic medications. Still, testing serum drug levels for certain first-generation antipsychotic medications seems to be most clinically useful in protecting against EPS. Although this practice is currently not a routine part of psychiatric care because EPS is a clinical diagnosis and a thorough history, physical examination, and mental status examination are currently the mainstay of clinical practice, there may be a role for drug level monitoring in certain cases.

Aside from clozapine, as discussed, there is less evidence for the role of blood testing in second-generation antipsychotic medications. For example, a study showed that risperidone blood levels varied greatly between patients receiving the same dose, suggesting a variety of physiologic, genetic, and environmental factors effecting blood levels. However, these variations in blood levels do not correlate with efficacy of the medication.[42,43] There is similarly inconclusive evidence for many other second generation antipsychotic medications.

For both first- and second-generation antipsychotic medications, there is no clear evidence for the role of urine drug testing in patients taking these medications.

In summary, TDM should be a part of treatment for patients taking clozapine, and can be considered in certain cases for patients taking first-generation antipsychotic medications. There is an overall lack of consistent evidence for the remainder of second-generation antipsychotic medications. There seems to be no well-defined role for urine drug testing for all antipsychotic medications in the assessment of therapeutic efficacy.

BENZODIAZEPINES

Benzodiazepines are a class of medications used for a variety of psychiatric disorders and symptoms, including anxiety disorders, alcohol withdrawal, insomnia, agitation, and catatonia, to name a few. While benzodiazepines have anticonvulsant, muscle relaxant, and amnesic properties, it is their sedative, hypnotic, and anxiolytic actions that are used to treat patients with psychiatric illness.[44]

Mechanism of Action

Benzodiazepines act on the central nervous system by binding to specific sites on the $GABA_A$ receptor, a ligand-gated channel that binds GABA, the major inhibitory neurotransmitter in the brain. When a benzodiazepine binds to the $GABA_A$ receptor, it alters the conformation of the receptor, increasing its affinity for GABA. This results in an influx of anions, leading to hyperpolarization, and thus inhibition of neuronal firing and subsequent central nervous system depression. The half-life for commonly used benzodiazepines range from 6 to 100 hours, and are divided into rapid, intermediate, and slow onset of action.

The most commonly used benzodiazepines are metabolized through the liver by the cytochrome P450 enzyme system. Aside from a few notable exceptions, benzodiazepines are metabolized initially by hepatic microsomal enzymes through various processes, including oxidation, hydroxylation, and demethylation. These products are then conjugated with glucoronic acid, which are readily excreted in the urine. Some benzodiazepines have active metabolites that produce clinically significant effects, whereas others do not. Notable exceptions to these metabolic steps are oxazepam, temazepam, and lorazepam, which are metabolized only by glucoronidation. As such, they have no active metabolites and are less sensitive to changes seen in liver disease and aging.

The clinical efficacy depends on the presence of at least a minimum effective concentration in the blood; however, there is great variability between benzodiazepines and between patients. For example, diazepam has a great volume of distribution, so a single dose will be active for only a short period. However, after repeated administration and saturation, owing to its long elimination half-life, it becomes bioavailable for a much longer time period. The opposite is true for many other benzodiazepines, which have low volumes of distribution and long elimination half-lives. At the furthest extreme are the rapid onset, high-potency, short half-life benzodiazepines. These properties make this subset of benzodiazepines very effective in producing sedative, anxiolytic, and hypnotic effects; however, they also are known to have a high abuse potential, cause tolerance, and pose a risk for withdrawal. As such, although a minimum concentration is at least needed to produce pharmacologic effects, a particular blood level in one individual may show efficacy, whereas the same level in another patient may not produce any effect at all, or worse, may cause intoxication or toxicity.[45]

Therapeutic Drug Monitoring

There is evidence showing a clear inconsistency between benzodiazepine blood level and clinical response. As such, TDM using blood levels does not play a role in guiding treatment with benzodiazepines. This is primarily owing to issues of tolerance and the variability of clinical response between patients.[46,47] Additionally, because the effects of benzodiazepines are rapid, treatment should instead be guided by immediate clinical impression rather than drug monitoring.

Although TDM using blood levels is not a routine part of care, urine drug screens can be used when there is concern for nonadherence or diversion. This should not be used indiscriminately, and should be guided by clinical judgment. For example, if a patient shows a lack of therapeutic effects under usual doses, a urine drug screen may help to inform the clinician about adherence. However, this is not a universal rule. There are many benzodiazepines that are not identified reliably on routine urine drug screens, so caution and sound clinical knowledge should be used when ordering urine drug screens.[48]

STIMULANTS

Attention deficit hyperactivity disorder (ADHD) is a childhood-onset disorder that affects a behavior, attention, and impulse control and is estimated to affect 3% to 8%

of children.[49] One of the mainstays of treatment for children with ADHD is a stimulant medication, which has been shown to be superior to intensive behavioral treatment and community care.[50] Although stimulants only have indications for ADHD and narcolepsy, they are also used off-label for the treatment of apathy and withdrawal in geriatric patients, antidepressant augmentation, and for SSRI-induced apathy and sexual dysfunction. Still, as compared with other psychiatric medications, stimulants have a narrow list of uses.

Although they are currently primarily used for ADHD, in the 1930s amphetamine was used medically for various pulmonary pathologies because they cause bronchodilation and respiratory stimulation, and then later for the treatment of depression. In 1954, methylphenidates were developed. In 1970, owing to their abuse potential, the FDA moved stimulant medications to schedule II, thus greatly limiting their use. Still, studies have consistently showed the child and adolescent patients with ADHD taking stimulants show a reduced risk of substance use disorders later in life.[51]

Mechanism of Action

Both amphetamines and methlyphenidates, the two main classes of stimulants used in psychiatry, generally are well absorbed orally, and have a short half-life. Peak blood levels are seen within a few hours after taking, and thus they need to be dosed several times per day. Blood level concentrations of sustained-release formulations peak an hour or two longer after their immediate release counterparts, and have a longer half-life, allowing for once a day dosing. Both the amphetamines and methylphenidates act by causing the release of norepinephrine, dopamine, and serotonin in monoamine neurons; however, they do so in slightly different ways. Amphetamines primarily cause the exocytosis of vesicles carrying monoamine neurotransmitters, whereas methylphenidates act by regulating both presynaptic and postsynaptic dopamine neurotransmitters in the prefrontal cortex and striatum.

Therapeutic Drug Monitoring

Although overdose, abuse, and central nervous system side effects are potential issues in patients taking stimulant medications, there is currently no role for TDM for several reasons. These medications are rapid onset and have short half-lives. As such, the medications' therapeutic effect and duration before metabolism and excretion is short lived. Symptoms instead should be monitored clinically, and dose adjustments should be made thoughtfully to target cognitive and behavioral symptoms while minding potential side effects such as headache, insomnia, and hypertension.

Many standard urine drug screens can detect amphetamine-derived stimulant medications. Similar to previous classes of medication, this may potentially be used to help the clinician when there is a question of adherence or diversion. However, given the rapid on–off of these medications, it should only be used in settings where the test can be administered within a few days after a dosing, and the clinician must still take into account the false-positive and false-negative results for these medications.

NONMEDICAL USE OF PSYCHIATRIC MEDICATIONS

In psychiatry, medication management plays an important role in treating many psychopathologies. Although most medications improve outcomes in patients with mental illness, certain classes of medications have the potential for nonmedical use, diversion, and addiction. Addressing the potential for addiction remains a core part of routine psychiatric care. There are psychiatric medications that have the potential to be misused. The classes of medications used in psychiatry that are most at risk for misuse are benzodiazepines, stimulants, and sleep aids. Before prescribing these medications, it is important for the psychiatrist to take a thorough substance use history, social history, and family history; and to remain open and nonjudgmental. If patients are at risk for nonmedical use but the benefit of treatment outweighs this risk, the medication may still be prescribed. In these cases, informed consent, consistent prescribing practices, and setting a treatment framework are of utmost importance. In certain cases, part of the treatment framework may include drug testing. If the psychiatrist and patient agree to urine drug testing, there are a few concepts that must be kept in mind. The frequency and randomness of the collection, the pharmacokinetics of the medication, and the limitations of the laboratory assay being used are just a few examples that may affect the usefulness of drug testing.[52]

In addition to these medications, there is limited but emerging evidence that other psychiatric medications have potential for nonmedical use as well. There are several case reports of quetiapine, particularly when combined with other known drugs of abuse.[53] Certain antidepressant medications have similar evidence. Case reports of bupropion abuse are emerging, via intranasal and intravenous administration.[54,55] There is also some evidence for abuse of TCAs, likely owing to their anticholinergic and antihistaminic properties.[56] More research is needed before TDM is a routine part of treatment in patients being prescribed these medications.

SUMMARY

Laboratory assessment is an invaluable tool for psychiatrists and has great potential to increase efficacy and decrease unwanted effects of psychiatric medications. However, the clinical laboratory should in no way be a substitute for a psychiatric examination. Because there is an incredible amount of variability in response to medications even at the same blood levels, laboratory values are meaningless without a clinical correlate, and are sometimes even meaningless with one. There is much research but mostly inconclusive evidence for the usefulness of blood levels improving outcomes, aside from the medications with well-established therapeutic windows, as discussed. These inconsistencies may reflect the heterogeneity of illnesses that we group under a single diagnosis, such as "major depressive disorder." For urine drug levels, in contradistinction to other fields of medicine (pain, addiction, emergency medicine, etc), we could not identify significant literature on how differences in levels affect clinical outcomes for those unique to psychiatry. When ordering laboratory tests, clinicians should already have in mind how any of the possible results would affect their patient's treatment. Laboratory assessment should be used to augment clinical judgment and should be used incisively. Psychiatry is a field that emphasizes longitudinal care and a therapeutic alliance with the patient. With the growing technological and scientific advances, psychiatrists would be best served by combining the good practices of clinical expertise with educated laboratory orders.

REFERENCES

1. Sadosty AT, Groleau GA, Atcherson MM. The use of lithium levels in the emergency department. J Emerg Med 1999;17(5):887–91.
2. Perrone J, De roos F, Jayaraman S, et al. Drug screening versus history in detection of substance use in ED psychiatric patients. Am J Emerg Med 2001;19(1): 49–51.
3. Rockett IR, Putnam SL, Jia H, et al. Declared and undeclared substance use among emergency department patients: a population-based study. Addiction 2006;101(5):706–12.

4. Schiller MJ, Shumway M, Batki SL. Utility of routine drug screening in a psychiatric emergency setting. Psychiatr Serv 2000;51(4):474–8.

5. Eisen JS, Sivilotti ML, Boyd KU, et al. Screening urine for drugs of abuse in the emergency department: do test results affect physicians' patient care decisions? CJEM 2004;6(2):104–11.

6. Kroll DS, Smallwood J, Chang G. Drug screens for psychiatric patients in the emergency department: evaluation and recommendations. Psychosomatics 2013;54(1):60–6.

7. Lukens TW, Wolf SJ, Edlow JA, et al. Clinical policy: critical issues in the diagnosis and management of the adult psychiatric patient in the emergency department. Ann Emerg Med 2006;47(1):79–99.

8. Gellar JL. The last half-century of psychiatric services as reflected in psychiatric services. Psychiatr Serv 2000;51(1):41–67.

9. Martin DJ, Garske JP, Davis MK, et al. Relation of the therapeutic alliance with outcome and other variables: a meta-analytic review. J Consult Clin Psychol 2000;68(3):438–50.

10. Cramer JA, Rosenheck R. Compliance with medication regimens for mental and physical disorders. Psychiatr Serv 1998;49:196–201.

11. Nose M, Barbui C, Gray R, et al. Clinical interventions for treatment non-adherence in psychosis: meta-analysis. Br J Psychiatry 2003;183:197–206.

12. Gelenberg AJ, Freeman MP, Markowitz JC, et al. Practice guideline for the treatment of patients with major depressive disorder third edition. Am J Psychiatry 2010;167(10):1.

13. Stahl SM. Stahl's essential psychopharmacology. The prescriber's guide. 4th edition. New York: Cambridge University Press; 2011.

14. Labbate LA, Fava M, Rosenbaum JF, et al. Handbook of psychiatric drug therapy. 6th edition. Philadelphia: Lippincott Williams & Wilkins Handbook Series; 2009.

15. Kirchheiner J, Nickchen K, Bauer M, et al. Pharmacogenetics of antidepressants and antipsychotics: the contribution of allelic variations to the phenotype of drug response. Mol Psychiatry 2004;9(5):442–73.

16. Hyman SE, Nestler EJ. Initiation and adaptation: a paradigm for understanding psychotropic drug action. Am J Psychiatry 1996;153(2):151–62.

17. Gelenberg AJ, Chesen CL. How fast are antidepressants? J Clin Psychiatry 2000; 61(10):712–21.

18. Kerr GW, Mcguffie AC, Wilkie S. Tricyclic antidepressant overdose: a review. Emerg Med J 2001;18(4):236–41.

19. Mauri MC, Fiorentini A, Cerveri G, et al. Long-term efficacy and therapeutic drug monitoring of sertraline in major depression. Hum Psychopharmacol 2003;18(5): 385–8.

20. Veefkind AH, Haffmans PM, Hoencamp E. Venlafaxine serum levels and CYP2D6 genotype. Ther Drug Monit 2000;22(2):202–8.

21. Amsterdam JD, Fawcett J, Quitkin FM, et al. Fluoxetine and norfluoxetine plasma concentrations in major depression: a multicenter study. Am J Psychiatry 1997; 154(7):963–9.

22. Asberg M, Crönholm B, Sjöqvist F, et al. Relationship between plasma level and therapeutic effect of nortriptyline. Br Med J 1971;3(5770):331–4.

23. Callaham M. Tricyclic antidepressant overdose. JACEP 1979;8(10):413–25.

24. Le bloc'h Y, Woggon B, Weissenrieder H, et al. Routine therapeutic drug monitoring in patients treated with 10-360 mg/day citalopram. Ther Drug Monit 2003;25(5):600–8.

25. Lundmark J, Bengtsson F, Nordin C, et al. Therapeutic drug monitoring of selective serotonin reuptake inhibitors influences clinical dosing strategies and reduces drug costs in depressed elderly patients. Acta Psychiatr Scand 2000; 101(5):354–9.

26. Hiemke C, Baumann P, Bergemann N, et al. AGNP consensus guidelines for therapeutic drug monitoring in psychiatry: update 2011. Pharmacopsychiatry 2011; 44(6):195–235.

27. Krishnan V, Nestler EJ. The molecular neurobiology of depression. Nature 2008; 455(7215):894–902.

28. Maurer HH, Bickeboeller-friedrich J. Screening procedure for detection of antidepressants of the selective serotonin reuptake inhibitor type and their metabolites in urine as part of a modified systematic toxicological analysis procedure using gas chromatography-mass spectrometry. J Anal Toxicol 2000;24(5):340–7.

29. Cade JF. Lithium salts in the treatment of psychotic excitement. Med J Aust 1949; 2(10):349–52.

30. Berridge MJ, Downes CP, Hanley MR. Neural and developmental actions of lithium: a unifying hypothesis. Cell 1989;59(3):411–9.

31. Stambolic V, Ruel L, Woodgett JR. Lithium inhibits glycogen synthase kinase-3 activity and mimics wingless signalling in Intact cells. Curr Biol 1996;6(12): 1664–8.

32. Gelenberg AJ, Kane JM, Keller MB, et al. Comparison of standard and low serum levels of lithium for maintenance treatment of bipolar disorder. N Engl J Med 1989;321(22):1489–93.

33. Bowden CL, Brugger AM, Swann AC, et al. Efficacy of divalproex vs lithium and placebo in the treatment of mania. The Depakote Mania Study Group. JAMA 1994;271(12):918–24.

34. Weisler RH, Kalali AH, Ketter T, et al. A multicenter, randomized, double-blind, placebo-controlled trial of extended-release carbamazepine capsules as monotherapy for bipolar disorder patients with manic or mixed episodes. J Clin Psychiatry 2004;65(4):478–84.

35. Bowden CL, Calabrese JR, Sachs G, et al. A placebo-controlled 18-month trial of lamotrigine and lithium maintenance treatment in recently manic or hypomanic patients with bipolar I disorder. Arch Gen Psychiatry 2003;60(4):392–400.

36. Abi-Dargham A, Laruelle M. Mechanisms of action of second generation antipsychotic drugs in schizophrenia: insights from brain imaging studies. Eur Psychiatry 2005;20(1):15–27.

37. VanderZwaag C, McGee M, McEvoy JP, et al. Response of patients with treatment-refractory schizophrenia to clozapine within three serum level ranges. Am J Psychiatry 1996;153:1579–84.

38. Roman M, Kronstrand R, Lindstedt D, et al. Quantitation of seven low dosage antipsychotic drugs in human post mortem blood using LC-MS-MS. J Anal Toxicol 2008;32:147–55.

39. Fitzgerald PB, Kapur S, Remington G, et al. Predicting haloperidol occupancy of central dopamine D2 receptors from plasma levels. Psychopharmacology (Berl) 2000;149:1–5.

40. Ulrich S, Wurthmann C, Brosz M, et al. The relationship between serum concentration and therapeutic effect of haloperidol in patients with acute schizophrenia. Clin Pharmacokinet 1998;34(3):227–63.

41. Robinson DG, Pollock BG, Mulsant BH, et al. Pharmacologic profile of perphenazine's metabolites. J Clin Psychopharmacol 2000;20(2):181–7.

42. Darby JK, Pasta DJ, Elfand L, et al. Risperidone dose and blood level variability: accumulation effects and interindividual and intraindividual variability in the nonresponder patient in the clinical practice setting. J Clin Psychopharmacol 1997;17:478–84.

43. Nyberg S, Eriksson B, Oxenstierna G, et al. Suggested minimal effective dose of risperidone based on PET-measured D2 and 5-HT2A receptor occupancy in schizophrenic patients. Am J Psychiatry 1999;156:869–75.

44. Buffett-Jerrott SE, Stewart SH. Cognitive and sedative effects of benzodiazepine use. Curr Pharm Des 2002;8:45–58.

45. Brunette MF, Noordsy DL, Xie H, et al. Benzodiazepine use and abuse among patients with severe mental illness and co-occurring substance use disorders. Psychiatr Serv 2003;54:1395–401.

46. Schulz M, Schmoldt A. Therapeutic and toxic blood concentrations of more than 800 drugs and other zenobiotics. Pharmazie 2003;58:447–74.

47. Greenblatt DJ, Shader RI, Franke K, et al. Pharmacokinetics and bioavailability of intravenous, intramuscular, and oral lorazepam in humans. J Pharm Sci 1979;68: 57–63.

48. Moeller KE, Lee KC, Kissack JC. Urine drug screening: practical guide for clinicians. Mayo Clin Proc 2008;83(1):66–76.

49. Biederman J. Attention-deficit/hyperactivity disorder: a selective overview. Biol Psychiatry 2005;57:1215–20.

50. A 14-month randomized clinical trial of treatment strategies for attention-deficit/hyperactivity disorder. The MTA Cooperative Group. Multimodal treatment study of children with ADHD. Arch Gen Psychiatry 1999;56(12):1073–86.

51. Biederman J, Wilens T, Mick E, et al. Pharmacotherapy of attention-deficit/hyperactivity disorder reduces risk for substance use disorder. Pediatrics 1999; 104(2):e20.

52. Heit HA, Gourlay DL. Urine drug testing in pain medicine. J Pain Symptom Manage 2004;27(3):260–7.

53. Malekshahi T, Tioleco N, Ahmed N, et al. Misuse of atypical antipsychotics in conjunction with alcohol and other drugs of abuse. J Subst Abuse Treat 2015; 48(1):8–12.

54. Baribeau D, Araki KF. Intravenous bupropion: a previously undocumented method of abuse of a commonly prescribed antidepressant agent. J Addict Med 2013;7(3):216–7.

55. Langguth B, Hajak G, Landgrebe M, et al. Abuse potential of bupropion nasal insufflation: a case report. J Clin Psychopharmacol 2009;29(6):618–9.

56. Haddad P. Do antidepressants have any potential to cause addiction? J Psychopharmacol 1999;13(3):300–7.

Clinical Toxicology and Its Relevance to Asthma and Atopy

Rauno Joks, MD[a],*, Martin H. Bluth, MD, PhD[b,c]

KEYWORDS

- Asthma • Bronchoconstriction • Opiate • Mast cell • Degranulation • Heroin
- Insufflation

KEY POINTS

- Both licit and illicit opiates have effects on the immune and neurologic components of asthma inflammation and clinical disease.
- How these effects summate determines the clinical output of this complex interplay, with either worsening or improvement of asthma.
- Laboratory toxicology/drug monitoring of patients can provide clinicians with objective information to facilitate appropriate prescribing and management determinations.

There are notable increases in the use of prescription pain relievers, substance use disorder treatment admission rates, and prevalence of asthma. The overall US prevalence of asthma increased from 7% of the general population in 2001 to 8% in 2010.[1] Select population demographics may have a greater prevalence in that the Black non-Hispanic population approaches 10% and the Puerto Rican subset of the Hispanic demographic has been reported at 16.5% in 2004.[1] The sales of prescription pain relievers in 2010 were 4 times those in 1999, and the substance use disorder treatment admission rate in 2009 was 6 times the 1999 rate.[2] The overdose death rate in 2008 was about 4 times the 1999 rate.[2] Fortunately, asthma death rates have leveled off in recent years.[1] However, increased asthma mortality rates are higher in women, Black persons, and adults.[1] The prevalence of asthma is greater for women (9.2%), than men (7.0%).[1] Women are more likely to have chronic pain, be prescribed prescription pain relievers, be given higher doses, and use them for longer periods than men.[3] Further, women may become dependent on prescription pain relievers more quickly than men.[3] Recent data from the Centers for Disease Control and

Disclosures: None.
[a] SUNY Downstate Medical Center, 450 Clarkson Avenue, Brooklyn, NY 11203, USA; [b] Department of Pathology, Wayne State University School of Medicine, 540 East Canfield, Detroit, MI 48201, USA; [c] Consolidated Laboratory Management Systems, 24555 Southfield Road, Southfield, MI 48075, USA
* Corresponding author.
E-mail address: Rauno.Joks@downstate.edu

Clin Lab Med 36 (2016) 795–801
http://dx.doi.org/10.1016/j.cll.2016.07.005
0272-2712/16/© 2016 Elsevier Inc. All rights reserved.

labmed.theclinics.com

Prevention have shown the greatest increase in epidemic of prescription drug over-doses from 2013 to 2014 occurred among non-Hispanic Black (8.2%), versus non-Hispanic White (8.0%) women and no change (0%) among Hispanics.[3] Taken together, both asthma and prescription pain reliever abuse are increasing and may disproportionately affect non-Hispanic Black women.

Drug overdose is the leading cause of accidental death in the in the United States, with 47,055 such deaths in 2014, with 18,893 overdose deaths related to prescription pain relievers.[4,5] There is a yin-yang interaction regarding the use of opiate analgesics with asthma pathophysiology and clinical course, which may be contributing to the current epidemic of opiate analgesic deaths.

In a recent review of hospitalizations among inner-city adults,[6] of 11,397 patients admitted in Chicago or Cleveland from 2005 to 2008, 3% were dependent on inhalational heroin. Heroin-dependent patients were 3 times more likely to be admitted for respiratory problems, compared with nondependent patients. This relationship was more striking for those with asthma exacerbations (odds ratio of 7.0).[6] Of 23 inner-city patients admitted to an inner-city intensive care unit with asthma exacerbations,[7] 56% describe asthma exacerbations associated with heroin insufflation. A 1996 review of fatal asthma in the same inner-city setting found that about a third of cases were confounded by substance abuse or alcohol,[8] which was roughly the same proportion as those dying from homicide. Asthmatic patients whose asthma death is confounded by opiate use are more likely to be older, have no immediate respiratory complaints before the event, and to be found dead.[9] Inhalation of heroin with cocaine has been linked to measurable airway hyperre-activity, which persists after the cessation of this substance abuse,[10] and, therefore, might contribute to ongoing bronchospasm and asthma activity.

These reports of the effects of illicit opiate use on asthma clinical disease activity are not complemented by studies of the effect of licit opiate use on asthma, which is an understudied area. In 2014 more people died of drug overdoses the United States than any previous year on record.[4] Approximately two-thirds of these involved opioids. These opioid deaths involve 2 trends: an increase in heroin use as well as a 15-year increase in deaths from prescription opiates, including fentanyl and tramadol. There is an increased availability of illicit fentanyl.[11] Although rare, licit fentanyl has been re-ported to cause asthma[12,13] and cough.[14]

The pediatric population warrants additional consideration. Asthma prevalence is greater in children in general than adults (8.6% for those younger than 18 years compared with 7.4% in adults) and is greater in select populations: 13.4% in the Black non-Hispanic populations and 23.5% in the Puerto Rican subset of the Hispanic pop-ulation.[1] Differences in physician gender and perception may bias referral to a pulmo-nologist compared with maintenance in a primary care setting as well as opioid prescribing habits for pediatric asthma and pain management.[15] Further, in a study of patients' opioid misuse, providers were more likely to assess African American pa-tients, younger patients, and patients with a history of illicit drug use as likely to have misused prescribed opioids. However, this perception was not correct; only the pa-tients who had a history of illicit drug use reported opioid misuse.[16]

In addition, in the pediatric population (12–17 years old), the prescribing rates for prescription opioids among adolescents and young adults nearly doubled from 1994 to 2007. In 2014, an estimated 28,000 adolescents had used heroin in the past year, and an estimated 16,000 were current heroin users. Most adolescents who misuse prescription pain relievers are given to them for free by a friend or relative; individuals often share their unused pain relievers, unaware of the dangers of nonmed-ical opioid use.[17] Thus, the relationship of opioid use and asthma in the pediatric pop-ulation may exacerbate the risks over and above the adult population.

There is a yin-yang effect of opiates on respiratory processes, which can result in poor outcomes but can also be of clinical benefit. Opioids are potent respiratory depressants,[18] which is the leading cause of death from their overuse.[19] Yet opioids are also useful in the management of cough[20] and dyspnea associated with heart failure and chronic obstructive pulmonary disease.[21,22] Stimulation of opioid receptors located in the airways has varying effects, from inhibition of tachykinergic and cholinergic mediated constriction to inhibition of mucous secretion.[23] Codeine has been isolated from Chinese herbal antiasthma proprietary remedies[24]; a benefit for such addition of codeine may arise, in part, from the antitussive properties of codeine.

Morphine sulfate has been shown to decrease airway hyperreactivity of mild asthmatics to the same degree as atropine[25] and decreases cholinergically mediated bronchoconstrictive responses to sulfites (sulfur dioxide).[26] A study of the safety of a novel inhalation delivery system for morphine for pain control found that asthmatic patients did not have worsening of their disease from delivery of morphine through a pulmonary route.[27] Similarly, morphine has been found to be safe in treating asthmatic patients who require ventilator support.[28]

Mast cell activation is a central process in asthma pathogenesis.[29] Opioids release histamine from mast cells to varying degrees; codeine, morphine, and meperidine have the greatest histamine-releasing capability, whereas tramadol, fentanyl, and remifentanil do not release histamine.[30] In a study using intradermal microdialysis of human skin, only codeine and meperidine induced mast cell activation with release of tryptase and histamine, whereas fentanyl and other derivatives did not.[31] As naloxone did not attenuate the degranulation and release of tryptase and histamine, the investigators suggested that it is unlikely that μ-opioid receptors are involved in the activation of mast cells.[31] However, intravenous morphine and nalbuphine given to patients for general anesthesia have been found to increase plasma histamine levels.[32] Histamine is released from porcine mast cells in response to oxycodone but not to morphine or hydromorphone[33]

Opiate-induced histamine release might help to understand the development of status asthmaticus in illicit drug users.[8,34] Inhalational studies of the effect of codeine on bronchoconstriction found a significant effect in 11 of 17 adult asthmatic subjects, who were also highly sensitive to histamine inhalation challenge.[35] This effect was not reproduced by codeine administered by mouth or spraying of the buccopharynx. Skin responses of these subjects to histamine and codeine were no different in those who responded to inhaled codeine when compared with those who did not.[35] The investigators suggested that the codeine effect might be directly due to μ receptors in the bronchi.

Studying the effects of naloxone, an opiate receptor agonist[36] on asthma provides an alternate approach to assessing the effect of opiates in asthma pathogenesis. The Food and Drug Administration approved a naloxone auto-injector on April 3, 2014 for adults and children, as a new therapy to treat opiate overdoses.[37] However, there are reports that opiate antagonism might worsen asthma and precipitate increased mast cell activation. Allegretti and colleagues[38] reported cases of deterioration of asthmatic patients with exacerbations who, after receiving naloxone, developed respiratory failure from status asthmaticus. Similarly, Tataris and colleagues[39] reported that 2 of 21 patients ($\sim$10%) with possible heroin-induced bronchospasm who received nebulized naloxone as a treatment had worsening of their bronchospasm. Such worsening of bronchospasm might be attributed to withdrawal-associated anxiety,[40] which itself might be associated with hyperventilation. As hyperventilation invokes the bronchoconstriction associated with exercise,[41] it may play a role in the anxiety-associated worsening of asthma.

Opiate withdrawal by injection of naloxone to morphine-dependent mice increases the concentration of mast cells in the thalamus.[42] Although the effects of opiates on immunoglobulin E (IgE) production are not known, in murine models chronic administration of naloxone is associated with decreased interleukin (IL)-4 production, with increases in IL-2 and interferon-γ production,[43] suggesting that this opiate antagonist induces a shift away from the T helper 2 (Th2) cytokines associated with IgE production.[44] In contrast, studies by Roy and colleagues[45] report that morphine increases anti-CD3/CD28 antibody induction of CD4+ T-cell IL-4 protein synthesis as well as IL-4 mRNA and GATA-3 mRNA accumulation.[45] Taken together, these findings strongly suggest that opiate use is associated with increased Th2 responses and may increase both IgE and allergic responses. This finding is in concert with observations of a patient who developed persistent exacerbation of underlying stable asthma after initiating fentanyl transdermal therapy for chronic low back pain. Laboratory investigations were remarkable for slightly elevated serum IgE levels and progressively increasing eosinophils, which resolved within 72 hours on removal of the offending agent. Testing for IgE to specific opioids may be helpful in diagnosis but are not readily available.[12]

It may be prudent to assess opioid ingestion in asthmatic patients, via urine drug testing (UDT), as a means to obtaining a patient's objective narcotic/analgesic drug footprint to assist in the diagnostic workup and before prescribing additional pharmacopeia. This relationship between opioids and asthma may be more pronounced in pediatric and adolescent medicine whereby Saroyan and colleagues[46] reported that 22% of patients prescribed analgesics were nonadherent. Factors associated with nonadherence included being prescribed opiates and older age ($\geq$18 years old). In those studies, 50% of those nonadherent patients were identified through self-report and 50% via UDT.

Taken together, there is a mixed effect of opiates on the pathophysiologic processes involved in the airway inflammation that results in clinical asthma. Although there is anecdotal evidence of worsening of asthma with illicit opiate use, there is a clinical benefit with antitussive effects and relief of dyspnea with licit opiate use short-term. Whether there is exacerbation of asthma and worsening of allergic responses when either licit or illicit opiate compounds are used long-term has yet to be determined. In concert with this understanding, toxicologic assays (UDT) to elucidate the relationship between use of an opiate, either licit or illicit, with asthma activity and allergic responses would further aid in monitoring the interaction between drug use and associated asthma and allergy.

REFERENCES

1. Available at: www.cdc.gov/asthma/asthmadata.htm. Accessed April 5, 2016.
2. Paulozzi LJ, Jones CM, Mack KA, et al, Division of Unintentional Injury Prevention, National Center for Injury Prevention and Control, Center for Disease Control and Prevention. Vital signs: overdoses of prescription opioid pain relievers – United States, 1999-2008. MMWR Morb Mortal Wkly Rep 2011;60:5.
3. Center for Disease Control and Prevention. Prescription painkiller overdoses: a growing epidemic, especially among women. Atlanta (GA): Centers for Disease Control and Prevention; 2013. Available at: http://www.cdc.gov/vitalsigns/prescriptionpainkilleroverdoses/index.html.
4. Rudd RA, Aleshire N, Zibbell JE. Increases in drug and opioid overdose deaths–United States, 2000-2014. MMWR Morb Mortal Wkly Rep 2016;64(50):1378–82.
5. Center for Disease Control and Prevention, National Center for Health Statistics, National Vital Statistics System, Mortality File. Number and age-adjusted rates of drug-poisoning deaths involving opioid analgesics and heroin: United States,

2000-2014. Atlanta (GA): Center for Disease Control and Prevention; 2015. Available at: http://www.cdc.gov/nchs/data/health_policy/AADR_drugpoisoning involving OA_Heroin US 2000-2014.pdf.

6. Choi H, Krantz A, Smith J, et al. Medical diagnoses associated with substance dependence among inpatients at a large urban hospital. PLoS One 2015;10(6): e0131324.

7. Krantz AJ, Hershow RC, Pruchand N, et al. Heroin insufflation as a trigger for patients with life-threatening asthma. Chest 2003;123:510–7.

8. Levenson T, Greenberger PA, Donoghue ER, et al. Asthma deaths confounded by substance abuse. An Assessment of fatal asthma. Chest 1996;110:604–10.

9. Hlavaty L, Hansma P, Sung L. Contribution of opiates in sudden asthma deaths. Am J Forensic Med Pathol 2015;36:49–52.

10. Boto de los Bueis A, Pereira Vega A, Sánchez Ramos JL, et al. Bronchial hyper-reactivity in patients who inhale heroin mixed with cocaine vaporized on aluminum foil. Chest 2002;121:1223–30.

11. Centers for Disease Control and Prevention. Increase in fentanyl drug confiscations and fentanyl-related overdose fatalities. HAN Health Advisory. Atlanta (GA): US Department of Health and Human Services, CDC; 2015. Available at: http://emergency.cdc.gov/han/han00384.asp.

12. Parmar MS. Exacerbation of asthma secondary to fentanyl transdermal patch. BMJ Case Rep 2009;2009 [pii:bcr10.2008.1062].

13. Otani S, Tokioka H, Fujii H, et al. A case of severe bronchospasm under epidural anesthesia with fentanyl. Masui 1997;46:1378–81.

14. Tweed WA, Dakin D. Explosive coughing after fentanyl injection. Anesth Analg 2001;92:1442–3.

15. Sabin JA, Greenwalt AG. The influence of implicit bias on treatment recommendations for 4 common pediatric conditions: pain, urinary tract infection, attention deficit hyperactivity disorder, and asthma. Am J Public Health 2012;102:988–95.

16. Vijayaraghavan M, Penko J, Guzman D, et al. Primary care providers' judgments of opioid analgesic misuse in a community-based cohort of HIV-infected indigent adults. J Gen Intern Med 2011;26:412–8.

17. Available at: http://www.asam.org/docs/default-source/advocacy/opioid-addiction-disease-facts-figures.pdf. Accessed April 5, 2016.

18. Weil JV, McCullough RE, Kline JS, et al. Diminished ventilator response to hypoxia and hypercapnia after morphine in normal man. N Engl J Med 1975;292:1103–6.

19. World Health Organisation (WHO). Community management of opioid overdose. Available at: http://www.who.int/substance_abuse/publications/management_opioid_overdose/en/.2014.

20. Chakravarty NK, Matallana A, Jensen R, et al. Central effects of antitussive drugs on cough and respiration. J Pharmacol Exp Ther 1956;117:127–35.

21. Foral PA, Maleskaer MA, Huerta G, et al. Nebulized opioids use in COPD. Chest 2004;125:691–4.

22. Baydur A. Nebulized morphine: a convenient and safe alternative to dyspnea relief. Chest 2004;125:363–5.

23. Groneberg DA, Fischer A. Endogenous opioids as mediators of asthma. Pulm Pharmacol Ther 2001;14:383–9.

24. Liu SY, Woo SO, Holmes MJ, et al. LC and LC-MS-MS analyses of undeclared codeine in antiasthmatic Chinese proprietary medicine. J Pharm Biomed Anal 2000; 22:481–6.

25. Eschenbacher WL, Bethel RA, Boushey HA, et al. Morphine sulfate inhibits bronchoconstriction in subjects with mild asthma whose response are inhibited by atropine. Am Rev Respir Dis 1984;130:363–7.

26. Field PI, Simmul R, Bell SC, et al. Evidence for opioid modulation and generation of prostaglandins in sulphur dioxide (SO)2-induced bronchoconstriction. Thorax 1996;151:159–63.

27. Otulana B, Okikawa J, Linn L, et al. Safety and pharmacokinetic of inhaled morphine delivered using the AERx system in patients with moderate-to-severe asthma. Int J Clin Pharmacol Ther 2004;42(8):456–62.

28. Pontopiddan H, Geffen B, Lowenstein E. Morphine for severe asthma? N Engl J Med 1973;288(1):50.

29. Djukanovic R, Hanania N, Busse W, et al. IgE-mediated asthma: new revelations and future insights. Respir Med 2016;112:128–9.

30. Prieto-Lastra L, Iglesias-Cadarso A, Reaño-Martos MM, et al. Pharmacological stimuli in asthma/urticarial. Allergol Immunopathol (Madr) 2006;34:224–7.

31. Blunk JA, Schmelz M, Zeck S, et al. Opioid-induced mast cell activation and vascular responses is not mediated by μ-opioid receptors: an in vivo microdialysis study in human skin. Anesth Analg 2004;98:364–70.

32. Doenicke A, Mass J, Lorenz W, et al. Intravenous morphine and nalbuphine increase histamine and catecholamine release without accompanying hemodynamic changes. Clin Pharmacol Ther 1995;58(1):81–9.

33. Ennis M, Schneider C, Nehring E, et al. Histamine release induced by opioid analgesic: a comparative study using porcine mast cells. Agents Actions 1991; 33(1–2):20–2.

34. Cygan J, Trunsky M, Corbridge T. Inhaled heroin-induced status asthmaticus. Five Cases and a review of the literature. Chest 2000;117:272–5.

35. Popa V. Codeine-induced bronchoconstriction and putative bronchial opiate receptors in asthmatic subjects. Pulm Pharmacol 1994;7:333–41.

36. Van Dorp E, Yassen A, Dahan A. Naloxone treatment in opioid addiction: the risks and benefits. Expert Opin Drug Saf 2007;6(2):125–32.

37. Merlin MA, Ariyaprakai N, Arshad FH. Assessment of the safety and ease of use of the naloxone auto-injector for the reversal of opioid overdose. Open Access Emerg Med 2015;2015(7):21–4.

38. Allegretti PJ, Bzdusek JS, Leonard J. Caution with naloxone use in asthmatic patients. Am J Emerg Med 2006;24(4):515–6.

39. Tataris KL, Weber JM, Stein-Spencer L, et al. The effect of prehospital nebulized naloxone on suspected heroin-induced bronchospasm. Am J Emerg Med 2013; 31(4):717–8.

40. Pinkofsky HB, Hahn AM, Campbell FA, et al. Reduction of opioid-withdrawal symptoms with quetiapine. J Clin Psychiatry 2005 Oct;66(10):1285–8.

41. Gotshall RW. Exercise-induced bronchoconstriction. Drugs 2002;62(12): 1725–39.

42. Taiwo O, Kovac K, Sperry L, et al. Naloxone induced morphine withdrawal increases the number and degranulation of mast cells in the thalamus of the mouse. Neuropharmacology 2004;46:824–35.

43. Panerai AE, Sacerdote P. Beta-endorphin in the immune system: a role at last? Immunol Today 1997;18:317–9.

44. Zhu J, Paul WE. Peripheral CD4 T cell differentiation regulated by networks of cytokines and transcription factors. Immunol Rev 2010;238(1):247–62.

45. Roy S, Wang J, Charboneau R, et al. Morphine induces CD4+ T cell IL-4 expression through an adenylyl cyclase mechanism independent of the protein kinase A pathway. J Immunol 2005;175(10):6361–7.
46. Saroyan JM, Evans EA, Segoshi A, et al. Interviewing and urine drug toxicology screening in a pediatric pain management center: an analysis of analgesic non-adherence and aberrant behaviors in adolescents and young adults. Clin J Pain 2016;32:1–6.

UNITED STATES POSTAL SERVICE® Statement of Ownership, Management, and Circulation
(All Periodicals Publications Except Requester Publications)

1. Publication Title	2. Publication Number	3. Filing Date
CLINICS IN LABORATORY MEDICINE	000 – 713	9/18/2016

4. Issue Frequency	5. Number of Issues Published Annually	6. Annual Subscription Price
MAR, JUN, SEP, DEC	4	$240.00

7. Complete Mailing Address of Known Office of Publication (Not printer) (Street, city, county, state, and ZIP+4®)

ELSEVIER INC.
360 PARK AVENUE SOUTH
NEW YORK, NY 10010-1710

Contact Person
STEPHEN R. BUSHING

Telephone (Include area code)
215-239-3688

8. Complete Mailing Address of Headquarters or General Business Office of Publisher (Not printer)

ELSEVIER INC.
360 PARK AVENUE SOUTH
NEW YORK, NY 10010-1710

9. Full Names and Complete Mailing Addresses of Publisher, Editor, and Managing Editor (Do not leave blank)

Publisher (Name and complete mailing address)

ADRIANNE BRIGIDO, ELSEVIER INC.
1600 JOHN F KENNEDY BLVD. SUITE 1800
PHILADELPHIA, PA 19103-2899

Editor (Name and complete mailing address)

LAUREN BOYLE, ELSEVIER INC.
1600 JOHN F KENNEDY BLVD. SUITE 1800
PHILADELPHIA, PA 19103-2899

Managing Editor (Name and complete mailing address)

PATRICK MANLEY, ELSEVIER INC.
1600 JOHN F KENNEDY BLVD. SUITE 1800
PHILADELPHIA, PA 19103-2899

10. Owner (Do not leave blank. If the publication is owned by a corporation, give the name and address of the corporation immediately followed by the names and addresses of all stockholders owning or holding 1 percent or more of the total amount of stock. If not owned by a corporation, give the names and addresses of the individual owners. If owned by a partnership or other unincorporated firm, give its name and address as well as those of each individual owner. If the publication is published by a nonprofit organization, give its name and address.)

Full Name	Complete Mailing Address
WHOLLY OWNED SUBSIDIARY OF REED/ELSEVIER, US HOLDINGS	1600 JOHN F KENNEDY BLVD. SUITE 1800 PHILADELPHIA, PA 19103-2899

11. Known Bondholders, Mortgagees, and Other Security Holders Owning or Holding 1 Percent or More of Total Amount of Bonds, Mortgages, or Other Securities. If none, check box ▶ ☐ None

Full Name	Complete Mailing Address
N/A	

12. Tax Status (For completion by nonprofit organizations authorized to mail at nonprofit rates) (Check one)
The purpose, function, and nonprofit status of this organization and the exempt status for federal income tax purposes:
☐ Has Not Changed During Preceding 12 Months
☐ Has Changed During Preceding 12 Months (Publisher must submit explanation of change with this statement)

13. Publication Title	14. Issue Date for Circulation Data Below
CLINICS IN LABORATORY MEDICINE	JUNE 2016

PS Form 3526, July 2014 [Page 1 of 4 (see instructions page 4)] PSN: 7530-01-000-9931   PRIVACY NOTICE: See our privacy policy on www.usps.com.

---

15. Extent and Nature of Circulation			Average No. Copies Each Issue During Preceding 12 Months	No. Copies of Single Issue Published Nearest to Filing Date
a. Total Number of Copies (Net press run)			202	196
b. Paid Circulation (By Mail and Outside the Mail)	(1)	Mailed Outside-County Paid Subscriptions Stated on PS Form 3541 (Include paid distribution above nominal rate, advertiser's proof copies, and exchange copies)	52	58
	(2)	Mailed In-County Paid Subscriptions Stated on PS Form 3541 (Include paid distribution above nominal rate, advertiser's proof copies, and exchange copies)	0	0
	(3)	Paid Distribution Outside the Mails Including Sales Through Dealers and Carriers, Street Vendors, Counter Sales, and Other Paid Distribution Outside USPS®	31	36
	(4)	Paid Distribution by Other Classes of Mail Through the USPS (e.g., First-Class Mail®)	0	0
c. Total Paid Distribution (Sum of 15b (1), (2), (3), and (4))		▶	83	94
d. Free or Nominal Rate Distribution (By Mail and Outside the Mail)	(1)	Free or Nominal Rate Outside-County Copies included on PS Form 3541	41	37
	(2)	Free or Nominal Rate In-County Copies Included on PS Form 3541	0	0
	(3)	Free or Nominal Rate Copies Mailed at Other Classes Through the USPS (e.g., First-Class Mail)	0	0
	(4)	Free or Nominal Rate Distribution Outside the Mail (Carriers or other means)	0	0
e. Total Free or Nominal Rate Distribution (Sum of 15d (1), (2), (3) and (4))		▶	41	37
f. Total Distribution (Sum of 15c and 15e)		▶	124	131
g. Copies not Distributed (See Instructions to Publishers #4 (page 83))		▶	78	65
h. Total (Sum of 15f and g)		▶	202	196
i. Percent Paid (15c divided by 15f times 100)			67%	72%

* If you are claiming electronic copies, go to line 16 on page 3. If you are not claiming electronic copies, skip to line 17 on page 3.

PS Form 3526, July 2014 (Page 2 of 4)

16. Electronic Copy Circulation		Average No. Copies Each Issue During Preceding 12 Months	No. Copies of Single Issue Published Nearest to Filing Date
a. Paid Electronic Copies	▶	0	0
b. Total Paid Print Copies (Line 15c) + Paid Electronic Copies (Line 16a)	▶	83	94
c. Total Print Distribution (Line 15f) + Paid Electronic Copies (Line 16a)	▶	124	131
d. Percent Paid (Both Print & Electronic Copies) (16b divided by 16c × 100)	▶	67%	72%

☒ I certify that 50% of all my distributed copies (electronic and print) are paid above a nominal price.

17. Publication of Statement of Ownership

☒ If the publication is a general publication, publication of this statement is required. Will be printed in the DECEMBER 2016 issue of this publication.

☐ Publication not required.

18. Signature and Title of Editor, Publisher, Business Manager, or Owner	Date
Stephen R. Bushing	9/18/2016

STEPHEN R. BUSHING - INVENTORY DISTRIBUTION CONTROL MANAGER

I certify that all information furnished on this form is true and complete. I understand that anyone who furnishes false or misleading information on this form or who omits material or information requested on the form may be subject to criminal sanctions (including fines and imprisonment) and/or civil sanctions (including civil penalties).

PS Form 3526, July 2014 (Page 3 of 4)   PRIVACY NOTICE: See our privacy policy on www.usps.com.

Moving?

Make sure your subscription moves with you!

To notify us of your new address, find your **Clinics Account Number** (located on your mailing label above your name), and contact customer service at:

Email: journalscustomerservice-usa@elsevier.com

800-654-2452 (subscribers in the U.S. & Canada)
314-447-8871 (subscribers outside of the U.S. & Canada)

Fax number: 314-447-8029

Elsevier Health Sciences Division
Subscription Customer Service
3251 Riverport Lane
Maryland Heights, MO 63043

*To ensure uninterrupted delivery of your subscription, please notify us at least 4 weeks in advance of move.

Printed and bound by CPI Group (UK) Ltd, Croydon, CR0 4YY

03/10/2024

01040397-0001